SECOND EDITION

INTRODUCTION TO HEALTH RESEARCH METHODS
A Practical Guide

Kathryn H. Jacobsen, MPH, PhD
Professor George Mason University
Fairfax, Virginia

JONES & BARTLETT
LEARNING

World Headquarters
Jones & Bartlett Learning
5 Wall Street
Burlington, MA 01803
978-443-5000
info@jblearning.com
www.jblearning.com

Jones & Bartlett Learning books and products are available through most bookstores and online booksellers. To contact Jones & Bartlett Learning directly, call 800-832-0034, fax 978-443-8000, or visit our website, www.jblearning.com.

Substantial discounts on bulk quantities of Jones & Bartlett Learning publications are available to corporations, professional associations, and other qualified organizations. For details and specific discount information, contact the special sales department at Jones & Bartlett Learning via the above contact information or send an email to specialsales@jblearning.com.

09453-4

Production Credits
VP, Executive Publisher: David D. Cella
Publisher: Michael Brown
Associate Editor: Lindsey M. Sousa
Senior Vendor Manager: Tracey McCrea
Senior Marketing Manager: Sophie Fleck Teague
Manufacturing and Inventory Control Supervisor: Amy Bacus
Project Management & Composition: Integra Software Services Pvt. Ltd.
Cover Design: Kristin E. Parker
Rights & Media Specialist: Merideth Tumasz
Media Development Editor: Shannon Sheehan
Cover Image: © neelsky/Shutterstock
Printing and Binding: Edwards Brothers Malloy
Cover Printing: Edwards Brothers Malloy

Library of Congress Cataloging-in-Publication Data
Names: Jacobsen, Kathryn H., author.
Title: Introduction to health research methods : a practical guide / Kathryn H. Jacobsen.
Description: 2nd edition. | Burlington, MA : Jones & Bartlett Learning, [2017] | Includes index.
Identifiers: LCCN 2016023372 | ISBN 9781284094534 (pbk.)
Subjects: | MESH: Biomedical Research—methods | Research Design
Classification: LCC R850 | NLM W 20.5 | DDC 610.72—dc23 LC record available at https://lccn.loc.gov/2016023372

6048

Printed in the United States of America

20 19 18 17 16 10 9 8 7 6 5 4 3 2

Contents

PREFACE

The goal of this book is to make the health research process accessible, manageable, and perhaps even enjoyable for new investigators. One of the reasons that engaging in health research is satisfying is that research is the necessary foundation for meaningful improvements in clinical and public health practice. Research helps us learn how to be healthier and how to help our families, friends, and communities improve and maintain their health. Without the building blocks provided by health research, we would not be able to identify and map areas that have a high rate of various diseases. We would not know about the risk factors for various disorders. We would not know which interventions are most effective for improving individual and community health.

But it is not just the outcomes that make research rewarding. The research process itself—the process of exploring the unknown and discovering answers to previously unanswered questions—can be exciting. This book is a practical, step-by-step guide to the research process.

All research projects follow the same steps: identifying a focused research question, choosing a study design, collecting data that will answer the question, analyzing the accumulated evidence, and disseminating the findings. The investigation proceeds through these same basic steps regardless of whether it involves conducting a clinical trial, organizing a neighborhood survey, analyzing an existing data set, or synthesizing the existing literature through meta-analysis. The same steps are followed whether the researcher is trained in medicine, nursing, public health, dentistry, physical therapy, occupational therapy, speech-language therapy, respiratory therapy, radiation technology, pharmacy, podiatry, dietetics and nutrition, athletic training, health policy, psychology, sociology, counseling, optometry, audiology, or any other clinical or social science discipline. And the steps are the same regardless of whether the investigator is an undergraduate student, a master's or doctoral candidate, or a seasoned professional.

Health research is an intentional process that requires fastidiousness and perseverance, but it is not complicated. Anyone who is willing to follow the steps outlined in this guidebook can conceptualize a research project and see it through to completion. This process can generate many personal benefits: the acquisition of new skills, the fulfillment of degree or work requirements, the satisfaction of personal curiosity, and even the opportunity to become a published author. And every project, no matter how modest, has the potential to contribute to expanding the knowledge base for the health sciences. That means that all researchers may eventually see their results translated into improved patient care, enriched organizational effectiveness, and enhanced community health. An increase in the number of active investigators who can conduct conscientious research and accurately communicate their findings to others will benefit us all.

This book is an invitation to make your own contribution to the evidence that will inform future decisions about preventing and treating disease, allocating health resources, and promoting health.

About the Author

Kathryn H. Jacobsen, PhD, MPH, is a professor of epidemiology and global health at George Mason University in Fairfax, Virginia. She has written more than 100 peer-reviewed articles and is also the author of *Introduction to Global Health* (Jones & Bartlett Learning).

What's New in the Second Edition

In this second edition of *Introduction to Health Research Methods*, every chapter from the 1st edition has been updated to improve content and clarity, and several new chapters and subsections have been added to provide more comprehensive coverage of health research methods. Step 1 ("Identifying a Study Question") presents additional strategies for deriving research ideas from theoretical frameworks and clinical practice experiences, and it includes new chapters on collaborating and mentorship. Step 2 ("Selecting a Study Approach") provides more examples and illustrations of the analytic strategies for each study design and features an expanded chapter on qualitative research theories and methods. Step 3 ("Designing the Study and Collecting Data") includes new subsections on reliability, validity, and research ethics plus a new chapter on writing grant proposals. Step 4 ("Analyzing Data") contains additional illustrations of how to calculate and interpret health statistics along with new chapters on regression analysis and other advanced analysis tools. Step 5 ("Reporting Findings") highlights many more strategies for writing success.

CHAPTER 1

The Health Research Process

Health research is the process of systematically investigating a single, well-defined aspect of physical, mental, or social well-being.

1.1 The Research Process

Research is the process of systematically and carefully investigating a subject in order to discover new insights about the world. No matter what the goals of a research project are or what methods are used to achieve those goals, the five steps of the research process are the same (**Figure 1-1**). The first two steps are to identify a study question and to select a general study approach. These two steps are often completed concurrently, because the approach selected may require the refinement of the study question. Once the objectives and the approach are set, the last three steps are to design the study and collect data, to analyze the data, and to write and share a report about the findings. These steps apply to nearly every research project. A research project is not finished until all five steps have been completed.

1.2 Health Research

Health research examines a broad spectrum of biological, socioeconomic, environmental, and other factors that contribute to the presence or absence of physical, mental, and social health and well-being. **Population health research**

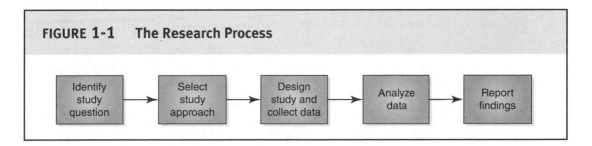

FIGURE 1-1 The Research Process

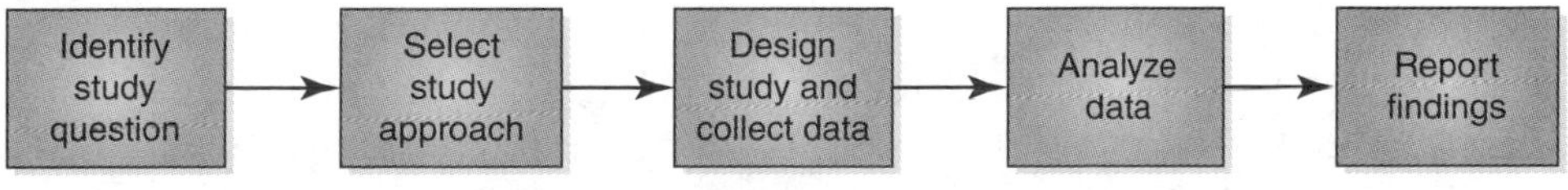

involves humans as the unit of investigation, rather than focusing on molecules, genes, cells, or other smaller biological components. Population health research ranges from clinical case studies with just a few individuals to global public health studies that may include many thousands of participants. Health research studies apply the tools from a diversity of fields. Some draw on the tools of the laboratory sciences, such as molecular biology, microbiology, immunology, nutrition, and genetics. Many use the tools of **demography** (the study of populations and population dynamics, such as birth and death rates), epidemiology, and various social sciences, including psychology, sociology, anthropology, and economics.

A distinction is made between routine practice activities and health research. It is not research when an epidemiologist working for a health department tracks down the source of an outbreak of gastroenteritis. However, that investigation may become a research project when the outbreak investigation team identifies an unusual food item as the cause of the outbreak, does additional survey and laboratory work to confirm their hypothesis, and then shares that discovery by writing a formal report describing their methods and results. It is not research when a clinician reads several articles about an unusual disease or completes other continuing education activities. It is research when a clinician conducts a systematic search of the literature, completes a novel synthesis of the compiled articles, and then writes and disseminates that summary. It is not research when an organization asks its clients to complete a customer satisfaction survey so that opportunities for quality improvement can be identified. However, it is research when a client survey uses a validated questionnaire and sampling methods, is approved by an ethics committee, answers a question that builds on the evidence base provided by previously published articles, and has its results shared through presentation or publication.

Some studies that are very specific to one population at one place and in one point in time are not particularly helpful for identifying broader patterns. However, most health researchers hope that their findings will reveal trends, relationships, and theories that are generalizable to other populations, places, and times. When these researchers complete the health research process by sharing their findings with others, they are contributing to the evidence base used for health policy and practice.

1.3 Health Research Purposes

Research in the population health sciences often seeks to answer questions about community health profiles, risk factors for disease, clinical effectiveness, and the impact of interventions. Some of the common reasons for initiating a health research study include:

- Needs assessment: What is the health status of this population? What are the major health concerns of members of this population? What health-related needs in this population are not being addressed? A population can be defined as any well-defined group of individuals, such as the patients of a particular hos pital, the clients of a particular organization, the residents living in a particular town, the students attending a particular school, or some other set of people.

- Risk assessment: What are the threats to health in this population? What are the risk factors for **morbidity** (illness), **mortality** (death), disability, and other health issues?
- Applied practice: How well are we preventing, diagnosing, and treating health concerns in the populations we serve? Similar questions can be asked by health professionals in a diversity of fields, including medicine, nursing, public health, physical therapy, occupational therapy, pharmacy, dentistry, optometry, clinical psychology, kinesiology, health policy, health administration and management, and others.
- Outcomes evaluation: Was this intervention successful at improving health status in this population? Alternative versions of this question might ask about the effectiveness of a procedure, process, project, program, policy, or other activity.

The goal of any single health research project is usually modest: to answer one well-defined question. When many researchers add their findings to the scientific literature, the cumulative information provides an evidentiary foundation for improving the health of individuals and communities.

1.4 Book Overview

Anyone who is committed to seeing a new and valid project through to completion can contribute to advancing health science. Health research does not require a license. It does not require a doctorate or a master's degree. It does not even require coursework in research methods, although that is certainly helpful. What research demands is perseverance and patience, honesty and integrity, carefulness and attention to detail, the willingness to learn new knowledge and develop new skills, openness to expert advice and feedback, and the ability to criticize and revise one's own work and writing. These are personal character traits that everyone can cultivate and develop.

This book is intended to serve as a handbook for population health researchers. The chapters are organized according to the five steps of the research process. The first section provides suggestions for selecting an appropriately focused research question and establishing good relationships with collaborators and mentors early in a project. The second section opens with a chapter that summarizes the various approaches to gathering data and then presents an overview of each of the main study designs used in the population health sciences. The third section describes the data collection process, and it emphasizes research ethics along with the methods for collecting new data. The fourth section summarizes common strategies for data analysis. The fifth section presents tips for writing success and a step-by-step guide for preparing a manuscript for review and publication. If the goal is to publish the findings of a study, it may be helpful to write throughout the research process. Thus, some readers may find it helpful to read some of the chapters from the fifth section of the book prior to finalizing their research plans.

This guidebook is not meant to be a compendium of everything that health researchers know about study design, data collection, and statistical analysis. Instead, it provides a comprehensive overview of the entire process. The best way to learn about health research is to do actual research and to learn firsthand how the research process works. As a research project unfolds, most researchers will benefit from consulting specialized references. Many excellent books, journal articles, technical reports, and other online and library resources contain the advanced information required for complex study designs and analytic techniques. It is also essential for the consulted resources to include human experts—professors, supervisors, colleagues, coauthors, librarians, statistical consultants, and others—who can provide insights gained from personal research experience and can direct new investigators to the background readings and other information that will be most helpful as they explore their selected research questions.

STEP 1

Identifying a Study Question

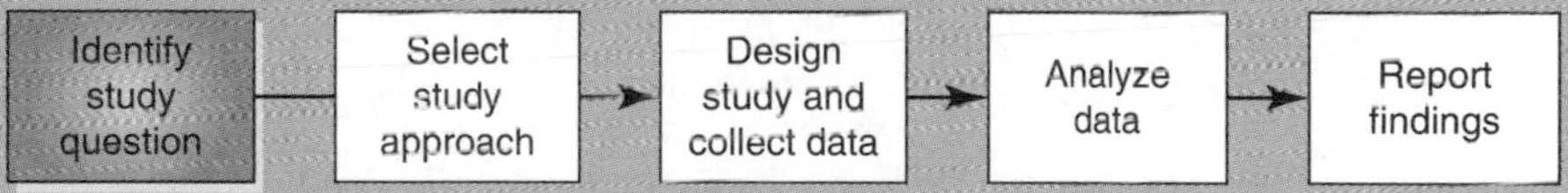

The first step in the research process is selecting the focus of the study. This section describes how to select a general topic, review the literature, refine the scope of the project, and work with collaborators.

- Selecting a general topic
- Reviewing the literature
- Focusing the research question
- Collaboration and mentorship
- Coauthoring

CHAPTER 2

SELECTING A GENERAL TOPIC

Selecting one workable study topic is the first step toward a successful research project. Many approaches can be used to identify potential research questions.

2.1 Practical Questions

Many research questions in the health sciences arise from observations made during applied practice. Consider the types of questions that different health practitioners might raise about trampoline injuries:

- An emergency room physician: "The trampoline injuries we've been seeing include a mix of limb fractures and head/neck trauma. Are the kids who present with trampoline-related arm fractures being screened for concussions? Are they being adequately treated for co-occurring conditions?"
- A physical therapist: "It seems like a lot more of the patients coming in for therapy this year are recovering from trampoline-related injuries. Has the rate of injuries really increased, or am I just noticing them more? Should I be telling my patients not to use home trampolines?"
- A health educator: "I'm working at a fitness center that offers trampoline workouts. Is this an effective way to improve cardiovascular fitness? What can we do to ensure the safety of our clients?"

Questions derived from practice often point toward an unmet demand for needs assessments, program evaluations, and clinical effectiveness studies. Any of these questions might be worth exploring in a new research project, assuming that a review of the literature shows that there is not yet consensus about the answers to these questions. Nonpractitioners looking for research ideas may find it helpful to reach out to clinical colleagues and other health professionals about possible collaborations.

When using practical experiences to frame research questions, remember that a good research question is one that ends in a question mark—that is, it is not a declaration or a value statement, but a genuine query. A good research question is also testable. **Testability** is present when the research question includes components that can be measured and examined.

2.2 Brainstorming and Concept Mapping

When a suitable research question does not arise from clinical practice, community observations, or personal experience, a **brainstorming** session can be a good starting point for identifying a research topic. The goal of brainstorming is to create a long list of possible research topics. This is not the stage for eliminating ideas because they do not appear feasible, and the ideas do not need to be well formed. The categories in **Figure 2-1** can be used to identify areas of personal interest. It can also be valuable to check with friends and colleagues about their ideas. Internet searches, journals, and books might reveal gaps in knowledge that are worthy of exploration. For example, many research articles end with a call for further research on a particular topic.

FIGURE 2-1 Brainstorming Questions

Area	Questions
Values	• What are my interests and personal values? • What research topics are personally meaningful? • Have some understudied conditions that I could explore significantly affected me, my family, my friends, or my patients/clients? • Have certain health issues sparked my passion because they reflect what I consider to be an injustice?
Skills	• What knowledge and skills do I already have?
Personal growth	• What new skills do I want to develop?
Connections	• What source populations and/or data sources might be available to me through professors, supervisors, colleagues, and other personal and professional contacts?
Job and/or course requirements	• What does my supervisor or professor want me to study?
Gaps in the literature	• What information is not currently available that would make a contribution to the discipline and/or to improving health practices or policies?

A related process is **concept mapping**. Begin by listing several diseases or population groups that might be interesting to study. Identify the related ideas that show up several times on the list and appear to be a central theme. Use circles and arrows to visibly group related topics to clarify the connections. Consider which of those broad areas might be worth exploring.

2.3 Keywords

A next step toward refining the areas of interest identified through brainstorming and topic mapping is compiling a list of related **keywords**. Jot down a long list of words that may help focus the research question. For example, a person who identifies an interest in child health in Africa might then list words like "malaria...children...Africa...bednets...Uganda...measles...vaccination...preschool children...malnutrition...vitamin A deficiency." A person who identifies an interest in aging might list words like "osteoporosis...falls...bedsores...physical therapy...calcium...bone density...home safety...rehabilitation...healthy aging...prevention." The goal is to identify a range of potential study foci within the major area of interest.

The ***MeSH*** **(*M*edical *S*ubject *H*eadings)** database, developed by the U.S. National Library of Medicine, can be helpful for identifying the full extent of a research area and also for narrowing the scope of a research area. Suppose, for example, that a potential area of interest is infection. The MeSH database suggests a variety of narrower topics related to infection, such as cardiovascular infections, sepsis, infectious skin diseases, and wound infection. Within the category of skin diseases, the MeSH database lists a variety of narrower topics, such as cellulitis, dermatomycoses (fungal skin infections), and bacterial skin diseases. Within the category of dermatomycoses, the MeSH database lists yet narrower topics, such as blastomycosis, cutaneous candidiasis, and tinea. Within these categories, MeSH offers even more refined points and still more refined points within successive subcategories.

Searching through the MeSH database can help a researcher in several ways. The researcher can move from a vague interest in infections or skin infections to a more focused interest in fungal skin infections or, even more specifically, ringworm infections. Alternatively, the MeSH database can be used to search for broader or related study ideas. A search for preeclampsia, for example, shows that preeclampsia is a type of pregnancy complication. It is related to other forms of pregnancy-induced hypertension, such as HELLP syndrome, which may be an equally interesting study topic for someone with an interest in obstetrics.

Once a list of keywords has been compiled, the researcher looks for the themes that emerge from them. Some topics may be easily eliminated because they do not fit the researcher's interests (Figure 2-1). Some keywords may stand out as particularly interesting to the investigator.

2.4 Exposure, Disease, Population (EDP)

Once several possible themes have been identified, each should be refined. Many topics in population health research can be expressed with the formula: [exposure] and [disease/outcome] in [population]. **Exposures** (**Figure 2-2**) and **diseases** (**Figure 2-3**) can encompass a wide variety of characteristics, some of which are:

- Social and environmental indicators
- Nutritional status
- Infections
- Chronic diseases
- Mental health status
- Quality-of-life measures
- Health service use

For experimental studies, the intervention being investigated is the exposure. The **population** is the group of individuals, communities, or organizations that will be examined (**Figure 2-4**).

The keywords compiled during brainstorming and concept mapping often fit into exposure, disease, and population categories. To use a "mad libs" style approach to creating a research question, the researcher should divide the keywords into three separate lists:

FIGURE 2-2 Examples of Types of Exposures

Socioeconomic Status	Health-Related Behaviors	Health Status	Environmental Exposures
• Income • Wealth • Educational level • Occupation • Age • Sex/gender • Race/ethnicity • Nationality • Immigration status • Marital status	• Dietary practices • Exercise habits • Alcohol use • Tobacco use • Sexual practices • Contraceptive use • Hygiene practices • Religious practices • Use of health care services	• Nutritional status • Immune status • Genetics • Stress • Anatomy and anatomical defects • Reproductive history • Comorbidities (existing health problems)	• Drinking water • Pollution • Radiation • Noise • Altitude • Humidity • Season • Natural disasters • Population density • Travel

FIGURE 2-3 Examples of Types of Diseases

Infectious and Parasitic Diseases	Noncommunicable Diseases (NCDs)	Neuropsychiatric Disorders	Injuries
• Candidiasis • Cholera • *Escherichia coli* • Hookworm • Malaria • Syphilis • Tuberculosis	• Asthma • Breast cancer • Cataracts • Diabetes • Hypertension • Osteoporosis • Stroke	• Alzheimer's disease and other dementias • Autism • Depressive disorders • Posttraumatic stress disorder • Schizophrenia	• Bone fractures • Burns • Crush injuries • Frostbite • Gunshot wounds • Near drownings • Poisonings

- One for exposures or interventions
- One for diseases or outcomes
- One for specific populations

These exposures, diseases (or other health-related **outcomes**), and populations—the "**EDPs**"—can then be combined to form potential study questions using a standard format of "Is [exposure] related to [disease/outcome] in [population]?" For example:

- Are exercise habits [exposure] related to the risk of bone fractures [disease] in adults with diabetes [population]?
- Is reproductive history [exposure] related to the risk of stroke [disease] among women living in rural Ontario [population]?

FIGURE 2-4 Examples of Types of Populations

- Australian children younger than 5 years old
- Women living in rural Ontario
- Adults with diabetes
- Teachers with at least 10 years of classroom experience
- Individuals newly diagnosed with influenza at St. Mary's Hospital in Newcastle
- Nongovernmental organizations working on issues related to HIV/AIDS in Uganda

- Is household wealth [exposure] related to the risk of hospitalization for asthma [disease] in Australian children younger than 5 years old [population]?

A literature review related to the candidate question will assist the researcher in determining what is already known about the topic and what new information a new study could contribute. Chapter 3 describes the literature review process.

2.5 PICOT

An alternative approach to framing a research question uses the acronym **PICOT**:

- What is the *P*atient/*P*opulation group that will be studied?
- What is the *I*ntervention that will be tested?
- What will the intervention be *C*ompared to?
- What is the *O*utcome of interest?
- What is the *T*imeframe for follow-up?

PICOT is especially helpful for addressing clinical research questions and designing intervention studies. One benefit of PICOT is that it points toward the selection of key indicators that would provide evidence for the success of the intervention.

CHAPTER 3

REVIEWING THE LITERATURE

After a general research area has been identified, background reading about the topic allows the aim and scope of the research idea to be refined.

3.1 Informal Sources

A starting point for learning about potential areas of inquiry is to read nontechnical documents and other files available on the Internet. Many major public health organizations, such as the World Health Organization (WHO) and the U.S. Centers for Disease Control and Prevention (CDC), have online factsheets about various diseases and risk factors for disease. Other international governmental organizations (including other agencies of the United Nations) and national governments also have factsheets, brochures, and websites that provide basic demographic, political, economic, geographic, and other health-related information about countries and regions. Newspapers and popular magazines may present compelling nontechnical articles about exposures, diseases, and/or populations that highlight what is interesting and important to know about a topic. The websites of disease advocacy organizations, personal websites, and other media may also be helpful in identifying and refining an important and meaningful study question. Informal sources that have not been peer-reviewed are not part of the formal scientific literature, so researchers must be cautious about any claims in these files that contradict more formal sources of scientific information. However, these initial background readings can provide a foundation for understanding the more technical scientific literature that will be read later as part of a thorough literature review.

3.2 Statistical Reports

When defining specific exposures, diseases, and/or populations of interest, it may be helpful to identify relevant statistics, such as the estimated prevalence of the exposure in a particular country, the annual global incidence of a disease, or the size of a particular population.

- For regional- and country-level population measures and comparisons, the World Bank's World Development Indicators database provides information about a wide range of topics.
- Additional statistical estimates can be found in the annexes of the annual reports issued by United Nations agencies, such as the World Health Organization's *World Health Statistics,* UNDP's *Human Development Report,* and UNICEF's *State of the World's Children*.
- The annual reports of private organizations like the Population Reference Bureau and the American Cancer Society include up-to-date statistical estimates and projections.
- For information about states, provinces, counties, cities, and other smaller governmental units, contact the relevant public health departments. This may be the best source of information about **vital statistics** like birth and death rates and other demographics indicators.
- The best place to find very specific information about health-related exposures and diseases may be in published scientific articles.

Although statistics may be readily found on the Internet, few are supported by citations and information about who collected the original data, how the data were collected, and even when the data were collected. When possible, trace the statistic back to its original source rather than relying on secondary reports. If the source of data is not clear, the statistic may not be trustworthy.

3.3 Abstract Databases

An **abstract** is a paragraph-length summary of an article, chapter, or book. Abstracts for journal articles in the health sciences usually provide a brief description of the study population (such as the sample size and the location of the study), the study design, and the key findings of the study. **Abstract databases** allow researchers to search thousands of abstracts for keywords or other terms. A careful and comprehensive search of at least one major abstract database is the most important component of a careful literature search.

Some abstract databases are available to the public at no cost. The most popular publicly available health science database is **PubMed**, which is a service of the U.S. National Library of Medicine of the National Institutes of Health, and provides access to more than 25 million abstracts. European PubMed Central (Europe PMC) is similar to PubMed but has more extensive coverage of European and Canadian journals. SciELO (the Scientific Electronic Library Online) and LILACS (Literatura Latino Americana e do Caribe em Ciências da Saúde) primarily focus on literature from Central and South America, and they allow searches to be conducted in English, Spanish, and Portuguese. African Journals Online (AJOL) allows searches of journals published by African institutions. Several other national and regional databases allow for searching in other languages.

Other health abstract databases are available from libraries via subscription, such as:

- CAB Direct, from the Centre for Agriculture and Biosciences International (CABI), which focuses on agriculture and nutrition

- CINAHL, the Cumulative Index to Nursing and Allied Health Literature
- Embase, a product of the large publishing company Elsevier
- ERIC, the Educational Resources Information Center, which is sponsored by the U.S. Department of Education
- MEDLINE, which is sponsored by the U.S. National Library of Medicine and features only journals that have applied for inclusion and passed through a review process
- PsycINFO, which is supported by the American Psychological Association (APA)
- Scopus, from Elsevier
- Web of Science, from the company Thomson Reuters, which includes journals from the sciences, social sciences, and arts and humanities as well as conference proceedings in the sciences

Additional search options are provided by the Cochrane Library and by companies that produce, manage, and distribute online journal collections such as EBSCO (which provides a variety of discipline-specific EBSCOhost databases like SPORTDiscus, which has extensive coverage of sports studies research), JSTOR, LexisNexis (which focuses on business and law), Ovid, and ProQuest. Some publishing companies offer databases of the articles published in their journals, including LWW Journals Online (from Lippincott, Williams & Wilkins, an imprint of the large publisher Wolters Kluwer), SAGE Journals Online, Elsevier's ScienceDirect, SpringerLink, Taylor & Francis Online, and the Wiley Online Library. A librarian can provide information about the best databases to use for particular research questions.

Even though these databases cover thousands of journals, many peer-reviewed journals are not included in any of them, especially journals not published in English. Therefore, a supplemental search with a general search engine like Google Scholar may be helpful for identifying additional relevant abstracts. A supplemental search is especially important when the topic of interest is narrow enough to yield only a small or moderate number of hits.

Abstract databases can be searched with keywords or MeSH terms, using Boolean operators like AND, OR, and NOT. Limits can be set so that results include only abstracts with particular publication years, languages, or other selected parameters. Databases can also be searched by article title, author (often using a last name and first initials format, such as "Baker JD" or "Patel AR"), and journal title. See Chapter 22 for more information about how to successfully search abstract databases.

3.4 Full-Text Articles

Abstracts provide a glimpse into the content of an article. However, the only way to truly understand a study is to read the full text of the article. Some articles are available online in their entirety as open-access files on journal websites, in digital archives like PubMed Central, or on the personal websites of the authors themselves. Most university libraries subscribe to thousands of online journals that allow patrons to access electronic versions of articles. Most university libraries also have a limited number of journals available in print form on their shelves, but a physical search of the stacks is unlikely to be required unless the article is relatively old. Universities often offer free or low-cost interlibrary loan services to affiliates, and these "loans" of journal articles usually take the form of electronic files or photocopies of the article that do not need to be returned. Research institutions from low- and middle-income countries can gain free access to hundreds of journals through the HINARI Access to Research in Health Programme, a service of the World Health Organization.

When none of these options yields a copy of the article of interest, another option is to contact the author directly and ask for a copy. Some database entries include the email addresses for article authors, and many journals provide contact information along with the abstract for the articles on their websites. At minimum, many database entries and most journal articles list the institutional affiliations of authors, and an Internet search for those institutions—or a search of social networking websites—will often yield contact information. There is no risk in writing to an author to politely request an electronic copy of an article. Most authors will be flattered that someone is interested in their work. At worst, the requester will get no response from the author. At best, the author might send an electronic copy of the article and an offer of further assistance within minutes of the request being sent.

3.5 Critical Reading

Once the researcher acquires a copy of the full-text article, a practical plan of action is to:

- Re-read the abstract.
- Look carefully at the tables and figures, which usually display the most important results.
- Read (or at least skim) the entire text of the article.
- Review the reference list for any additional sources that the reviewer should read.

Chapter 32 provides a checklist for the particular information to look for within each section of a paper that follows the standard outline for scientific reporting.

All articles should be evaluated carefully. Critical reading involves asking a series of questions about the **internal validity** of a study in order to ascertain how well a particular study was designed, conducted, interpreted, and reported and to assess how likely it is that the resulting paper presents the truth about a particular research question in a particular population at a particular place and time. For example, a reader should ask:

- What was the goal of the study? Were the methods appropriate for the goal? Was the main study question answered?
- Were the methods used to collect and analyze data scientifically valid? For example, did a study collecting new survey data select an appropriate sample population, recruit an adequate number of participants, use a validated questionnaire, and apply appropriate statistical tests? Was the study conducted ethically? Have the authors acknowledged and discussed the limitations of the study methods?

- Do the results seem reasonable? What types of bias in the design, conduct, analysis, and interpretation of the study might have caused some of the results to be inaccurate?
- Are all of the study's conclusions supported by the study's results? If a study was attempting to answer a question about causality, does the article provide sufficient evidence to support that claim?

Critical reading also requires questioning the **external validity** of the study, which is the likelihood that the results of a study with internal validity can be generalized to other populations, places, and times. Questions about external validity (also called **generalizability**) might include ones like:

- How well do the findings of this study fit with existing knowledge about the topic? Have **replication studies** in diverse populations supported the generalizability of the findings?
- For experimental studies, how likely is it that the observations from the trial would occur in everyday life outside laboratory conditions?
- To what other populations might the results apply? For example, are results from a study in Canadian men ages 30–49 likely to be applicable to Mexican men ages 30–49, Canadian women ages 30–49, and/or Canadian men ages 50–69?

3.6 Annotated Bibliographies

One of the common approaches used to track the articles identified during a literature review is the creation of an **annotated bibliography**. An annotated bibliography includes, at minimum, a full reference for the document being reviewed and a brief summary of the article or report. Researchers may also find it helpful to take notes about how a published report relates to the proposed new research project. The goal is not to replicate a document's abstract. The goal is to summarize the content most pertinent to the new investigation.

Some annotated bibliographies for a new research project are compiled in a document file where summary paragraphs can be typed in for each source. Some reference management software programs include a field where personal notes can be added to a record, and this can be used to log annotations about a document. Sometimes it is easiest to extract the most relevant information from each source into a spreadsheet, with separate columns for essential details about the study design, study population, definitions used for exposures and outcomes, statistical results, study limitations, interpretations, and/or the reader's evaluations of internal and external validity.

3.7 What Makes Research Original?

Every researcher is looking for an "original" topic. This can be a paralyzing prospect for anyone who thinks that originality requires the discovery of a newly emergent disease in a previously unrecognized people group on a remote island.

Such remarkable discoveries are occasionally featured in the news, but even a cursory review of the literature proves that the vast majority of original research is far less dramatic. For a research project to demonstrate **originality**, it needs to have only one substantive difference from previous work. That could be a new exposure of interest, a new disease of interest, a new source population, a new time period under study, or a new perspective on a field of exploration.

Figure 3-1 illustrates this point. An original research project could look at a new potential risk factor (E_2) for a disease (D_1) that is already well studied in a population (P_1). It could look at whether an exposure (E_1) that is known to increase the risk of one disease (D_1) in a population (P_1) also increases the risk of a second disease (D_2). Or it could see whether the association between an exposure (E_1) and a disease (D_1) observed in one or more parts of the world (P_1 and P_2) is also true in another part of the world (P_3). Or a research project using a meta-analysis approach could aim to synthesize everything that has already been published on the association between an exposure (E_1) and an outcome (D_1).

For example, a literature review might find that several studies have shown that older adults (the population) who take 30-minute walks several times a week (the

FIGURE 3-1 Ideas for New Studies

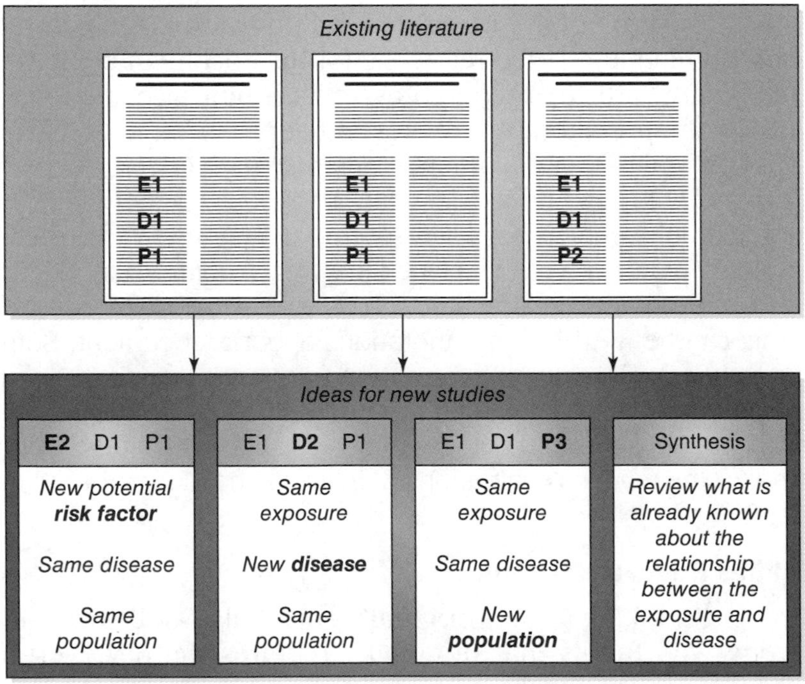

exposure) score higher on memory tests (the disease or outcome) than adults who do not routinely walk for exercise. A proposed new study could ask:

- Is playing table tennis (a new exposure) effective at improving memory in older adults (the same outcome and population)?
- Do older adults who walk several times a week (the same exposure and population) improve their balance (a new disease or outcome)?
- Does walking (the same exposure) improve memory (the same outcome) in children (a new population)?

Once a researcher identifies a possibly novel research question, a more complete review of the literature can help confirm that the area has not already been examined.

Some new investigators struggle to find a research topic that has not been previously explored in the literature, but a recognition that most research is about incremental steps forward opens up infinite options for new explorations. The main challenge when selecting a research question is the need to limit each research project to just one focused area. Very few studies create entirely new areas of research, but every research project has the possibility of contributing to advancing a field of research when it addresses **gaps in the literature** (that is, missing pieces of information that a new study could fill) and builds on previous work.

CHAPTER 4

FOCUSING THE RESEARCH QUESTION

After identifying a general research topic, the researcher needs to develop a specific research goal and a workable research plan.

4.1 Study Approach

The decision about the exact study question must be made in conjunction with the decision about the study approach to use. At a minimum, a choice must be made early in the research process about how data will be gathered (**Figure 4-1**):

- **Primary study**: New data will be collected from individuals.
- **Secondary study**: An existing data set (or data extracted from existing records) will be statistically analyzed.
- **Tertiary study**: The existing literature will be reviewed.

Each of these three major study approaches has its own critical considerations (**Figure 4-2**).

- If new data will be collected, the researcher has great freedom in selecting study topics but may struggle to recruit adequate numbers of participants.

FIGURE 4-1 Primary, Secondary, and Tertiary Research

Research Approach	Study Plan
Primary	Collect and analyze new data
Secondary	Analyze existing data
Tertiary	Review and synthesize the literature

FIGURE 4-2 Key Considerations

Study Approach	Key Questions to Ask
• Collection and analysis of new data	• What are possible source populations? • Will it be possible to recruit enough participants?
• Analysis of existing data	• What are possible sources of usable data files? • What questions can be explored with the available data?
• Review of the literature	• Does the researcher have access to adequate library resources? • Can the researcher reasonably expect to acquire *all* of the needed articles?

- If existing data will be analyzed, then a pertinent and valid source of data must be identified. The researcher must be prepared to select a study question based on the content of the available data files (and knowledge of which variables in the data set have not already been explored by others).
- If the plan is to synthesize current knowledge by conducting a literature review, the researcher must be prepared to track down the full text of all relevant articles. Researchers with a university affiliation need to check with the university library about its policies (and possible fees) for acquiring articles that are not part of the university's collections. Researchers without a university affiliation must consider the costs involved in accessing all of the required articles.

4.2 Conceptual and Theoretical Frameworks

Many research projects benefit from the development of a conceptual model that will inform the design, implementation, and interpretation of the study. A **conceptual framework** is often sketched out using boxes and arrows that illustrate the various relationships that will be evaluated during the study. A variety of established **theoretical frameworks** that are based on extensive reviews of the published literature can inform the components and flows of the conceptual framework for a new research study. For example, several popular theories describe the factors that influence individual health beliefs and behaviors. Conceptual and theoretical frameworks are especially common in the nursing, social science, and educational research literature.

4.3 Study Goal and Specific Objectives

The literature review and consideration of a study approach should lead to the selection of one very specific study topic that can be stated in terms of a single overarching study goal or study question. **Figure 4-3** lists several types of common study goals in the health sciences. A **study goal** often includes the specific exposure, disease, and population that will be the focus of the study.

After finalizing the overarching study goal, the researcher should identify three or more **specific objectives**, **specific aims**, or **hypotheses** that stem from the main study goal. Each of these specific objectives should take the form of a measurable question or a "to" statement that uses action verbs. Each should represent a logical step toward answering the main study question. For example, the study goal may be "to assess the impact of lead poisoning on school performance in kindergarten students in southeast Michigan." The three specific objectives for this study might be:

1. To measure the prevalence of high blood lead levels in a random sample of kindergarten students in southeast Michigan
2. To determine whether children in that sample with high blood lead levels have lower scores on academic tests than children with lower blood lead levels
3. To estimate the total impact of high blood lead levels on kindergarten performance in southeast Michigan by applying the rates in the sample population to the total population of the region

All three of these specific objectives relate to the overall goal of the study, and together they provide a clear pathway for achieving the main goal. Most published

FIGURE 4-3 Examples of Study Goals

- To describe the incidence or prevalence of a particular exposure or disease in one well-defined population
- To assess the perceived health-related needs of a community
- To compare the levels of exposure or disease in two or more populations
- To identify possible risk factors for a particular disease in a population
- To test the effectiveness of a new preventive intervention, diagnostic test, assessment method, therapy, or treatment
- To evaluate whether an intervention shown to be successful in one population is equally successful in a second population
- To examine the impact of a program or policy
- To synthesize or integrate existing knowledge

scientific papers list the study goal and specific objectives in the last paragraph of the introduction section. The specific aims of already published papers related to the topic are often helpful resources when refining the research objectives of a new study.

4.4 Checklist for Success

A consideration when narrowing the focus and clarifying the aims of a new research project is the likelihood that the project can actually be successfully completed. **Figure 4-4** summarizes some of the critical questions to ask before committing to a particular project. These concepts are also captured by the acronym **FINER**, which reminds researchers that a good research project is:

- *F*easible
- *I*nteresting
- *N*ovel
- *E*thical
- *R*elevant

FIGURE 4-4 Questions Essential to the Success of the Project

Area	Questions
Purpose and significance	• What will the study contribute? • What will be new and noteworthy about the study? • Can the importance and necessity of this project be justified? • How will the study enhance the body of knowledge in its discipline? • Who will benefit from the study besides the researcher? • How will the study help individuals and/or communities live healthier lives? • How might the study contribute to improving health practices and/or policies?
Scope and feasibility	• Is the scope of the intended project reasonable and manageable—neither too broad nor too narrow? • Can the proposed study question actually be answered? • Can the researcher answer the proposed study question?

FIGURE 4-4 (continued)

Area	Questions
Capacity and collaborators	• Does the researcher have the knowledge and skills needed to conduct the study? • Does the researcher have access to collaborators who have the expertise needed for the project? (See Chapter 5 for information on assembling a support team.)
Money and materials	• Are there adequate financial resources to conduct the study? • Does the researcher have access to equipment, space, and other physical requirements? • Given the resources available, can the researcher reasonably expect to conduct a scientifically rigorous and valid study?
Time	• Does the researcher have the time to conduct this study? • Does the researcher have the time to make this an excellent study that does not waste health resources?
Population or data	• If the plan is to collect new data from individuals, does the researcher have access to a reasonable source population and an adequate number of participants? • If the plan is to analyze existing data or to write a review paper, does the researcher have access to a reasonable existing data set and/or to an extensive library collection?
Ethics	• Will the researcher be making good use of the resources available? • Has the researcher considered the relevant ethical issues, especially those related to the collection and use of individual-level data? (See Chapter 21 for the ethical issues that should be considered.) • Is the researcher prepared to conduct culturally appropriate and scientifically rigorous research?
Target audience	• Who is likely to be interested in the findings? • Is the resulting paper likely to be publishable?

CHAPTER 5

Collaboration and Mentorship

New researchers should assemble a team of collaborators and mentors early in the research process.

5.1 Collaborators and Consultants

Scientific research is rarely completed by one person working alone, even if the lead investigator may spend many hours working independently on various aspects of a project. Although some papers in the health sciences have only one author, the typical paper has about four coauthors and some have dozens of coauthors. Most projects are headed by a **lead researcher**, defined here as the researcher who will do the majority of the work. (Sometimes, the term "lead researcher" is instead used to refer to the **senior researcher**, an experienced researcher who guides the work of a newer investigator.) Once the lead researcher has committed to doing a research project, it is helpful to assemble a team of collaborators who can help ensure that the project conducted is:

- Scientifically valid
- Ethical and culturally appropriate
- Time- and cost-efficient

For students, the first step is identifying a professor or other experienced researcher to serve as a mentor. For early career professionals, one or more senior colleagues may be willing to serve as formal or informal mentors. Mentors can help the lead author identify and connect with other potential collaborators, such as experts on the study population, experts on the exposure or disease being examined, experts on the study design or methods being used for the project, and technical experts such as statisticians and laboratory specialists. For international research projects, at least one local researcher at the study site should be a coinvestigator who is involved in every step of the research process, including the identification of the study question, the design of the study, and the collection of data.

Some of the individuals the lead researcher communicates with may become core members of the research team and earn coauthorship. Others may play a more limited role as consultants. The lead author should have a conversation with all potential contributors about the amount of time they can dedicate to the project and their expectations regarding compensation and authorship. For example, a statistical consultant may ask to be paid by the hour to help a researcher think through analysis options as a non-coauthor, or the statistician may waive the consulting fee but request coauthorship in return for the development of a data analysis plan, or another arrangement may be requested. The lead author should maintain a record of all the statistical consultants, laboratory technicians, interviewers, librarians, and others who contribute in a meaningful way to the project. When appropriate, these individuals who do not earn coauthorship can be thanked in the acknowledgments sections of manuscripts that benefited from their contributions. (Always ask for permission to thank people by name, because some people prefer not to have their names published.)

5.2 Finding Research Mentors

Sometimes a new investigator does not have a choice about who will supervise a project because the supervisor is assigned by an employer or an academic program director. In this situation, the individual may find it helpful to seek out a team of several mentors who can provide supplemental guidance and advice during the project. (If these individuals may earn coauthorship as a result of their mentorship, their project-specific involvement must be approved by the assigned primary supervisor prior to involving them in the project. The supervisor does not need to approve other mentorship roles, such as those that relate to general professional development.) Student researchers writing theses or dissertations may need to identify a primary mentor and then recruit several additional established scholars to serve on their research committees. New investigators who work in a unit or study in a program that does not have a research requirement may have to seek out their own supervisors and mentors for projects.

Research **mentorship** is a formal or informal relationship in which an experienced mentor offers professional development advice and guidance to a less experienced mentee. When seeking research mentorship, it is important to find mentors who are a good match to the needs and personality of the mentee. New investigators seeking mentorship can identify potential advisors by:

- Asking colleagues, classmates, professors, and others about experienced researchers who might be helpful mentors based on shared research interests, the type(s) of mentorship the new investigator is seeking, and whether the communication style of the potential mentor is a good match to that of the mentee
- Searching the profiles of researchers at the new investigator's home institution (or potential collaborating institutions) to see who is actively conducting and publishing research on relevant topics

- Emailing the individuals identified as potential mentors to share a CV (or résumé) and request an in-person meeting to discuss possible research collaboration opportunities

The new investigator should be prepared for the contacted individuals not to respond or to reply with a message indicating that they are not currently accepting new mentees, interns, or research assistants. Even if a meeting is scheduled, not all conversations will yield a mentor–mentee relationship. An invitation to meet is not an agreement to serve as a mentor. However, all conversations have the possibility of pointing the new investigator to useful resources, including contact information for other individuals who might be well suited to serve as mentors.

5.3 The Mentor–Mentee Relationship

Some formal research mentorship programs require both mentors and mentees to sign an agreement letter that spells out the commitments of both parties, but most mentorships are less formal. A new investigator should not agree to enter into a mentor–mentee relationship until after gaining an informed understanding of several key matters:

- The potential mentor's time availability
- The mentor's preferred frequency and style of communication (such as how often emails will be exchanged and how often telephone calls or in-person meetings will be scheduled)
- The roles and responsibilities the mentor agrees to take on
- The resources the mentor agrees to provide, if the mentee expects the mentor to supply full or partial funding for a project, access to laboratory or computing facilities and equipment, or other types of material support
- The expectations the mentor has of the mentee

Once a research relationship is established, there are many things a mentee can do to ensure that the partnership is a productive and pleasant one. Research supervisors appreciate when mentees:

- Communicate often
- Ask questions
- Complete assigned tasks satisfactorily and on time
- Are honest about what they have done and what they plan to do
- Maintain meticulous research records
- Express gratitude for the contributions of the supervisor

5.4 Professional Development

No one senior researcher, or even a team of research coaches, can provide all of the professional mentorship that a rising researcher requires. Individuals hoping to establish a long-term research trajectory benefit from engaging in a diversity of networking and professional development activities, including:

- Participating in journal clubs that read and discuss recently published research articles
- Becoming active in professional organizations that host research symposia, publish academic journals, and/or provide other opportunities for participating in research-related activities
- Attending and presenting at local, regional, national, and/or international research conferences, and using this time for networking with established researchers
- Enrolling in training programs, which may range from half-day workshops to years-long fellowships

CHAPTER 6

COAUTHORING

Decisions about coauthorship should be made early in the research process.

6.1 Coauthorship

Good coauthors adhere to the highest ethical and professional standards in how they design studies, interact with collaborators and study participants, analyze data, and report their findings. They ask lots of questions so that they fully understand the research project's protocols, the roles and responsibilities of all collaborators, and the decisions made about manuscript drafts. They pay attention to details, and they provide valuable feedback to the lead author and other members of the research team. They are committed to developing their technical writing skills. They disclose potential conflicts of interest. They accept responsibility for their own contributions and for the project as a whole. They treat all members of the research team with respect. And they respond quickly to research communications and never miss a deadline.

Most researchers serve as "middle" coauthors—ones who are not listed first or last in the order of coauthors—before moving into a lead author role for the first time. Being a supporting member of a research team provides an opportunity to become familiar with academic writing and publishing and to develop the habits of good coauthorship. Students working for professors are often hesitant to ask if they will be listed as coauthors on the manuscripts that result from the projects they are supporting. Similar uncertainty might arise for those who are consulted about a research project because they have special technical or other skills but who are not asked to be involved in drafting the subsequent paper. Anyone who is contributing to a project and wants to be considered for inclusion in the authorship list should have a conversation with the lead author as early as possible in the research process so that roles and responsibilities can be clarified.

Lead authors should construct the list of coauthors for a report, poster, or paper based on widely accepted disciplinary standards. All decisions about coauthorshop should be transparent, and they should be communicated to all contributors, both those who are expected to earn coauthorship and those who will be acknowledged but not considered coauthors.

6.2 Authorship Criteria

The **International Committee of Medical Journal Editors (ICMJE)** has established criteria for authorship in the health sciences that most journals in the field have adopted. According to the criteria listed in ICMJE's *Recommendations for the Conduct, Reporting, Editing, and Publication of Scholarly Work in Medical Journals* (as updated in December 2014), to earn **coauthorship** a researcher must meet **all four** of the following conditions:

- Making substantial contributions to conception and design of the study and/or data collection, analysis, or interpretation
- Drafting the article and/or providing critical revisions of intellectual content
- Approving the final version of the article that is submitted and published
- Accepting responsibility for the integrity of the paper

A contributor does not have to engage in all parts of the study—designing the study and collecting the data and analyzing it—to be a coauthor. Participating in a meaningful way in any one of these parts of the study fulfills the first condition. However, participating in design, conduct, and analysis is not sufficient to earn authorship. Authorship requires participation in the writing of the research report. The second ICMJE authorship condition is that all coauthors must make a consequential intellectual contribution to the written product stemming from the research investigation, either by drafting part of the manuscript or by critically revising it. The third condition is intended to ensure that no one is listed as an author against his or her will or without his or her knowledge. A manuscript should not be submitted to a journal until all the coauthors have consented to the submission and agree to accept responsibility for the integrity of their contributions.

According to these guidelines, as examples:

- A person who conducts interviews for the project but does not contribute further would not be eligible for authorship. However, an interviewer who also writes a paragraph for the discussion section would meet authorship criteria.
- A hospital laboratory technician who analyzes blood samples of patients included in a clinical study but makes no further contributions would not be eligible for authorship. A lab tech who analyzes the samples and writes part of the methods section describing laboratory techniques would be a coauthor.
- A data entry assistant who makes no additional contributions to the project would not be considered an author. A data manager who runs statistical tests and creates a results table for the manuscript would meet authorship criteria.
- A technical editor who cleans up the grammar and spelling in a manuscript does not earn authorship. An editor who raises important questions about the interpretation of the results and the meaning of the work may be eligible for authorship.
- Senior researchers who provide funding and supervision for a project usually qualify for authorship, but supervision alone—when not accompanied by involvement in study design or interpretation as well as writing or editing—is not sufficient to justify coauthorship. Just like any other contributor, sponsors and supervisors must make a meaningful intellectual contribution to a project to merit authorship.

These rules are intended to ensure that everyone who has done the work of a coauthor receives recognition for that work and accepts responsibility for it. There should be no **ghost authorships**, in which someone who has made a substantial intellectual contribution is not appropriately recognized. There should be no **gift authorships**, in which someone is given honorary coauthorship without having significantly contributed to the work. Anyone who contributes to a paper without earning coauthorship can be named in an acknowledgments section but not listed as a coauthor.

6.3 Authorship Order

For most disciplines in the health sciences, the **first author** (or **lead author**) is the person who was the most involved in writing the manuscript. Although this is often the person who took the lead in the whole study process from design through analysis and writing, this is not always the case. Sometimes the person who designed the study and collected the data is unable to conduct the analysis and to write up the results, or that person (often a senior researcher) turns the responsibility of writing the manuscript over to someone else who is subsequently listed as the first author. Sometimes multiple people are involved in study design and data acquisition, and one person is asked by the group to take the initiative to generate a draft paper. Sometimes organizations make data sets available to researchers for secondary analysis, and the organizations may not request authorship for any of the employees involved in study design or data collection. In all of these situations, the person who does most of the writing is often designated as the first author. When there is any doubt as to who is making the most significant contribution, the decision about who will be first author should be made in consultation with all of the people who took a major role in conducting the study.

The remaining authors are usually listed in order of contribution, which is usually defined in terms of time dedicated to the project as well as intellectual contribution. The person who contributes the second most amount of time and energy to the project is listed as second author, and so on. When many coauthors are involved, it is sometimes difficult to quantify the relative contributions of, say, the seventh and eighth authors. In this situation, the coauthors should be consulted about their preferences, but the best solution may be to list authors with equal contributions in alphabetical order.

The one exception to the rule about listing authors in order of contribution is that the **senior author**—usually the primary research supervisor for a student or research group—is often listed as the **last author**, even if he or she was heavily involved in all aspects of the work and might otherwise be the second author. Not every paper has a senior author. However, students are usually required to have a professor or other approved supervisor oversee their work, and it is usually helpful for relatively inexperienced researchers to seek out a senior investigator to serve as a mentor. The senior author may or may not be heavily involved in the day-to-day details of the study but meets the authorship criteria by providing clarity and direction along the way and by providing critical feedback on the manuscript. Additionally, the senior author can serve as a mediator if disputes about authorship or other issues arise. An experienced researcher will be able to provide insight into disciplinary standards and can prevent or resolve many of the issues that might befuddle a newer researcher.

6.4 Decisions About Authorship

In order to avoid last-minute debates over which individuals have made important contributions to a research project, it is helpful to decide ahead of time what the roles and responsibilities of each member of the research team will be and how they will earn coauthorship if that is the intended outcome. There should be no surprise about who is being included or excluded as an author. The lead researcher (or senior researcher) should check with each contributor about expectations. Ideally, this conversation should take place before anyone begins work on project-related tasks. If everyone agrees that a person expected to make only a minor contribution will not earn coauthorship, make sure that the person is not asked to write any part of the paper or to provide critical feedback on a draft. If everyone agrees that someone will be a coauthor, make sure that the person has the opportunity to make an important intellectual contribution to the paper.

Decisions about who will be listed as a coauthor on a report, poster, or paper, as well as the order in which those persons will be listed, should be made as early as possible in the research process. Publications are an important metric of success in the sciences and academia, and authorship is often the only reward for the time put into a project. As a result, authorship decisions can be very stressful. They can trigger strong emotional responses, and they can sometimes harm relationships among researchers. Lead researchers therefore need to be transparent with everyone involved in the project not only about who will and will not be contributing in ways that merit coauthorship, but also about the role each person will be playing. A growing number of journals now require a description of what each coauthor contributed to a manuscript and how each met the authorship criteria. It might be helpful to draft that statement before writing any other part of the paper, so that anyone who sees the draft knows what is expected of each coauthor.

Sometimes the list of expected contributors might change during the project. Perhaps a new collaborator is needed to run advanced statistics or to provide an expert's perspective on the policy implications of the work. In such cases, all coauthors need to be immediately informed about the addition. When the addition of new collaborators significantly alters another contributor's position in the order of authors, perhaps bumping a person from second to fourth author, the affected person must be consulted and an agreement reached before any promises are made to the new coauthors.

Any disputes over authorship criteria or the order of authors are usually best referred to the senior author on the paper. The written guidelines for authorship from ICMJE, relevant professional societies, and/or the target journal may also be helpful for resolving disputes. Coauthors with concerns should speak with the lead author first, before appealing to the senior author or other authorities.

STEP

2

Selecting a Study Approach

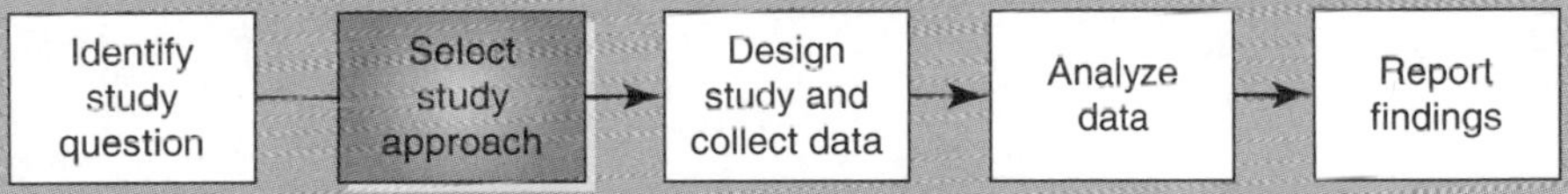

The second step in the research process is selecting a general study approach. This section provides an overview of several of the most common primary study designs.

- Case series
- Cross-sectional surveys
- Case-control studies
- Cohort studies
- Experimental studies
- Qualitative studies
- Correlational studies

CHAPTER 7

OVERVIEW OF STUDY DESIGNS

Many good study designs exist for clinical and population health research. Eight designs are especially common in health science research.

7.1 Types of Study Approaches

Eight study designs are listed in **Figure 7-1**. These designs will be discussed in detail in the following chapters. The figure does not represent a comprehensive list of all types of studies. Many research projects use variations of one of these approaches, and in others a hybrid of two approaches might be suitable. A diversity of designs can be valid and helpful approaches for the collection and analysis of new data, the analysis of existing data, and the reviewing of the literature in the health sciences.

The design selected must be appropriate for the goals of the study. For example, if the goal is to see whether an intervention is effective, an experimental design is likely to be the only suitable one. If the goal is to understand populations, to describe patterns, or to ask research questions that are not focused on causality, the best design may be an observational one, such as a cross-sectional or cohort study. Often, the best study approach is the analysis of existing quantitative data rather than the collection of new data from individual participants. Sometimes the best approach is a systematic review or meta-analysis. Sometimes several different study approaches can be appropriate for exploring the relationship between an exposure and a disease. In these situations, it is helpful to consider other factors during decision-making, including the expected duration and cost of the study, the populations available for inclusion in the study, and the possible availability of existing data.

7.2 Primary, Secondary, and Tertiary Studies

A first critical decision is whether to collect new data from individuals (a primary analysis), use existing data (a secondary analysis), or write a review article (a tertiary analysis) (**Figure 7-2**). Primary studies are often time consuming because they require the collection of new data from participants. However, primary studies

FIGURE 7-1 Summary of Study Approaches

Study Approach	Goal
Case series	Describe a group of individuals with a disease
Cross-sectional survey	Describe exposure and/or disease status in a population
Case-control study	Compare exposure histories in people with disease (cases) and people without diseases (controls)
Cohort study	Compare rates of new (incident) disease in people with different exposure histories or follow a population forward in time to look for incident diseases
Experimental study	Compare outcomes in participants assigned to an intervention or control group
Qualitative study	Seek to understand how individuals and communities perceive and make sense of the world and their experiences
Correlational (ecological) study	Compare average levels of exposure and disease in several populations
Review/meta-analysis	Synthesize existing knowledge

also give the researcher control over important details like the selection of a source population and the content and wording of the questionnaire. The obvious advantage of secondary and tertiary analyses is that a researcher may be able to move quickly from the definition of the study question to the analysis of related data. However, only a limited number of data sets and publications are available for analysis. Also, these sources might not include either the exact variables or the particular population of greatest interest to the researcher.

7.3 Study Duration

The time required for collecting and analyzing data varies from study to study. Some primary studies call for the collection of all needed information from participants at one point in time. Others require participants to be followed for weeks, months, or even years (**Figure 7-3**). The timeline for a secondary study might be very short if an entire data file and the relevant supporting documentation (such as copies of the questionnaire and codebook) can be downloaded from a website. Or secondary data collection might become labor intensive if old hospital charts have to be retrieved, read (often after deciphering somewhat illegible and faded handwriting), coded, and entered into

FIGURE 7-2 Primary, Secondary, and Tertiary Study Approaches

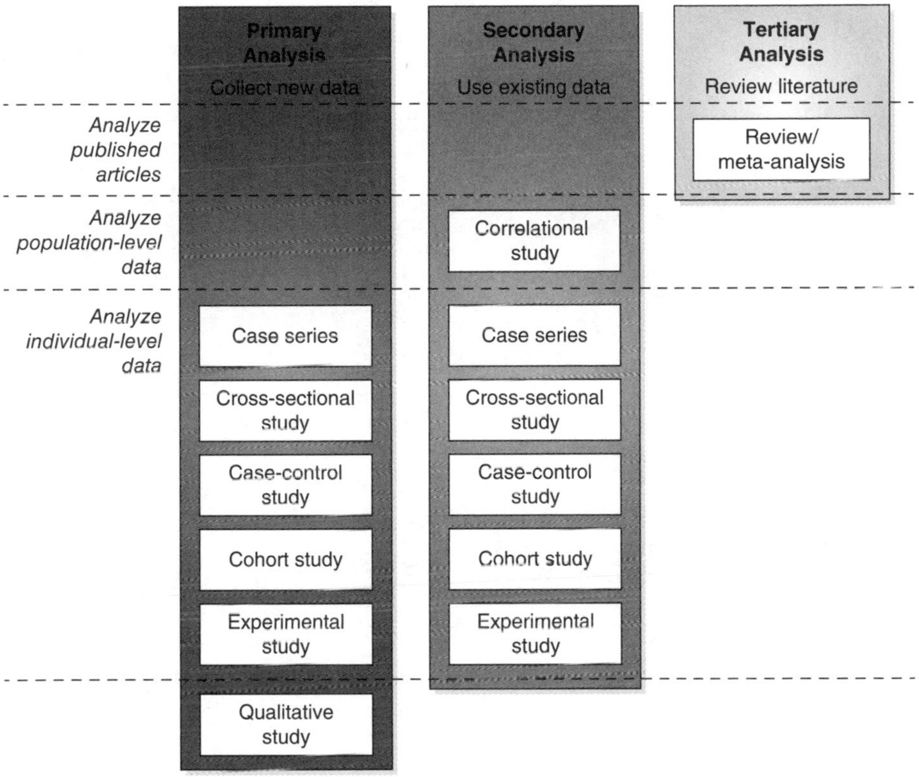

a database. The duration of tertiary studies is highly dependent on library access and on the number of publications that need to be acquired, read, and summarized.

7.4 Primary Focus: Exposure, Disease, or Population?

Most study designs are oriented toward a particular kind of population (**Figure 7-4**). All interventional studies and many cohort studies focus on individuals with a particular exposure—one that is assigned in experimental trials and merely observed in cohort studies. Case series and case-control studies both focus on individuals ("cases") with a particular disease. Cross-sectional studies and some types of cohort studies seek to recruit a study population that is representative of a well-defined larger population. Researchers who have relatively easy access to a group of individuals with a particular exposure or disease or to a unique population group often choose a study approach based on the design's appropriateness for the available participants.

FIGURE 7-3 Time Frame for Primary Data Collection

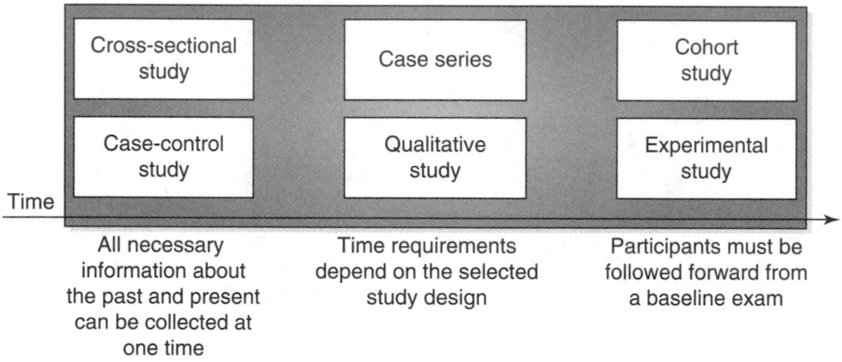

FIGURE 7-4 Population Selection for Each Study Approach

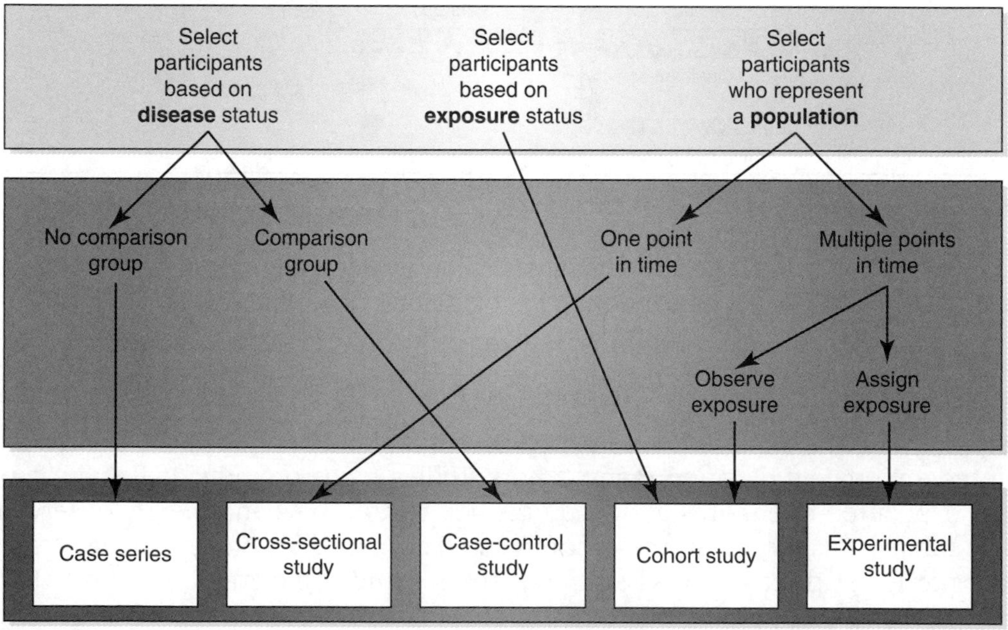

CHAPTER 8

Case Series

A case series describes a group of patients who have the same disease condition or who have undergone the same procedure.

8.1 Overview

A **case report** describes one patient. A **case series** describes a group of individuals with the same disease or who have undergone the same procedure (**Figure 8-1**). A case series can only be written and disseminated when a researcher has access to an appropriate source of cases and when there is a compelling reason to write about those cases. This study approach can be useful for:

- Describing the characteristics of and similarities among a group of individuals with the same signs and/or symptoms of disease
- Identifying new syndromes and refining case definitions
- Clarifying typical disease progression
- Describing atypical presentations of a disease or unusual complications from a treatment
- Developing hypotheses for future research

Some case series for rare conditions may require only a handful of participants. Others may include several hundred or even several thousand individuals.

8.2 Case Definitions

A researcher conducting a case series must select one disease of interest, determine what will be new and interesting about the study, and identify an appropriate and available source of cases. The next step is to establish a clear **case definition** that spells out inclusion and exclusion criteria. Participants may be selected from clinical locations that use **ICD codes** (that is, diagnoses based on the International Classification

FIGURE 8-1 Key Characteristics of a Case Series

Objective	Describe a group of individuals with a disease
Primary study question	What are the key characteristics of the cases in this study population?
Population	All individuals in the study must have the same disease or be undergoing the same procedure.
When to use this approach	A source of cases is available, and no comparison group is required or available.
Requirement	An appropriate source of cases is available.
First steps	1. Specify what new and important information the analysis will provide. 2. Identify a source of cases. 3. Assign a case definition. 4. Select the characteristics of the study population that will be described.
What to watch out for	A lack of generalizability
Key statistical measure	Only descriptive statistics are required.

of Diseases, known more formally as the International Statistical Classification of Diseases and Related Health Problems). If so, the ICD number can be part of the case definition, but a code alone is rarely sufficient to cover all inclusion and exclusion criteria. A more comprehensive case definition will include a disease description plus any relevant **person, place, and time ("PPT")** characteristics (**Figure 8-2**). Case definitions are also essential for any outbreak investigation, no matter which study approach is used to investigate the epidemic.

8.3 Special Considerations

A case series might be constructed from primary data acquired by interviewing cases about their experiences using a questionnaire and/or qualitative techniques. The data might be supplemented or confirmed with a review of the participants' medical records. Alternatively, a case series can be—and often is—based solely on secondary data, usually acquired from a review of patient charts.

When medical records will be consulted as part of the data collection process, it is often helpful to create a questionnaire that guides the extraction of information from these files. One of the limitations of relying on patient charts is that they

FIGURE 8-2 Sample Case Definitions

Category	Example 1	Example 2
Disease/ procedure	Whooping cough (ICD-10 code A37)	Liver transplantation
Person	Any person with a confirmed case of whooping cough, defined as an acute cough of any duration with isolation of Bordatella pertussis from a clinical specimen or a cough lasting 2 or more weeks with paroxysms of coughing, inspiratory "whoop," or posttussive vomiting and contact with a laboratory-confirmed case of pertussis	Adult patients (ages 18 and older at the time of transplant), excluding those who were not receiving their first liver transplant and those who received multi-organ transplants
Place	Residents of Big City whose diagnoses were reported to the Big City Health Department (which requires notification of all diagnoses of pertussis)	Patients who had transplant surgery at the Oakville Regional University Medical Center
Time	First sought clinical care between January 1 and March 31, 2016	Recipients of liver transplants between January 1, 2006, and December 31, 2014, who were followed for a minimum of 2 years post-transplant

usually contain only information deemed at the time of examination to be clinically relevant. The medical information in patient files is not recorded for research purposes, so records are unlikely to contain all the information that researchers would like to know. Many signs and symptoms, patient comments, and clinician observations are not routinely recorded. As a result, the absence of a specific note about a symptom or history does not necessarily mean that the exposure was not present, just that it was not recorded. A data extraction tool should include space to indicate the absence of a desired piece of information in the record. During the analysis and interpretation stage of the research project, the researcher should carefully consider the amount and type of missing information.

Case series studies come with special requirements to protect patient privacy. All case series projects require approval by a research ethics committee, as well as informed consent from participants and/or the careful use of existing records. Researchers must pay close attention to protecting the identities of participants. This is especially important when the disease or procedure is relatively rare and/or when the place and time characteristics are so narrow that individuals familiar with the source community might be able to recognize the participants. In most situations, all potentially identifiable information must be removed prior to publication.

All clinicians and researchers whose work might be enhanced by the use of photography must adhere to patient privacy laws and regulations as well as the policies of the medical centers where they work. When photographs will be used as part of a published article or public presentation, the researcher usually must acquire informed consent to share the patient's image in this way. Many journals require written proof of consent from patients before images with potentially identifiable features are published. Documentation of consent may be required even when there are no identifying marks in the image that could reveal the participant's identity.

8.4 Analysis

Most case study reports do not require any numbers beyond simple counts and percentages, but some may benefit from the use of well-defined measures of morbidity and mortality. For example, the **case fatality rate** is the proportion of persons with a particular disease who die as a result of that condition. (This is different from the **mortality rate**, which is the percentage of members of a population who die of any condition during a specified time period. It is also different from the **proportionate mortality rate**, which is the proportion of deceased members of a population whose death was attributable to a particular cause.) When the sample size is sufficiently large, statistical tests may be used to compare subpopulations of cases or to compare before-and-after measures for the same individual participants.

Although many case series studies do not have any time dimension, some follow patients for days, months, or even years. In this type of study approach, the case series becomes, functionally, a cohort study in which all participants are defined by their disease status. Chapter 12 discusses cohort study approaches.

CHAPTER 9

Cross-Sectional Surveys

A cross-sectional survey provides a snapshot of the health status of a population at one point in time. Cross-sectional surveys, sometimes called prevalence studies, are among the most popular study approaches in the health sciences because they allow for the rapid collection of new data.

9.1 Overview

The goal of a **cross-sectional survey**, also called a **prevalence study**, is to measure the proportion of a population with a particular exposure or disease. This determination should be made over a short period of time based on a representative stample of a population (see **Figure 9-1**). Cross-sectional surveys are used to:

- Describe communities
- Assess population needs
- Support program planning
- Monitor and evaluate programs
- Establish baseline data prior to the initiation of longitudinal studies

Cross-sectional surveys are one of the most common study designs used in **epidemiology**, the study of the distribution and determinants of health in populations.

9.2 Representative Populations

In some ways, cross-sectional studies use the simplest study design. The researcher just asks an adequate number of people—usually a few hundred—to complete a short questionnaire, and then those data are analyzed. However, there is one very important requirement: The participants must be reasonably representative of some larger population. **Representativeness** means that the researchers cannot simply ask friends, the fans attending a youth football game, or individuals attending one chiropractic clinic to complete a survey and then assume that the results of

FIGURE 9-1 Key Characteristics of Cross-Sectional Surveys

Objective	Describe the exposure and/or disease status in a population
Primary study question	What is the prevalence of the exposure and/or disease in the population?
Population	The study participants must be representative of the population from which they were drawn.
When to use this approach	Time is limited and/or the budget is small.
Requirement	The exposures and outcomes are relatively common, and the researchers expect to be able to recruit several hundred participants.
First steps	1. Define a source population. 2. Develop a strategy for recruiting a representative sample. 3. Decide on the methods to be used for data collection.
What to watch out for	Non-representativeness of the study population
Key statistical measure	Prevalence

the survey will be generalizable to all town residents. If the results are intended to reflect the profile of an entire town or other population group, then the study's sampling strategy must recruit a population that is as diverse as the town. Chapter 16 has more detailed information about populations for a cross-sectional survey, and Chapter 17 explains how to estimate sample size requirements.

9.3 KAP Surveys

One commonly used type of cross-sectional study is a **KAP survey** that asks participants about their *k*nowledge, *a*ttitudes (or beliefs or perceptions), and *p*ractices (or behaviors). A KAP survey may be conducted with a representative sample of the patients of a hospital system or clinical practice, the clients of a community organization or business, the students or employees of a school district, the residents of a neighborhood or city, or the members of some other well-defined population. KAP surveys can be particularly helpful for identifying gaps between what people know and how they act on that knowledge. For example, the adults in a KAP survey might demonstrate high knowledge about the benefits of exercise on cardiovascular health but at the same time indicate that they exercise rarely because a variety of perceived barriers prevent them from being as physically active as they know they ought to be for maximum fitness.

9.4 Repeated Cross-Sectional Surveys

A **repeated cross-sectional study** re-samples and re-surveys representatives from the same source population at two or more different time points. For example, a cross-sectional survey might be conducted annually as part of a national health surveillance program. This is the method used for many of the largest studies conducted by the U.S. CDC, including the Behavioral Risk Factor Surveillance System (BRFSS), the National Health and Nutrition Examination Survey (NHANES), and the U.S. National Health Interview Survey (NHIS). A repeated cross-sectional study design does not track the same individuals forward in time. Instead, a new set of participants is sampled from the source population each time a survey is conducted. Some people may happen by chance to be selected for more than one round of surveying, but their answers to the different surveys are not linked. Repeated cross-sectional surveys can reveal trends in population-level metrics over time, but they do not allow for the examination of individual-level changes. (A longitudinal cohort study is used to study individual participants over a lengthy period of time.)

9.5 Analysis: Prevalence

Cross-sectional surveys measure the prevalence of various exposure histories, disease states, and demographic characteristics in one well-defined population at one point in time (or over a short duration of time, with all data collected within a few days, weeks, or months). The most common way to report results for a cross-sectional survey is simply to report the **prevalence rate**, which is the percentage of the population with a given trait at the time of the survey.

Comparative measures can also be used. For example, **prevalence rate ratios** compare the prevalence of a characteristic in two population subgroups by taking a ratio of their prevalence rates, such as comparing the prevalence rate in males to the rate in females or comparing the rate in older adults to the rate in younger adults. Because a cross-sectional survey has no time dimension, it cannot be used to assess causality. An exposure can be said to be "associated" or "related" to a disease, but a cross-sectional survey cannot show that an exposure caused a disease.

CHAPTER 10

Case-Control Studies

A case-control study compares the exposure histories of people with and without a particular disease in order to identify likely risk factors for the disease.

10.1 Overview

Individual participants in a **case-control study** are selected for inclusion in the study based on their disease status (**Figure 10-1**). Participants with the disease of interest are classified as **cases**. Those without the disease are classified as **controls**. Both cases and controls are asked the same set of questions about past exposures (**Figure 10-2**). A case-control study is often the best study approach for identifying possible risk factors for a disease. This is especially true when the disease is uncommon, and a study of the general population would be unlikely to yield more than a few cases. A special type of statistic—an odds ratio—is used to identify likely risk factors.

10.2 Finding Cases and Controls

Because case-control studies require an adequate number of cases in order to be valid, the first step in designing a case-control study is to identify an appropriate and accessible source of individuals with the disease of interest. Hospitals, specialty clinics, physicians' offices, public health agencies, disease registries, and disease support groups may be able to assist researchers in identifying individuals who are likely to meet the study's case definition.

Regardless of the source, in most situations these organizations will not release any information about individuals until a research project has received approval from an appropriate ethics oversight committee. When patient health information is disclosed, the researcher must exercise extreme care to protect the privacy of potential participants and the confidentiality of their personal information.

FIGURE 10-1 Key Characteristics of Case-Control Studies

Objective	Compare exposure histories of people with a disease (cases) and people without that disease (controls)
Primary study question	Do cases and controls have different exposure histories?
Population	Cases and controls must be similar except for their disease status.
When to use this approach	The disease is relatively uncommon, but a source of cases is available.
Requirement	A source of cases is available.
First steps	1. Identify a source of cases. 2. Assign a case definition. 3. Decide what type of control population will be appropriate for the study. 4. Decide whether cases and controls will be matched.
What to watch out for	Recall bias
Key statistical measure	Odds ratio (OR)

All cases must have the same disease, disability, or other health-related condition, and the study's case definition must specify exactly what characteristics must be present or absent for a person to be deemed a case. Clinical manuals and publications stemming from previous studies of the disease can be helpful references for

FIGURE 10-2 Framework for a Case-Control Study

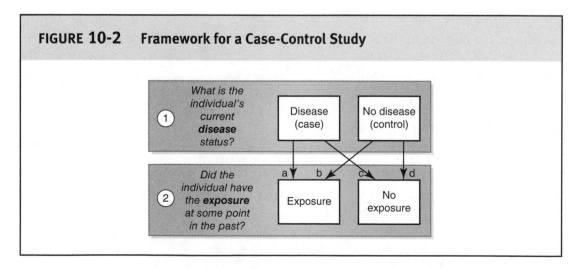

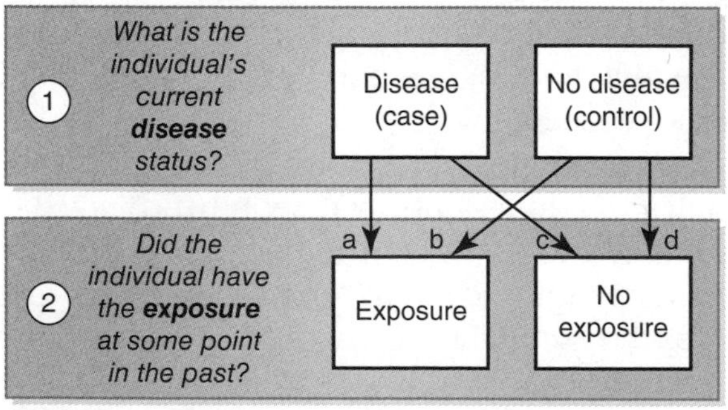

drafting and refining the inclusion and exclusion criteria. The case definition should include person, place, and time (PPT) characteristics.

Next, an appropriate source of controls must be selected. Depending on the goals of the study, controls may be recruited from, among other sources:

- Friends and relatives of cases
- Hospital or clinic patients without the disease of interest
- The general population

A **control definition** should spell out all of the eligibility criteria for members of the comparison population. Controls must be similar to cases except for their disease status, so the inclusion and exclusion criteria for cases that do not specifically relate to the disease must also apply to controls. For example, if cases must be males between 25 and 39 years of age, controls must also be men in this age group.

Individuals who do not meet the case definition or the control definition must be excluded from the study. Excluded individuals may not meet one of the person, place, or time criteria for inclusion, or they may have an intermediate or indeterminate disease status that prevents them from meeting either the case or the control definition.

Chapter 16 provides additional details about the selection of cases and controls for case-control studies.

10.3 Matching

Early in the study design process, a decision must be made about whether and how to match cases and controls. There are three often-used options for **matching**: no matching, frequency (group) matching, and matched-pairs (individual) matching.

Some studies use no matching. They simply assume that similar inclusion and exclusion criteria for cases and controls will result in case and control populations that have similar distributions according to sex, age group, socioeconomic status, and other characteristics that may be confounders of the association between the key exposure and the disease.

Some studies use **frequency matching** (also called **group matching**) for a few variables to ensure comparable case and control populations. For example, suppose a study is using hospitalized cases and controls. For each case, the researcher may select one control from the hospital registration files who was admitted the same week as the case, who is the same sex as the case, and who is within ±3 years of the age of the case. Alternatively, frequency matching can be used to identify two, three, or more controls for each case. (The process of estimating the sample size required for different ratios of cases to controls is described in Chapter 17.) For group matching like this, the goal is to recruit a control population that is similar to the case population. Individual cases are not linked to individual controls during analysis, so the analysis uses the same approaches as those used for unmatched case-control studies.

Some studies use **matched-pairs matching** (also called **individual matching**). Each case is personally linked to a particular individual control. This approach is common in genetic studies that link each case to a genetic sibling or another close genetic relative for analysis. This kind of matched-pairs approach requires a special type of analysis that is discussed at the end of this chapter.

For both frequency matching and matched-pairs matching, it is important not to overmatch. The variables used as matching criteria cannot be considered as exposures during analysis. For example, suppose cases and controls are frequency matched based on the date of hospital admission, sex, and age. The case and control populations will therefore, by design, have the same proportion of admissions in April, the same percentages of males and females, and about the same mean age. As a result of this forced similarity, the study will not be able to examine whether cases are more or less likely than controls to require hospitalization in a certain month, to be males, or to be octogenarians. Additionally, when there are more matching characteristics, it can be difficult to find controls who meet all of the matching criteria. The study population may end up being quite different from the general population because of the strict eligibility requirements, and this may limit the external validity of the study. **Overmatching** may also result in a statistical bias that obscures the relationship between an exposure and the disease.

10.4 Special Considerations

Once the key decisions about the study design are made, planning for data collection may begin, as described in the third section of this book. Researchers must think carefully about possible sources of **bias**, a systematic error in the design, conduct, or analysis of a study that can cause the results of a study not to accurately reflect the truth about the source population. Each type of study design has particular types of bias that are most likely to be problematic, but careful study design and implementation can minimize the associated problems. Researchers must keep two considerations in mind when designing the survey instrument for case-control studies.

First, each participant must be asked questions that confirm whether the respondent is a case, a control, or neither. The questions must ensure that only confirmed cases and controls are included in the analysis. Adhering to strict definitions for what constitutes a case and what constitutes a control minimizes the risk of **misclassification bias**.

Second, researchers must be aware of the risk of **recall bias**, which occurs when cases and controls systematically have different memories of the past. This type of risk is particularly important in case-control studies. Participants are often asked to recall events from the distant past that cannot be confirmed by documents from when the exposure would have occurred. Cases may be searching for answers to questions about why they have become ill. As a result, they may have more vivid memories of participation or lack of participation in activities perceived to be risky or beneficial. For example, adult cases in a study of night blindness may report that they rarely ate carrots as children. They may say this not because they never ate carrots but because they assume that they would have good vision as adults if they had eaten lots of vegetables high in vitamin A when they were younger. Alternatively, cases may overestimate childhood carrot intake. They may wonder why they developed night blindness when they have such fond memories of happily munching on carrot sticks every day at lunch in grade school. The reality may be that they ate carrots only once a month. Controls, on the other hand, are unlikely to have spent much time thinking about risk factors for poor eyesight. They may recall eating carrots sometimes rather than rarely or often.

Because of recall bias, a study of nightblindness might find a significant difference in the reported childhood consumption of carrots by cases and controls even if in reality there was no difference in the average diet of the two groups. Alternatively, the survey may fail to capture a true difference in dietary history. Although there is no way to prove that recall bias is occurring because of systematically different memories among cases and controls, the results of case-control studies must be interpreted cautiously in light of the possibility that differential recall may have influenced the findings.

10.5 Analysis: Odds Ratios (ORs)

Researchers considering using a case-control study approach must become familiar and comfortable with the concepts of odds and odds ratios. The odds ratio is the measure of association that readers will expect to be reported for a case-control study. **Odds** are most familiar from their connection with betting. A horse with an equal chance of winning a race (50% likely to win) or of losing a race (50% likely to lose) is said to have "even odds," or odds of 1 (50%/50%). Similarly, a case-control study compares the likelihood of having had a particular exposure to not having had it (**Figure 10-3**). If 50% of the participants in a study report a history of exposure and 50% report no past exposure, then the odds of exposure are 50%/50%, or 1. If 25% report having the exposure and 75% do not, then the odds are 25%/75%, or 0.33. If 2% report being exposed in the past and 98% report not being exposed, then the odds are 2%/98%, or 0.02.

The main measure of association for case-control studies compares the odds of exposure among cases to the odds of exposure among controls. This is called an **odds ratio (OR)**. A **contingency table** (sometimes called a **crosstab**) is a row-by-column table that displays the counts of how often various combinations of events happen. **Two-by-two (2×2) tables** are used in case-control studies to compare two dichotomous (yes/no) variables. **Figure 10-4** shows a sample 2×2 table for a case-control study. In the 2×2 table for an unmatched case-control study, the columns are for disease status (case = yes, and control = no) and the rows are for exposure status (exposed = yes, and unexposed = no). All of the participants in the study are assigned to one of the four resulting boxes: *(a)* cases with an exposure history, *(b)* controls with an exposure history, *(c)* cases with no exposure history, and *(d)* controls with no exposure history. As a check, the total number of cases

FIGURE 10-3 Odds

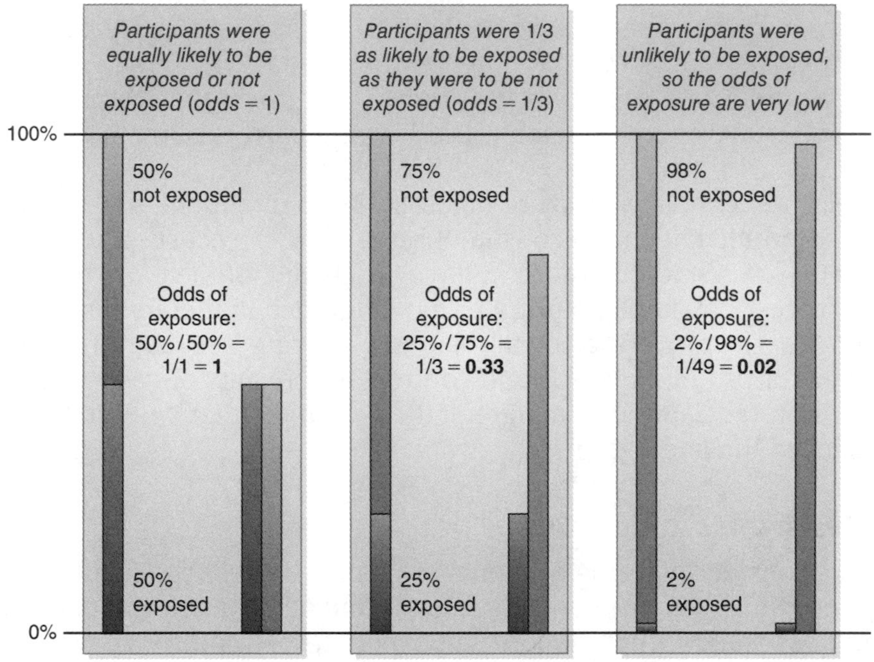
Participants were equally likely to be exposed or not exposed (odds = 1)
Participants were 1/3 as likely to be exposed as they were to be not exposed (odds = 1/3)
Participants were unlikely to be exposed, so the odds of exposure are very low
100%
0%
50% not exposed
Odds of exposure: 50%/50% = 1/1 = 1
50% exposed
75% not exposed
Odds of exposure: 25%/75% = 1/3 = 0.33
25% exposed
98% not exposed
Odds of exposure: 2%/98% = 1/49 = 0.02
2% exposed

FIGURE 10-4 Odds Ratio (Point Estimate)

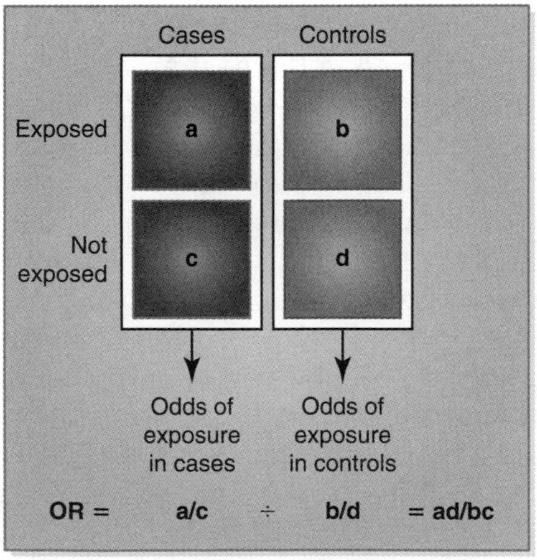
Cases
Controls
Exposed
Not exposed
a
b
c
d
Odds of exposure in cases
Odds of exposure in controls
OR = a/c ÷ b/d = ad/bc

in the study should be $a + c$, the total number of controls in the study should be $b + d$, and the total number of participants should be $a + b + c + d$.

The odds of exposure in cases are the number of cases with the exposure (a) divided by the number of cases without the exposure (c). The odds of exposure in controls are the number of controls with the exposure (b) divided by the number of controls without the exposure (d). Basic algebra shows that the equation for the odds ratio of $(a \div c)/(b \div d)$ can be simplified to

$$\mathrm{OR} = \frac{ad}{bc}$$

This calculation is the **point estimate** for the odds ratio, and it provides a starting point for understanding the relationship between the disease and exposure status in the study population.

- OR = 1: the odds of exposure were the same for cases and controls.
- OR > 1: cases had higher odds of exposure than controls, implying that the exposure was risky.
- OR < 1: cases had lower odds of exposure than controls, implying that the exposure was protective.

The 95% confidence interval shows whether an OR is statistically significant (**Figure 10-5**). (Chapter 17 provides additional information about how to interpret confidence intervals and how they are related to sample size.)

FIGURE 10-5 Interpretation of the Odds Ratio Based on Its 95% Confidence Interval

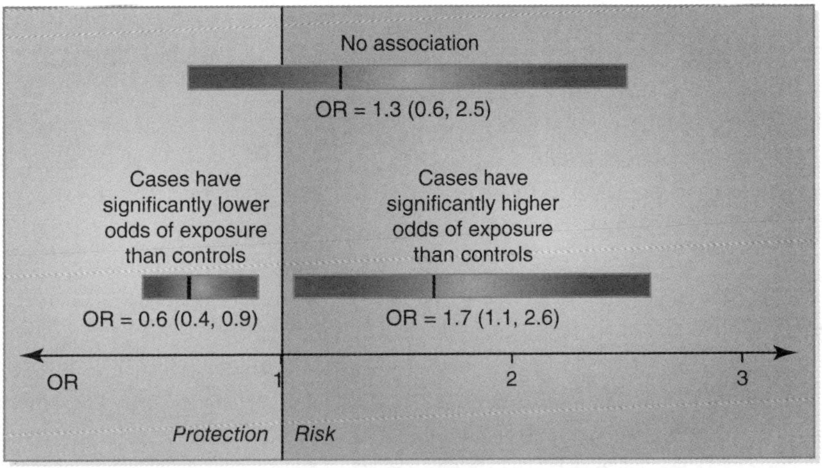

- When the entire 95% confidence interval is less than 1, the OR is statistically significant, and the exposure is deemed to be protective in the study population.
- When the entire 95% confidence interval is greater than 1, the OR is statistically significant, and the exposure is deemed to be risky in the study population.
- When the 95% confidence interval (95% CI) overlaps OR = 1, the OR is said to be not statistically significant in the study population. This is because the lower end of the confidence interval is less than 1, suggesting protection, while the higher end of the confidence interval is greater than 1, suggesting risk. In this situation, the exposure and disease are deemed to have no association in the study population. This may reflect a true absence of a relationship between the exposure and the disease, but it may also indicate that the sample size was too small. Power calculations can be used to verify whether the sample size was sufficient to detect differences in the odds among cases and controls if a difference really did exist.

Chi-square tests are derived from the same tables used to calculate odds ratios. When the 95% confidence interval does not overlap 1, the *p*-value for the Chi-square test will be $p < 0.05$, which is statistically significant. When the 95% confidence interval for an OR overlaps the number 1, the *p*-value for the Chi-square test will be $p > 0.05$, which indicates no association.

Once the counts for *a, b, c,* and *d* are known, computer- and Internet-based statistical programs (such as statistical software packages or the OpenEpi.com website) can be used to calculate the point estimate for the OR (the value of *ad/bc*), along with its corresponding 95% confidence interval. Sample output is shown in **Figure 10-6**. One example has an odds ratio of 1.588 and a 95% confidence interval of (1.027, 2.453), implying that the exposure was risky since the entire 95% CI is greater than 1. The Chi-square *p*-value of $p < 0.05$ confirms this conclusion. The other example has an odds ratio of 1.158 (0.650, 2.066). Since the 95% CI overlaps 1, the association is not statistically significant. The correct conclusion in this example is that there is no association between the exposure and the disease. The Chi-square *p*-value of $p > 0.05$ confirms this conclusion. Logistic regression models can be used to calculate odds ratios that adjust for possible confounding variables.

For a case-control study, it is incorrect to say that "the exposed had a higher (or lower) rate of disease than the unexposed" because the rates of disease in exposed and unexposed participants are not known. Case-control studies recruit participants because they have or do not have a disease. Usually about 50% of participants in a case-control study are cases even if cases make up less than 1% of the community from which the study population was drawn. As a result, the prevalence of disease among exposed persons in the study population could be 70% even when the prevalence of disease among exposed persons in the community from which participants were drawn is less than 1%. Because the study population is usually not representative of the community as a whole, case-control studies are unable to estimate rates of disease among the exposed and unexposed.

FIGURE 10-6 Examples of Odds Ratio Calculations

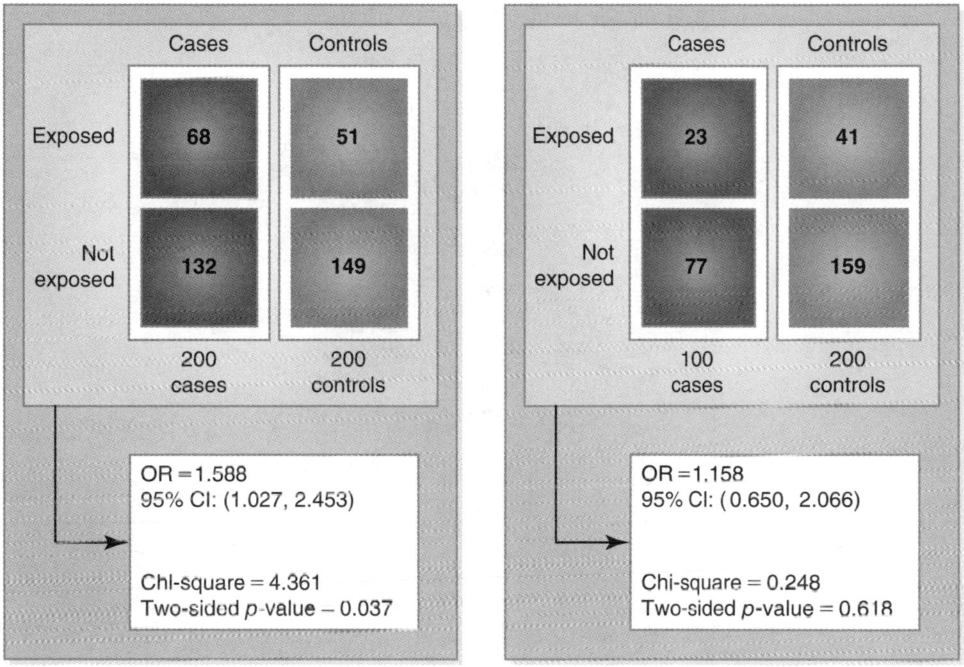

Case-control studies are, however, able to examine odds of exposure among the diseased and the not diseased. For case-control studies, the orientation should always be from disease status to exposure history, and from odds rather than risks or rates. Accordingly, the results should always be phrased to indicate that cases had greater (or lesser) odds of exposure than controls.

10.6 Matched Case-Control Studies

Individually matched case-control studies require the calculation of a matched-pairs odds ratio that uses a special kind of 2×2 table that shows how often pairs of cases and controls had the same or different exposure histories (**Figure 10-7**). When both the case and control in a matched pair have the same history of exposure or no exposure, their experiences are **concordant** (cells *a* and *d*). Concordant pairs do not provide much useful information about the potential relationship between the exposure and the disease. However, when the exposure histories for a pair are **discordant** (cells *b* and *c*), they provide an indication about whether the exposure is likely to be risky or protective. A ratio of the number of times the case was exposed and the control was not (*b*) to the number of times the control was exposed and the

FIGURE 10-7 Matched-Pairs Odds Ratio

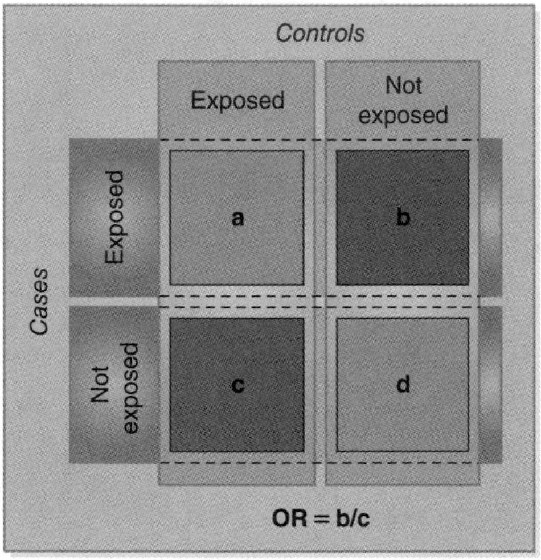

case was not (*c*) provides an estimate for a special type of **matched-pairs odds ratio** ($OR_{mp} = b/c$).

- When $b/c > 1$ and the 95% confidence interval (which is calculated using all four categories in the figure, including the concordant pairs) does not overlap 1, cases were more likely than controls to have been exposed. This implies that the exposure is risky.
- When $b/c < 1$ and the 95% confidence interval does not overlap 1, cases were less likely than controls to have had the exposure. This implies that the exposure is protective.
- When the 95% confidence interval for b/c includes 1, then there is no statistically significant association between the disease and the exposure.

For additional information about how to analyze individually matched (matched-pairs) case-control studies, consult a reference that specifically addresses matched-pairs methods and analysis.

CHAPTER 11

Cohort Studies

A cohort study follows participants through time to calculate the rate at which new disease occurs and to identify risk factors for the disease.

11.1 Overview

A **cohort** is a group of similar people followed through time together (**Figure 11-1**). Health research makes use of several types of cohort-based study approaches. All **cohort studies** are observational (not experimental) studies with at least two measurement times:

- An initial survey that determines the baseline exposure and disease status of all participants

FIGURE 11-1 Key Characteristics of Cohort Studies

Approach	Prospective or Retrospective Cohort	Longitudinal Cohort
Objective	Compare rates of new (incident) disease over time in people with and without a particular well-defined exposure.	Follow a representative sample of a well-defined population forward in time to look for new (incident) diseases associated with a diversity of exposures.
Primary study question	Is exposure associated with an increased incidence of disease?	Is exposure associated with an increased incidence of disease?

FIGURE 11-1 Key Characteristics of Cohort Studies (continued)

Approach	Prospective or Retrospective Cohort	Longitudinal Cohort
Population	Participants must be similar except for exposure status.	Participants must be available for follow-up months or years after enrollment.
	Because the goal is to look for incident disease, no one can have the disease of interest at the start of the study.	The study participants must be reasonably representative of the population from which they were drawn.
Use this approach when	An exposure is relatively uncommon but a source of exposed individuals is available.	The goal is to examine multiple exposures and multiple outcomes and time is not a concern.
Do not use unless	A source of individuals with the exposure is available.	There is adequate time and money for the study.
First steps	1. Identify a source of individuals with the exposure. 2. Decide what type of unexposed individuals will be an appropriate comparison group.	1. Select a source population. 2. Select the exposures and outcomes that will be assessed. 3. Decide how often data will be collected. 4. Develop a strategy for minimizing the burden of participation and maximizing benefits and incentives.
Watch out for	Loss to follow-up (prospective studies) or missing records (retrospective studies)	Loss to follow-up
	Information bias in which the exposed participants are more thoroughly examined for disease than unexposed participants	Potential data management challenges if a lot of information is collected at many points in time
Key statistical measure	Incidence rate ratio (RR, also called the relative risk)	Incidence rate ratio (RR, also called the relative risk)

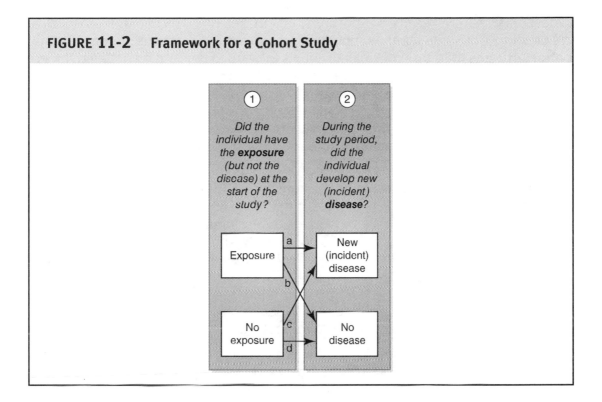

FIGURE 11-2 Framework for a Cohort Study

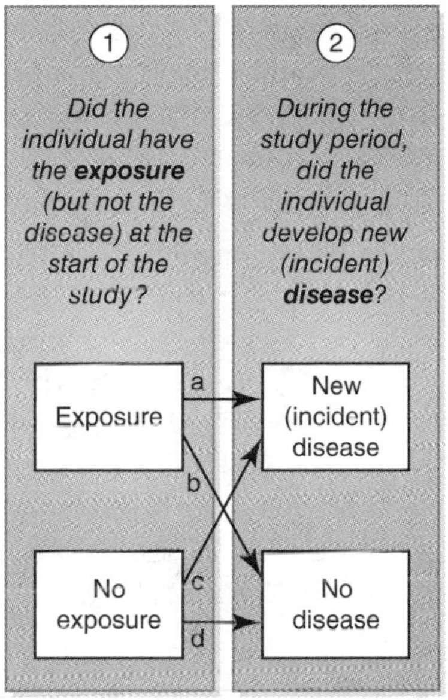

- One or more follow-up assessments that determine how many participants have developed a new (incident) disease since the initial examination (**Figure 11-2**).

Because information is collected from individuals at multiple points in time, researchers can know with certainty which exposures were present in individual participants before the onset of new disease. This information allows for the identification of potentially causal exposures.

11.2 Types of Cohort Studies

Cohort studies can take many forms. For simplicity, this chapter will group cohort study designs into three categories: retrospective, prospective, and longitudinal. Because the word "prospective" (which means future-oriented) can be used as an adjective for any cohort study, the published literature is somewhat inconsistent in how these particular terms are used. Any study that follows participants forward in time can be considered to be a **prospective study**. However, the epidemiological approaches for these three types of cohort studies are distinct.

Both **retrospective cohort studies** (sometimes called **historic cohort studies**) and **prospective cohort studies** recruit participants based on their exposure status. One group of participants is recruited because they are known to have had a particular exposure. A second group is recruited because they are known not to have been exposed. Recruiting based on exposure status makes retrospective and prospective cohort studies the optimal study approaches for uncommon exposures. **Longitudinal cohort studies** follow a group of individuals forward in time but do not recruit them based on exposure status. Instead, participants are recruited based on membership in a well-defined source population. Longitudinal cohorts may follow all the residents of one town, a representative sample of members of one professional organization, or a cohort of students recruited from the same university.

For retrospective and prospective cohort studies, the members of the two comparison groups should be similar except for their exposure status. For example:

- A retrospective cohort study might compare industrial workers exposed to a certain chemical to workers in a plant that does not use the chemical. It would not be valid to compare factory workers to office managers.
- A prospective cohort study might compare health outcomes in children with high blood lead levels and low blood lead levels who attend the same elementary school. It would not be as helpful to examine the impact of blood lead levels if the exposed students were from one primary school and the unexposed were from another school. Any differences in health observed might be due to differences in socioeconomic status rather than lead exposure.

The key difference between retrospective and prospective studies is when the baseline measurements are established (**Figure 11-3**). Retrospective cohort studies use documented baseline information collected at some point in the past and follow the cohort to another point in the past or to the present. Retrospective studies establish baseline information from birth records, school records, medical files, occupational records, or other sources that may be decades old. Then the researcher matches the baseline records to later files or to information solicited directly from the same individuals in the present. For example, a retrospective cohort study might track down two groups of young adults in equal numbers: those born at a particular hospital in a particular year who had low birthweights and those born in the same hospital in the

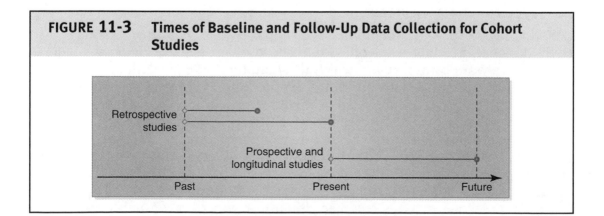

FIGURE 11-3 Times of Baseline and Follow-Up Data Collection for Cohort Studies

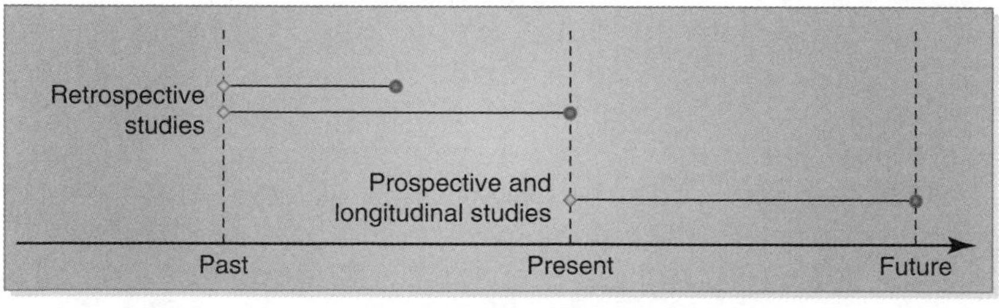

same year who had normal birthweights. The aim could be to see how birthweight influenced adult health status. Similarly, a retrospective study might track down the causes of death after discharge from the armed services of soldiers whose military records indicate whether they served or did not serve in a particular deployment zone.

Prospective and longitudinal cohort studies have a different time orientation than retrospective studies. Prospective and longitudinal studies collect baseline data about exposures and outcomes in the present and follow the cohort to some point in the future.

Because all cohort studies examine incident (new) disease, retrospective and prospective studies must be able to demonstrate that the outcome of interest was not present in any members of the cohort at baseline. A retrospective cohort study that looks at the causes of death after the baseline assessment will have no trouble proving that the outcome—death—was not present at the time of the initial assessment. It is more challenging to conduct a retrospective study when the outcome of interest is a condition that may have been present at baseline but not documented.

Individual participants in longitudinal studies are usually assessed at baseline for several exposures and diseases. Then they are followed forward in time to determine the incidence rate for one or more outcomes of interest. A participant with a history of breast cancer at the baseline exam would need to be excluded from any analyses of breast cancer incidence. However, that person could be included in studies of heart disease incidence if she did not have heart disease at the baseline exam.

Longitudinal studies may use a **fixed population** in which all participants start the study at the same time and no one is allowed to join later. Alternatively, they may use a **dynamic population** (also called an **open population**) with rolling admission and replacement of dropouts (**Figure 11-4**). For dynamic populations, the time to follow up is usually based on individual participants' dates of enrollment rather than on a fixed calendar date.

FIGURE 11-4 Longitudinal Studies

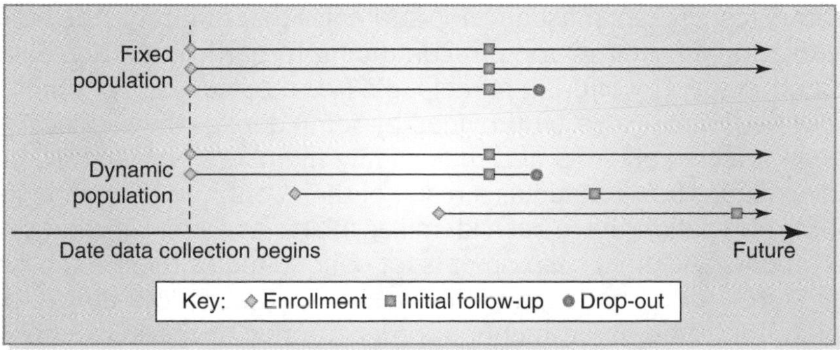

Several variants of longitudinal studies measure the same individuals repeatedly over time, as longitudinal cohort studies do. These studies may be called **time series studies** or **panel studies**. Surveillance systems that are designed to monitor whole populations over an extended period of time, often using continuous data collection rather than discrete time points, may also use a cohort approach. However, studies that measure individuals randomly sampled from the same populations at different points in time (that is, repeated cross-sectional surveys) are not using a cohort study approach, because they do not necessarily capture the same individuals in each round of questioning.

11.3 Special Considerations

For a prospective cohort study that will recruit participants based on exposure status, the first step is to identify two accessible source populations: one for individuals with the exposure of interest and one for those without the exposure. For a longitudinal cohort study, the first step is to select a source population. For a retrospective study, the first step is to identify a source of existing records that can provide baseline data of adequate quality. In some situations, existing records may provide all required follow-up data, and no contact with the individuals whose files are being examined is required. (For some historic studies, this is the only option available because all of the "participants" are already deceased.) For retrospective studies that require contact with individuals, a method for contacting the people identified in historic records must be developed, tested, and shown to result in a reasonable participation rate.

Alternatively, if the goal is to conduct secondary analysis of existing data, the first step is to identify an existing source of data. The secondary analysis of existing data is the most cost-effective way to examine study questions when a completed or ongoing cohort study has assessed the exposures and outcomes of interest and electronic data files are available to outside researchers for analysis.

For prospective and longitudinal cohort studies, decisions must be made about how often follow-up data collection will take place and how long the study (or at least the first wave of the study) will continue. Because **loss to follow-up** of participants before the end of the study period is a major concern of studies that follow participants forward in time, researchers must develop strategies that minimize the burden of participation while maximizing interest in continuing to participate. Some studies may increase retention rates by offering participants free medical tests or other incentives. Sufficient motivation may also be provided by reminders of the significant impact of the disease on affected persons and their family members or by notifications of the important discoveries being made as a result of their continued participation.

Once source populations have been identified, plans for data collection can be made. Survey instruments and other assessments for cohort studies must establish exposure and disease status for all participants at baseline and at follow-up. All participants must complete the same assessments in order to prevent the information bias that might result when exposed participants are more thoroughly examined for disease than unexposed participants. A strong data management system must be established to link baseline and follow-up data while maintaining the confidentiality of the information provided by participants. Data management is discussed in Chapter 26.

11.4 Analysis: Incidence Rate Ratios (RRs)

The goal of cohort studies is to observe the incidence of new disease or other new outcomes. The **incidence rate** is the number of new cases of disease in a population during a specified period of time divided by the total number of persons in the population who were at risk during that period. Individuals who already have the disease of interest at the start of the study period are not at risk of getting new disease, so they are removed from the denominator (**Figure 11-5**). For example, suppose a cohort study examined the incidence of disease over 1 year in a population with 50 members and that 7 of those 50 already had the disease at the start of the year. In that situation, the denominator should be 43 rather than 50. If 4 of those 43 are diagnosed with the disease during the year, then the incidence rate is 4/43, or 93 cases per 1000 people per year. Incidence rates are usually converted to units of "per 1000," "per 10,000," or the like so that they can be more easily compared.

FIGURE 11-5 Incidence

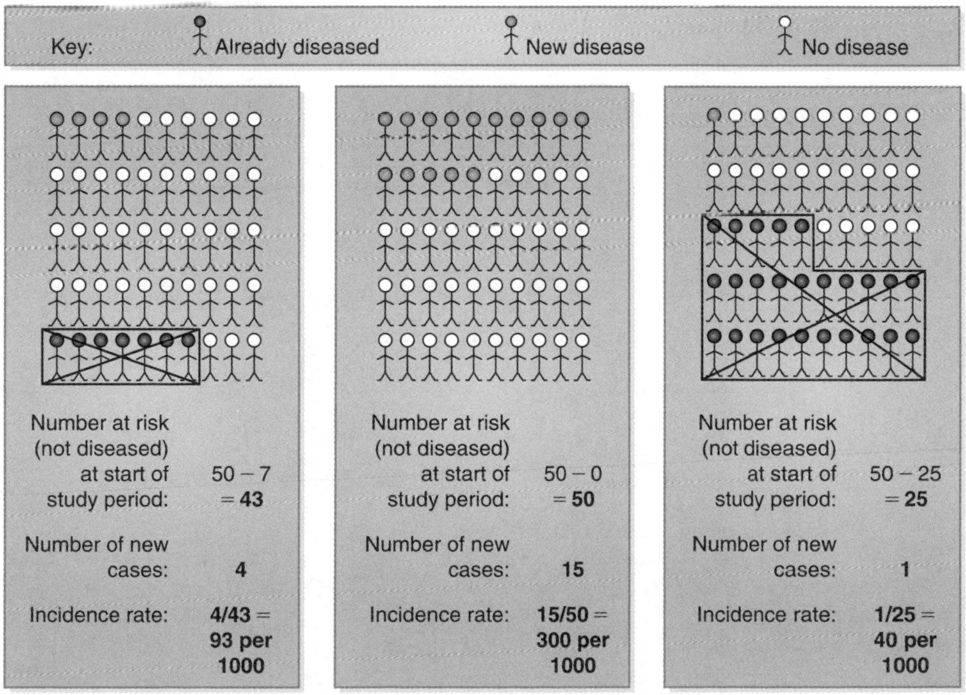

Some cohort studies, especially those with dynamic populations and those that run for many years, use person-time as a denominator. **Person-time** is a way of accounting for individuals in the study population being observed for different lengths of time. Person-time can be expressed in units of person-years, person-months, or even person-days. Suppose that a study recruits 10 individuals at baseline (**Figure 11-6**). After 4 years, 6 of the 10 participants are still active in the study and have not been diagnosed with the disease of interest. Together, these 6 individuals have contributed 24 person-years of observation during the first 4 calendar years of the study. Suppose that 2 of the 10 original participants are diagnosed with the disease of interest at their annual study examinations. One person is diagnosed 2 years into the study, and the other 4 years into the study. Together, these 2 individuals contributed 6 person-years of observation to the study. However, once they are diagnosed and no longer able to develop incident disease, they are no longer able to contribute further person-years to the denominator for the calculation of incidence. Two other participants also leave the study and are **censored** (removed from analysis). One drops out of the study after the second year but before the third year; this participant is considered to have contributed 2 person-years of observation. Another dies after the first year and contributes only that 1 person-year of observation. In total, over 4 calendar years, the 10 original participants experience 2 incident cases of disease

FIGURE 11-6 Person-Year Analysis

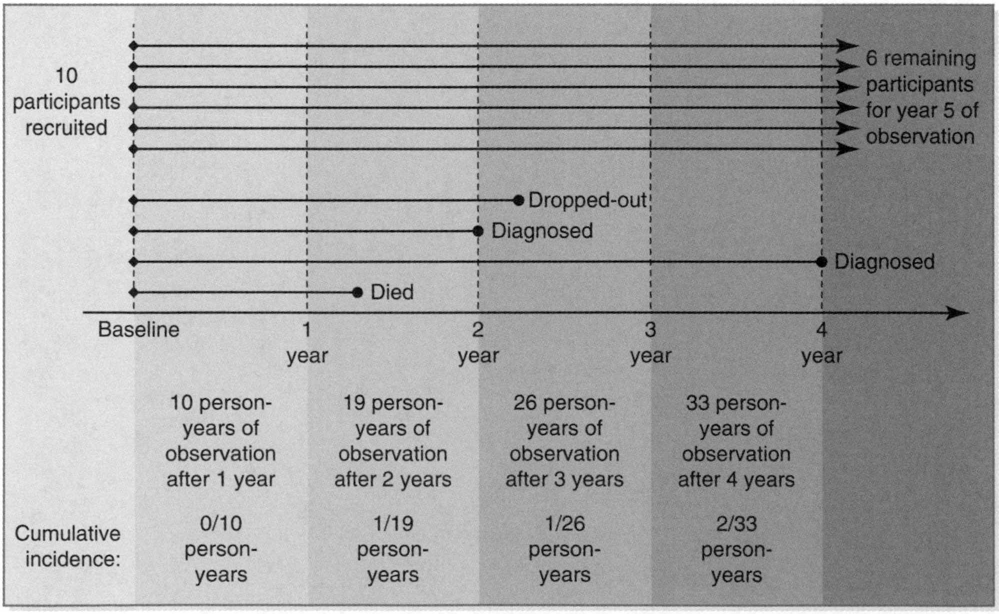

over 33 person-years of observation. For the calculation of incidence rate ratios and other measures that rely on the comparison of incidence rates, it does not matter whether the incidence rates are measured per 1000 participants (Figure 11-5) or per 1000 person-years (Figure 11-6), as long as all incidence rates in the equation use the same units.

There are several ways to compare the rates of new disease in the exposed and unexposed members of a cohort. **Excess risk**, or **attributable risk (AR)**, is the absolute difference in the incidence rate (see **Figure 11-7**). For example, if 10% of the unexposed and 15% of the exposed became ill during the study period, then the excess risk in the exposed was 15% – 10% = 5%. This number represents the additional rate of disease in the exposed that can be attributed to the exposure. The calculation assumes that the exposed would have had the same rate as the unexposed if they had not had the exposure. This assumption is one of the reasons why the exposed and unexposed populations in a cohort study must be similar except for their exposure status.

The **attributable risk percent (AR%)** is the proportion of incident cases among the exposed that are due to the exposure. The percentage is calculated by comparing the excess risk to the incidence rate in the exposed. For the preceding example, the AR% is 5% ÷ 15% = 33%. The interpretation of this result is that one-third of the cases of disease in the exposed could have been prevented if the exposure was removed.

FIGURE 11-7 Attributable (Excess) Risk

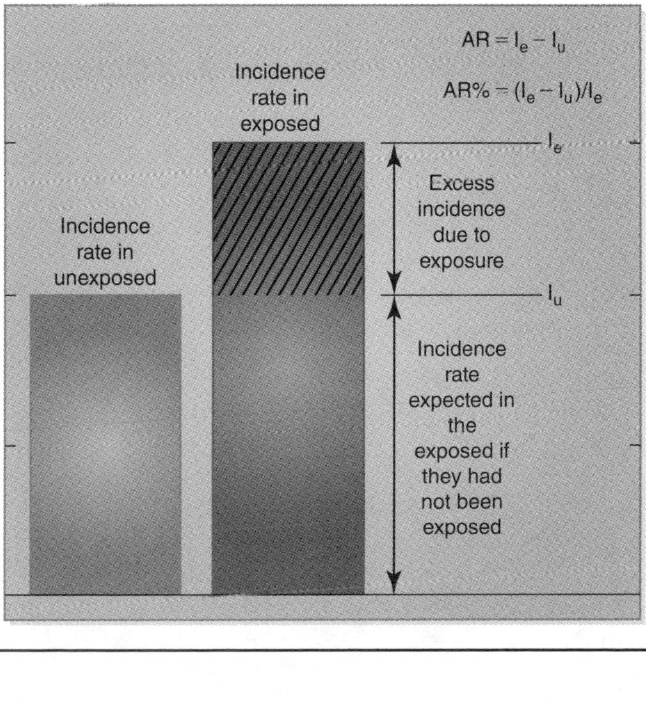

FIGURE 11-8 Rate Ratio (Point Estimate)

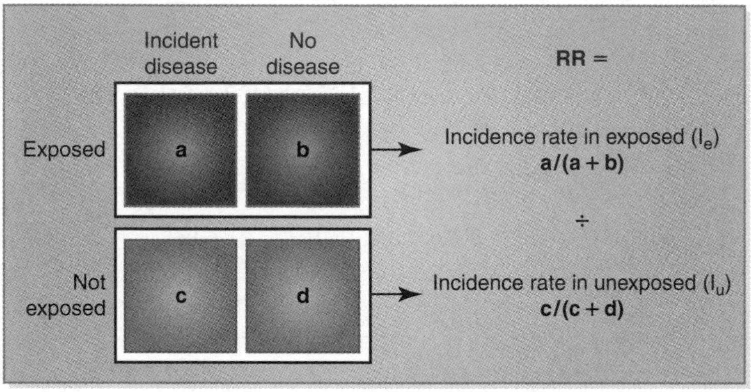

The most common measure of association for cohort studies is the **incidence rate ratio (IRR)**. This is usually simply called the **rate ratio (RR)**, and it is also reported as the **relative rate**, **risk ratio**, and **relative risk**. The RR compares the incidence rate among the exposed to the incidence rate in the unexposed (**Figure 11-8**). The point estimate for the RR is calculated as:

$$RR = \frac{a/(a+b)}{c/(c+d)}$$

The point estimate for the RR provides an initial interpretation for the incidence rate ratio.

- R = 1 (or close to 1): the incidence rate was the same (or about the same) in the exposed and in the unexposed.
- RR > 1: the incidence rate was higher in the exposed than in the unexposed, suggesting that the exposure was risky.
- RR < 1: the incidence rate was lower in the exposed than in the unexposed, suggesting that the exposure was protective.

The 95% confidence interval indicates whether the RR is statistically significant (**Figure 11-9**). (Chapter 17 provides additional information about how to interpret confidence intervals and how they are related to sample size.)

- When the entire 95% confidence interval is less than 1, the RR is statistically significant and the exposure is deemed to be protective in the study population.
- When the entire 95% confidence interval is greater than 1, the RR is statistically significant and the exposure is deemed to be a **risk factor** for the disease in the study population.

FIGURE 11-9 Interpretation of the Rate Ratio Based on Its 95% Confidence Interval

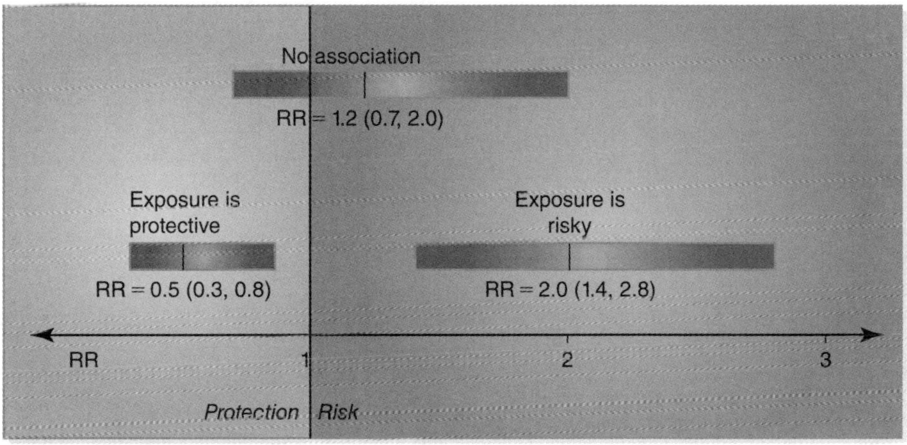

- When the 95% confidence interval (95% CI) overlaps RR = 1, the association between the exposure and the outcome is not statistically significant. This is because the lower end of the confidence interval is in the protective range (RR < 1), and the higher end is in the risky range (RR > 1), so there is no clear association between the exposure and the disease. The appropriate conclusion is that there is no evidence for an association between the exposure and the disease in the study population. This conclusion must be verified by power calculations that examine whether the sample size was sufficient to make this conclusion.

For the protective example in Figure 11-9, it would be accurate to report that "participants with the exposure were half as likely to develop the disease as those without the exposure." For the risky example in Figure 11-9, the report could state that "participants with the exposure were twice as likely to develop the disease as participants without the exposure."

Computer- and Internet-based statistical programs are available for the calculation of statistics that can be derived from a 2×2 table (**Figure 11-10**), such as the:

- Incidence in the exposed
- Incidence in the unexposed
- Excess risk or attributable risk (AR)
- Attributable risk percent (AR%)
- Incidence rate ratio (RR)
- Confidence intervals for the incidence rate, AR, AR%, and RR
- Chi-square statistic and its associated *p*-value

FIGURE 11-10 Examples of Rate Ratio Calculations

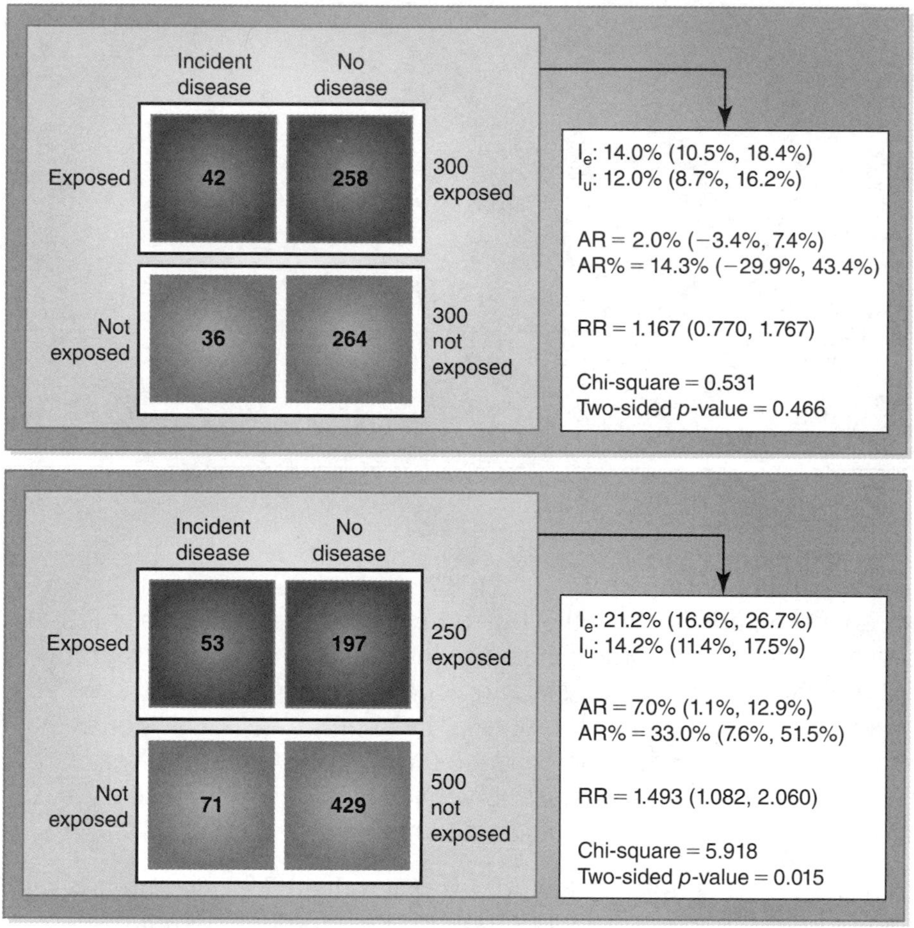

The top example in Figure 11-10 has an incidence rate ratio of 1.167, a 95% confidence interval of (0.770, 1.767), and a *p*-value of $p = 0.466$. This RR is not statistically significant because the 95% confidence interval overlaps 1. The Chi-square *p*-value of $p > 0.05$ confirms the conclusion of no association. The bottom example has an RR of 1.493 (1.082, 2.060) and a *p*-value of $p = 0.015$. This is a statistically significant result, one that implies risk because the entire 95% CI is greater than 1. The Chi-square *p*-value of $p < 0.05$ confirms the conclusion of statistical significance. Linear regression models and other statistical techniques can be used to calculate rate ratios that adjust for possible confounding variables.

CHAPTER 12

EXPERIMENTAL STUDIES

An experimental study assigns participants to intervention and control groups in order to test whether an intervention causes an intended outcome.

12.1 Overview

Experimental studies (also called **intervention studies**) assign participants to receive a particular exposure (**Figure 12-1**). This is the primary distinction between an experimental study and other study designs. **Observational designs** (such as cross-sectional, case-control, and cohort studies) do not "do" anything to participants; they simply ask for a report on participants' experiences. An observational study may ask whether participants eat or do not eat an apple a day, run or do not run on a treadmill for at least 30 minutes three times each week, take or do not take a particular medicine twice a day, or have seen or have not seen an ad for a health promotion campaign. In contrast, an experimental study may assign some or all study participants to eat one red delicious apple daily, run on a treadmill every other day, take a pill every 12 hours, or read a health brochure.

Experimental studies are the gold standard for assessing causality. They are used for clinical trials of new therapies for individuals with various illnesses, field trials of individual-level preventive interventions like vaccinations, and community trials (often cluster randomized trials) of public health and environmental interventions. Because the researcher assigns participants to receive a particular exposure, the exact dose, duration, and frequency of the exposure are known. The researcher knows when the exposure occurred, so the health status of each participant before and after the exposure can be compared. The researcher can therefore assess whether the exposure may have caused a particular outcome.

A typical experimental study design in the health sciences is a **randomized controlled trial (RCT)** in which:

- Some participants are randomly assigned to an active intervention group.
- The remaining participants are assigned to a control group.

FIGURE 12-1 Key Characteristics of Experimental Studies

Objective	Compare outcomes in participants assigned to an intervention or control group
Primary study question	Does the exposure cause the outcome?
Population	Similar participants are randomly assigned to an intervention or control group.
When to use this approach	Assessing causality
Requirement	The experiment is ethically justifiable.
First steps	1. Decide on the intervention and eligibility criteria. 2. Define what will constitute a favorable outcome. 3. Decide what control is an appropriate comparison for the intervention. 4. Decide whether blinding will be used to prevent participants and/or the researchers who will assess outcomes from knowing whether a participant has been assigned to the intervention or the control group. 5. Select the method for randomizing participants to an intervention or control group.
What to watch out for	Noncompliance
Key statistical measure	Efficacy

- All participants from both groups are followed forward in time to see who has a favorable outcome and who does not (**Figure 12-2**).

All experimental studies require careful definitions of:

- The intervention
- What type of control is appropriate
- How participants will be assigned to exposure groups
- What constitutes a favorable outcome for the trial

Experimental studies also all require careful consideration of the ethical challenges associated with assigning participants to an exposure, even if that exposure is expected to improve health status.

12.2 Describing the Intervention

The first step in an experimental study is to carefully define the intervention that participants assigned to the active intervention group will receive and to decide

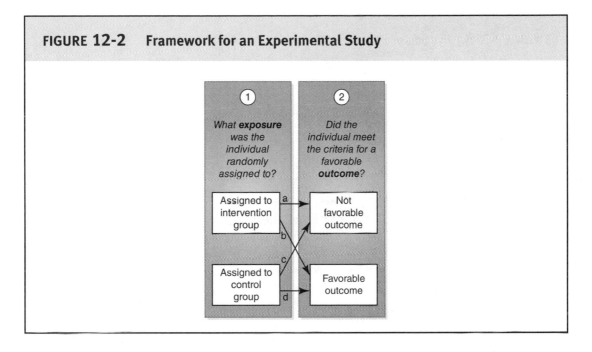

FIGURE 12-2 Framework for an Experimental Study

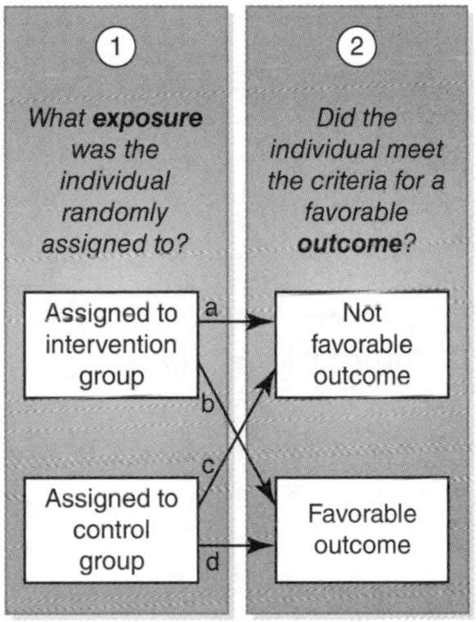

on the person, place, and time (PPT) criteria for the study. The description should state exactly:

- What the intervention will be
- The eligibility criteria for participants
- Where and how participants will receive the intervention
- When, how often, and for what duration participants will receive the intervention

For example, a new drug trial will declare very strict requirements for the composition of the pill to be ingested, how often it will be taken, for how many weeks it will be taken, and who will meet the case definition for eligibility to participate. A new strength-building intervention will provide detailed descriptions of the exercise procedures and how they will change in intensity over the study period, how participants will be coached or supervised, where participants will engage in the exercises, how long the study period will last, and what inclusion and exclusion criteria will apply to potential volunteers.

12.3 Defining Outcomes

Most experimental studies are **superiority trials** that aim to demonstrate that a new intervention is better than some type of control (**Figure 12-3**). "Better" could mean that an intervention is more effective than a current therapy at curing existing disease, or it could mean that a new intervention is more effective than a placebo at preventing

FIGURE 12-3 Types of Success

Goal	Success
Superiority trial	The intervention is better than the control.
Noninferiority trial	The intervention is not worse than the control.
Equivalence trial	The intervention is equal to the control.

new disease from occurring. In some studies, "better" could mean that a less expensive intervention is as good as, or no worse than, a more expensive intervention and is therefore economically more favorable. Because the term "better" can be defined in so many ways, the researcher must carefully define what constitutes a favorable outcome for an individual participant and for the experimental study as a whole. These measures of success must be stipulated prior to the initiation of the study.

The first step is defining a favorable outcome for an individual. For example, an individual participant's success in a weight-loss program could be defined as the loss of at least 10% body weight and the maintenance of the lower weight for at least 6 months (**Figure 12-4**). Alternatively, success could be defined as the loss of at least 15 pounds over a 2-month intervention period or as achieving a body mass index (BMI) of less than 30 by the end of the study period.

If the goal of a study is to test whether a new drug is better than a sugar pill at improving the quality of life of those with a particular disease condition, the definition of "improved quality of life" should be carefully considered and validated. This can be done by means of clinical examinations and/or survey instruments designed to assess various aspects of quality of life. If the goal is to evaluate whether a new vaccine prevents infection, then laboratory tests should be used to confirm the presence or absence of past, recent, and/or current infection.

These measures of individual success can then be translated into measures of study success. For example, a weight-loss study could be considered a success if the proportion of participants with favorable individual-level outcomes is significantly greater in the intervention group than in the control group.

12.4 Selecting Controls

Experimental studies usually assign some participants to the active intervention and the remainder to a control group (**Figure 12-5**). One commonly used type of control is a **placebo**, an inactive comparison that is similar to the therapy being tested. Examples of placebos are a sugar pill used as a control for a pill with an active medication, a saline injection used as a control for an injection of an active substance, and a sham procedure that is designed to look and feel like a real clinical procedure used as a

FIGURE 12-4 Examples of Favorable Outcomes

Intervention	Intended Outcome	Favorable Outcome for an Individual	Unfavorable Outcome for an Individual	Favorable Outcome for the Study Population
New diet- and exercise-based weight-loss Program	Significant weight loss	The loss of ≥10% body weight and maintenance of lower weight for ≥ 6 months	The loss of <10% body weight or failure to maintain weight loss of ≥10% or more for ≥ 6 months	The proportion of those who lose at least 10% of their body weight and maintain that loss for at least 6 months is higher in the intervention group than in the control group.
New drug therapy	Improvement of the quality of life for those with a particular disease condition	Improvement in quality of life	Failure to demonstrate improvement in quality of life	The rate of improvement in the drug therapy (intervention) group is higher than the improvement rate in the placebo (control) group, according to a carefully defined and validated set of criteria for what constitutes improvement.
New preventive vaccine	The prevention of infection	Incident infection does not occur	Incident infection occurs	The incidence of infection in the vaccinated (intervention) group is lower than the incidence of infection in the unvaccinated (control) group, as confirmed by laboratory testing.

FIGURE 12-5 Examples of Types of Controls

Type of Control	Active Intervention	Comparison
Placebo/inactive comparison	Active pill	Inactive pill
	Injection of an active substance	Injection of saline solution
	Acupuncture needles inserted at acupuncture points	Acupuncture needles inserted at locations in the body that are not acupuncture points (sham acupuncture)
	Some other active ingredient	An inactive substance that is indistinguishable from the active intervention in terms of appearance, odor, taste, texture, and delivery mechanism
Active comparison/ standard of care	New therapy	Current best therapy for the condition being studied
	New therapy	Current standard therapy
	New therapy	Some other existing therapy
	Current therapy plus new therapy	Current therapy alone
Dose-response	Some dose of a medication	Alternate doses of the medication
	Some duration of a therapy	Alternate durations of the therapy
No intervention	New intervention	Participants assigned to the control group are asked to maintain their usual routines.
Self	New intervention	Each participant's status before the intervention is compared to his or her own status after the intervention.
	New intervention	Each participant receives the new intervention for some duration and the comparison for some duration, preferably in a random order.

control for that active procedure. The mere act of taking a pill or receiving some other form of therapy, even if it is inert or inactive, is often enough to make recipients feel better. Placebo-controlled studies allow the effect of the active therapy to be examined separately from the boost in health status that people may experience simply by participating in a clinical trial or receiving some other intervention.

Not all experimental studies use placebos. When the goal of the experiment is to test whether a new therapy is better than (or at least equivalent to) a current one, it is appropriate to compare the new therapy to some existing **standard of care**, whether that is the best therapy currently available or the therapy that is used most often in the location where the study is being conducted. Sometimes the new therapy may be given in addition to the existing therapy.

Sometimes the goal is to determine how much of an intervention is required. For example, should the dose of a substance be changed? (Is 100 mg of a medication as effective as 200 mg?) Or should the duration of therapy be reconsidered? (Is 4 weeks of physical therapy as effective as 8 weeks?) In such cases, varying doses and durations may be tested and compared to one another. Sometimes different interventions are compared in various combinations within one randomized controlled trial using a **factorial design** (**Figure 12-6**).

Although experimental studies sometimes include a control group of participants who are randomly assigned to maintain their usual routines, this method is usually not preferred. The approach raises ethical concerns about discouraging the adoption of healthier lifestyles during the course of the study. It also raises concerns

FIGURE 12-6 Examples of RCT Approaches

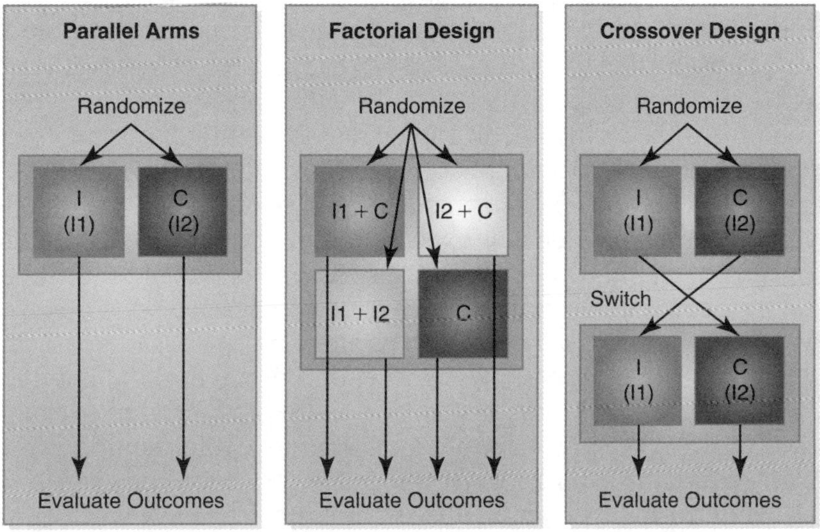

about a type of bias called the **Hawthorne effect** that can occur when participants in a study change their behavior for the better because they know they are being observed. For example, suppose a researcher is initiating a study of a new weight-loss program and plans to randomly assign participants either to the new therapy or to a usual routine group. In this situation, simply informing the controls that they will be weighed at the start and end of the study period will be enough to spur a sizable proportion of the control group to initiate an exercise program, start eating a healthier diet, or take other steps to lose weight. These changes may interfere with the accurate measurement of the impact of the new intervention.

When there are ethical concerns about the appropriateness of not assigning all participants to a potentially life-saving intervention, it may be possible for participants to serve as their own controls. A **before-and-after study** is a non-randomized experimental study that measures the same individuals before and after an intervention. Some experimental studies use a **crossover design** in which the researcher assigns some participants first to the active intervention and then the control and assigns other participants first to the control and then to the active intervention. (Both groups may take a break, called a **washout period**, between the two arms of the experiment in order to reduce the **carryover effects** of the first treatment biasing the apparent results of the second treatment.) Each participant's status before the intervention is compared to his or her own status after the intervention. However, the results of crossover experimental designs may not be as clear-cut as placebo studies because time alone can lead to significant improvements or declines in health status, especially among those who are severely ill.

12.5 Blinding

Blinding, sometimes called **masking**, occurs when participants in an experimental study, and perhaps some research team members, do not know whether a participant is in the active intervention group or the control group, which would be a type of observer bias. In a **single-blind study**, participants are unaware of their exposure status. In a **double-blind study**, neither the participants nor the persons assessing the participants' health status know which participants are in the active and control groups.

Blinding minimizes the **information bias** that can occur if participants or assessors are able to evaluate outcomes differently based on the results they expect for an exposure. For example, blinding prevents participants in the active intervention group from reporting more favorable results because they expect a positive outcome. Blinding also prevents assessors from recording more favorable results, either intentionally or unconsciously, for participants in the active intervention group, which would be a type of **observer bias**.

Blinding is usually possible only when all participants are assigned to similar exposures. If participants in both the active intervention group and the control group are taking pills (of the same color, shape, size, and taste) or if both are getting injections, a blinded study may be possible. In contrast, if the active intervention is a special diet and the controls eat their usual diets, if the active group will participate in exercise classes and the controls will be on their own, or if the active intervention will include both diet and exercise components and the control only a diet plan, then a blinded study may not be possible. To minimize the likelihood of bias in studies that are not blinded, it is helpful to identify objective outcome measures (such as laboratory tests) rather than subjective outcome measures (such as participants' self-reported feelings).

12.6 Randomization

Randomization when assigning participants to an exposure group in an experimental study reduces several types of possible bias. For example, randomization minimizes the problems that could occur if participants were able to choose the intervention or control group they preferred. Some people would prefer to know they were getting the active intervention, while others with less risk tolerance might prefer to be in a control population. Self-selection might significantly alter the results of the intervention. Randomization also mitigates the **allocation bias** that might occur when people with different backgrounds, such as different exposure histories, are not equally distributed across treatment arms. (Randomization does not remove the **selection bias** that occurs when the people who volunteer to participate in a study are not representative of the source population as a whole.)

A variety of approaches can be used to randomly allocate participants to an active intervention group or a control group (**Figure 12-7**).

- **Simple randomization** uses a coin toss, a random number generator, or some other uncomplicated procedure to assign each individual to one of the groups.
- **Block randomization** randomly assigns groups of people to an intervention group and other groups of people to a control group. For example, if there were 10 elementary schools in a county, all of the students in 5 of those schools could be randomly assigned to the intervention group and all of the students in the other 5 schools could be randomly assigned to the control group.

FIGURE 12-7 Examples of Types of Randomization

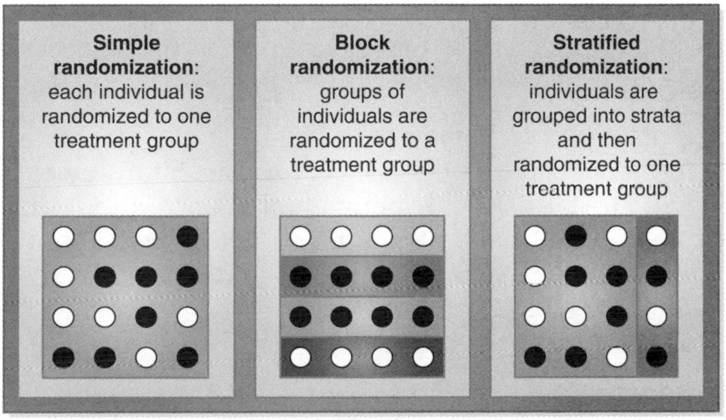

- **Stratified randomization** randomly assigns individuals within certain subgroups to a particular exposure. This type of randomization is useful when simple randomization may not result in enough members of certain subgroups being randomized to each of the exposure groups. For example, suppose that 75% of the volunteers for a study are female and only 25% are male. To ensure that enough males are assigned to the intervention group, two separate randomization processes could be used, one for females and one for males. This would ensure that 50% of the females are assigned to the intervention group along with 50% of the males.

Reference books that focus specifically on experimental studies provide additional details about methods for randomization.

Some experimental studies use non-randomized approaches because randomization is unethical or is not feasible. **Quasi-experimental designs** assign participants to an intervention or control group using a non-random method. Aside from using a non-random method to assign participants to exposure groups, most quasi-experimental studies use methods similar to those of randomized studies. Most quasi-experimental studies use both pre- and post-intervention tests to compare the two arms of a controlled study. However, some quasi-experimental studies have no control group, and some use only a post-intervention assessment (with or without a control group).

Some research studies are considered to be **natural experiments** because the researchers do not have any control over the interventions. For example, a researcher may seek to understand the impact of a devastating tornado on the health of residents of the affected community. Or suppose that a hospital announces that it will implement a new infection control policy. A researcher would not have the authority to assign some patients to one infection control strategy and other patients to a different policy. However, inpatients hospitalized during the year after the policy update could be considered to be the active intervention group for a study examining the effectiveness of the new policy in reducing healthcare-associated infections, and inpatients who stayed at the hospital during the year before the policy change could be considered to be the control group. These are not true experimental studies because the "interventions"—a natural disaster and a policy change—are not ones that can be manipulated by a researcher. These questions can be examined with observational study approaches.

12.7 Ethical Considerations

All research with human participants or their identifiable personal data raises ethical concerns that researchers must address, but experimental studies involve a particularly high level of ethical risk. In experimental studies, the researcher assigns participants to exposures that the participants do not choose and may have been unlikely to encounter had they not volunteered to participate in a research project. This means that a number of issues must be considered before initiating an experimental study (**Figure 12-8**). For example:

- The principle of **equipoise** states that experimental research should be conducted only when there is genuine uncertainty about which treatment will work better.

FIGURE 12-8 Examples of Ethical Issues in Experimental Studies

Study Stage	Examples of Questions to Ask
Study topic selection	• Is the study really necessary (equipoise)? • Is an experimental design truly necessary?
Recruitment	• Is the source population an appropriate and justifiable one? • Is the inducement to participate appropriate and not coercive?
Randomization	• Do participants truly understand that they might not receive the active intervention? • Is it appropriate to use a placebo? Is it appropriate to use some other control?
Data collection	• How will adverse outcomes be monitored and addressed? • When might an experiment need to be discontinued early?
Follow-up	• What happens if a participant experiences study-related harm after the conclusion of the study? • Will participants have continuing access to the therapy if it is shown to be successful?

- The principle of distributive justice implies that the source population must be an appropriate one and that the research must not exploit individuals from populations that are unlikely to have continued access to the therapy if it is found to be successful.
- The principle of respect for persons requires that all participants volunteer for a study without being unduly influenced by the prospect of being compensated for their participation. Respect also requires that all participants understand what it means to be a research subject, including the possibility of being assigned to a control group instead of the new intervention.
- The principles of beneficence and nonmaleficence require that researchers balance the likely benefits and risks of the study. For example, researchers must make a careful decision about when to use placebo or another type of control, must put in place a monitoring system for adverse reactions, and must identify the conditions under which an experiment would be discontinued early either because the exposure proves to be risky or because the new intervention appears to be so beneficial that keeping it from the control group would be unethical. An **adverse event** is a negative reaction to an intervention or another bad outcome related to a study.

Chapter 22 discusses additional ethical principles that must be considered when planning and conducting research with human subjects. Research ethics committee review is required for all experimental studies, as explained in Chapter 23.

12.8 Analysis

Experimental studies use many of the same measures of association that cohort studies do, including rate ratios, attributable risks (excess risk or risk reduction), attributable risk percentages, measures of survival, and various types of regression models. Cohort studies use these measures to examine the impact of an unassigned exposure on the incidence of disease. Experimental studies use the statistics to quantify the impact of an assigned exposure on the likelihood of having a favorable or an unfavorable outcome.

There are also several measures that are specific to experimental studies.

- Efficacy is the proportion of individuals in the control group who experience an unfavorable outcome who could have been expected to have a better outcome if they had been assigned to the active group instead of the control group (**Figure 12-9**). A high efficacy is an indicator that an intervention is successful. More precisely, **efficacy** refers to results under ideal circumstances, such as when an experiment is conducted in a controlled laboratory setting and all participants are fully compliant with the protocol. **Effectiveness** is calculated with the same equation as efficacy, but refers to results obtained under less than ideal circumstances. For example, in a "real world" setting, some participants might skip some doses of

FIGURE 12-9 Efficacy and NNT

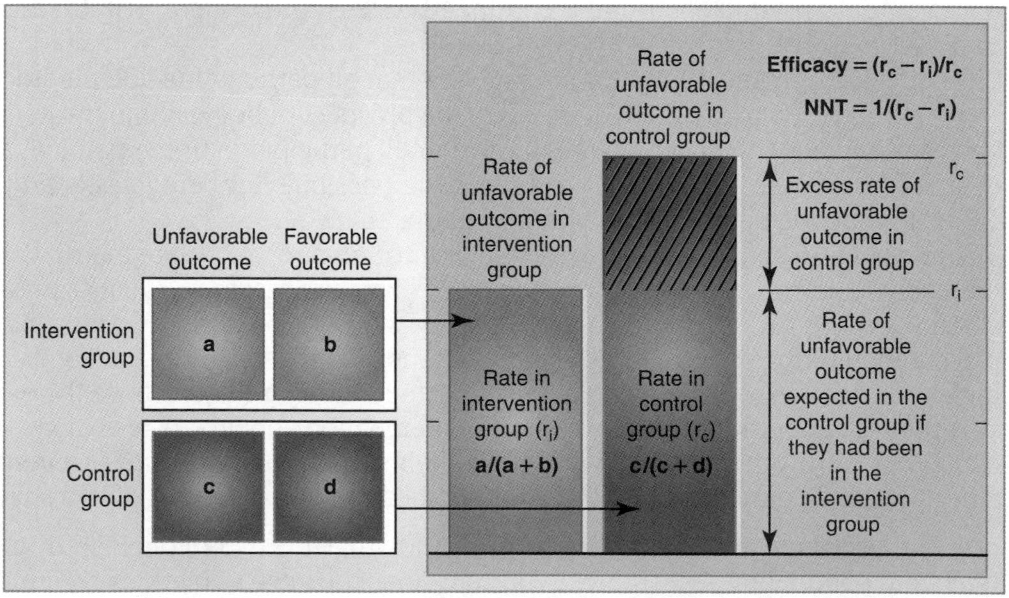

an experimental drug, or they might not take the doses at the exact specified times, or they might not store the pills at the ideal temperature.

- The **number needed to treat (NNT)** is the expected number of people who would have to receive a treatment to prevent an unfavorable outcome in one person (or, alternately stated, to achieve a favorable outcome in one person). A small NNT indicates a more effective intervention. If a drug is intended to prevent stroke and has an NNT of 5, then 5 people have to take the drug for one year (or some other specified time period) to prevent one of the 5 from having a stroke. If the drug has an NNT of 102, it means that 102 people have to take the drug to prevent one of the 102 from having a stroke.
- A related concept is the **number needed to harm (NNH)**, which is the number of people who would need to receive a particular treatment in order to expect that one of them would have a particular adverse outcome. A large NNH indicates a safer intervention. NNT and NNH are often used for cost-effectiveness analysis. **Efficiency** is an evaluation of the cost-effectiveness of an intervention that is based on both its effectiveness and resource considerations.

A related consideration for experimental studies is whether to use a **treatment-received approach**, which limits analysis to the participants who were fully compliant with their assigned intervention, or to use a **treatment-assigned approach** (or **intention-to-treat approach**) that includes all participants even if they were not fully compliant with their assigned intervention. Treatment-received analysis allows for the calculation of efficacy, because the only participants included in the analysis are those who never missed taking a pill at the prescribed time, never missed a scheduled clinical exam, and were otherwise exemplary study subjects. Treatment-assigned analysis is better at measuring real-world (rather than ideal-world) effectiveness.

No matter which analytic approach is used, the research protocol should include specific plans for promoting compliance and minimizing dropouts. The flow of participants through the study, from the recruitment and enrollment stages through the analysis stage, should be included in reports of findings for any experimental study (**Figure 12-10**).

12.9 Screening and Diagnostic Tests

The goal of some studies of screening or diagnostic tests is to compare two assessments that are supposed to measure the same thing. In most situations, this goal involves comparing a new test to an existing one. For example, a new blood antigen test for a type of cancer might be compared to biopsy results. Positive and negative biopsy results would serve as the "gold standard" or **reference standard** against which the blood test would be evaluated. The hope is that the blood test—which would likely be cheaper, quicker, and less invasive than a biopsy—will yield results similar to those from the biopsy. Many comparative studies of laboratory-based tests can be considered observational because they do not require the researchers to do anything to the participants other than collect a biological specimen.

FIGURE 12-10 Flow of Participants in an Experimental Study

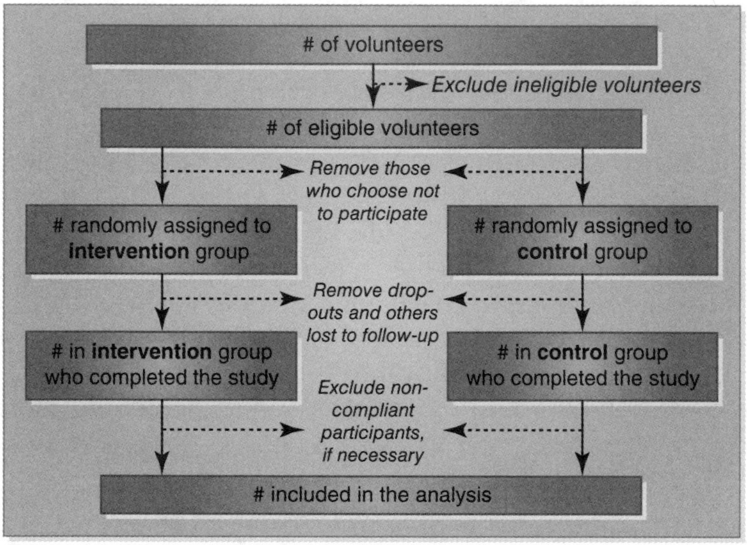

However, some tests involve experimental procedures (such as biopsies in individuals who might otherwise forego this kind of testing because they are almost certain to yield negative results) and are appropriately classified as experimental.

Studies of new screening and diagnostic tests should have a clear set of eligibility criteria. They may call for intentionally seeking out some individuals known to have the disease of interest and some known to be disease free. An appropriate reference standard must be identified, and a rationale for any **cutpoint** for the new test and reference test should be determined. For example, the protocol should specify the concentration of antigens in the blood that will indicate a positive versus a negative test result. A system should be put in place to ensure that the examiners—the clinicians or laboratory scientists conducting the assessments—are blinded to the "actual" status of the participants as indicated by the reference test.

Figure 12-11 shows how to calculate the sensitivity, specificity, positive predictive value, and negative predictive value of a new screening or diagnostic test in comparison to a reference standard. The **sensitivity** is the proportion of people who actually have a disease (according to the reference standard) who test positive using the new test. The **specificity** is the proportion of people who do not have the disease who test negative with the new test. The **positive predictive value (PPV)** is the proportion of those who test positive with the new test who actually have the disease (according to the reference standard). The **negative predictive value (NPV)** is the proportion of

FIGURE 12-11 Screening and Diagnostic Test Results

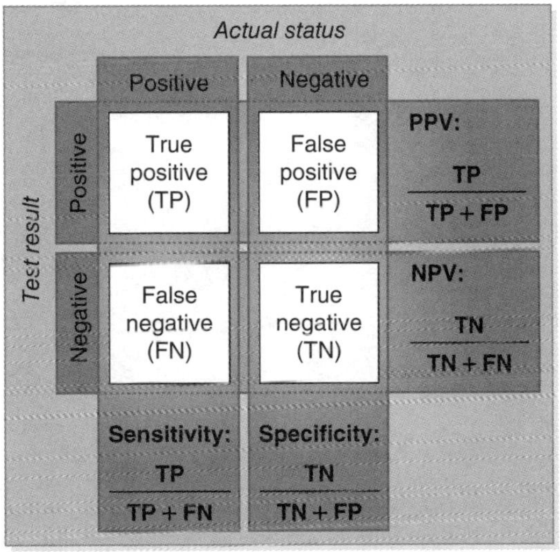

those who test negative who actually do not have the disease. A good screening or diagnostic test will have high values for each of these measures—ideally 100% for all four calculations.

For tests with a flexible cutoff point for defining positive and negative test results, there is always a trade-off between sensitivity and specificity (**Figure 12-12**). Increasing the sensitivity decreases the specificity. Increasing the specificity decreases the sensitivity. Consider the use of systolic blood pressure as an indicator of hypertension. If the cutoff for being classified as having clinically high blood pressure is dropped from 160 mm Hg to 140 mm Hg, the sensitivity will increase (since a higher percentage of people with hypertension will be classified as hypertensive) but the specificity will decrease (since a lower percentage of people without hypertension will be correctly classified as not being hypertensive). **Receiver operating characteristic curves**, or **ROC curves**, plot 1 – specificity (that is, the number one minus the specificity, which must fall between 0 and 1) on the x-axis and sensitivity on the y-axis for a variety of cutoff points. ROC curves and the **area under the curve (AUC)** can be used to graphically examine the accuracy of a diagnostic test.

Three other measures are also commonly used for screening tests. The **diagnostic accuracy** is the percentage of the participants who were either true positives or true negatives (that is, the percentage for which both the reference test and the new test yield the same result). An ideal test will have 100% diagnostic accuracy. The **positive likelihood ratio (LR+) test** examines whether a new test is good at predicting the presence of disease. The LR+ is calculated as the probability that an individual with

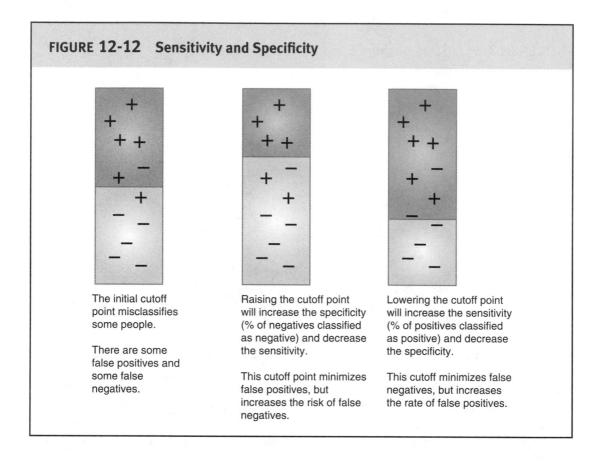

FIGURE 12-12 Sensitivity and Specificity

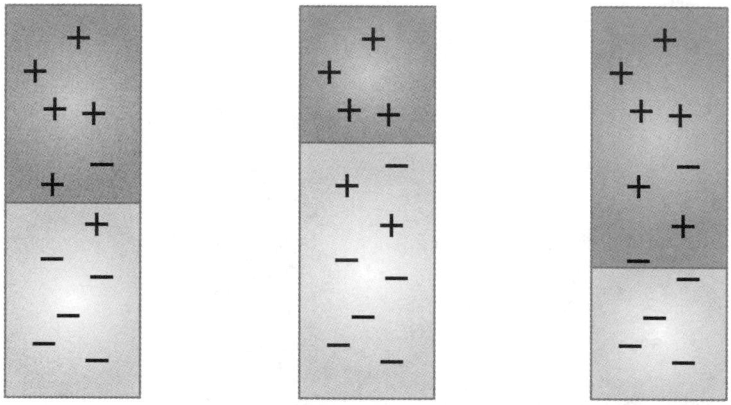

The initial cutoff point misclassifies some people.

There are some false positives and some false negatives.

Raising the cutoff point will increase the specificity (% of negatives classified as negative) and decrease the sensitivity.

This cutoff point minimizes false positives, but increases the risk of false negatives.

Lowering the cutoff point will increase the sensitivity (% of positives classified as positive) and decrease the specificity.

This cutoff minimizes false negatives, but increases the rate of false positives.

the disease has a positive test divided by the probability that an individual without the disease has a positive test. This is equivalent to:

$$LR+ = \frac{sensitivity}{1 - specificity}$$

A larger LR+ (such as LR > 10) indicates a good test. The **negative likelihood ratio (LR–) test** examines whether a new test is good at predicting the absence of disease. The LR– is calculated as the probability that an individual with the disease has a negative test divided by the probability that an individual without the disease has a negative test. This is equivalent to:

$$LR- = \frac{1 - sensitivity}{specificity}$$

A smaller LR– (such as LR < 0.1) indicates a good test.

CHAPTER 13

QUALITATIVE STUDIES

A qualitative study looks for the themes and meanings that emerge from observation of and interaction with key informants.

13.1 Qualitative Research Theories

Qualitative research seeks to answer questions like "why?" and "how?" that numbers-focused **quantitative research** cannot adequately answer (**Figure 13-1**). In the health sciences, many qualitative research projects aim to improve health promotion programs and clinical processes or to provide a foundation for social change. Other qualitative studies seek to understand how people experience health and illness as individuals and as members of communities, why they engage in (or do not engage in) various health-related behaviors, and how they make health-related decisions.

Qualitative data collection is not a detached, structured process based on a random sample of individuals. Instead, researchers have intense contact with a selected group of informants. These **key informants** are often identified through purposive sampling. The researchers are allowed to express empathy with informants and, when appropriate, to be **participant observers** who gain access to and understanding of a community by immersing in its practices. Because qualitative researchers are so closely engaged with participants, they need to reflect on how their backgrounds might bias their observations, and they need to be transparent about these potential biases when reporting findings.

A carefully considered approach is used to gather and interpret qualitative data. For example:

- **Phenomenology** seeks to understand how participants understand, interpret, and find meaning in their own unique life experiences and feelings.
- **Grounded theory** is an inductive reasoning process that uses observations to develop general theories that explain human behavior.

FIGURE 13-1 Comparing Typical Qualitative and Quantitative Research Approaches

	Quantitative	Qualitative
Main types of questions answered	Who? Where? When? What?	Why? How?
Participants	A large randomly-sampled population	A small purposively-recruited population
Data collection approach	Structured	Unstructured or semi-structured
Common data collection methods	Surveys	Participant observations, in-depth interviews, and focus groups discussions
Types of questions asked	Close-ended (fixed response options)	Open-ended (flexible response options)
Data collected	Numeric data	Textual data (words, images, and objects)
Goal of data analysis	Test existing hypotheses	Formulate new theories
Outcomes reported	Statistics	Themes and patterns

- **Ethnography** aims to develop an insider's view (an **emic perspective**), rather than an outsider's view (an **etic perspective**), of how members of a particular cultural group see their world.

Qualitative researchers also often identify a foundational framework that guides their study designs and interpretations. These paradigms explain how a researcher defines reality and truth (**ontology**) and how that researcher knows what is real and true (**epistemology**). For example:

- **Post-positivism**: Researchers aim to experimentally test theories about how the world works, but they acknowledge that the unpredictability of human behavior limits the validity of some empirical methods.
- **Critical theory**: Researchers consider reality to be dependent on social and historical constructs. Reality can be uncovered by identifying and challenging power structures.
- **Constructivism**: Researchers have a relativist perspective that considers reality for each individual to be a function of that person's lived experiences. There are many realities, not just one reality.

- **Transformative paradigm**: Researchers assume that reality can be changed when research addresses social justice issues. Research conducted under this framework is change-oriented and values advocacy, collaboration, and the empowerment of marginalized populations. For example, **action research** is designed to allow participants to work together to solve a social problem.
- **Pragmatism**: Researchers assume that reality is situational, and that it is acceptable to use any and all research tools and frameworks to try to understand a particular problem so it can be addressed. The goal of research is to solve problems, and the focus is on the outcomes of the research project rather than the theories and processes that guide it.

13.2 Qualitative Research Techniques

A set of somewhat flexible techniques is used to ensure the comprehensiveness of information collected during qualitative studies. Data collection may involve a combination of listening and watching, with field notes recording both verbal and nonverbal cues. Participants may be asked to use a **think-aloud protocol** or **talk-aloud protocol** to describe their thoughts and actions while they complete a task. They may be invited to complete a **photovoice** project in which participants take photographs that they feel represent their communities and then share what aspects of their lived experiences they intended to capture in those images. **Narrative inquiry** examines autobiographies, personal letters, family stories, interview tapes, and other records to understand how people frame their identities and social relationships.

Before initiating any qualitative study, researchers should consult specialty references or experts in qualitative methods to ensure that rigorous and appropriate methods will be used to answer the study question. Researchers should carefully consider how best to acquire and document the informed consent of participants and how to maintain the confidentiality of personally identifiable information about participants. The rules for human subjects research, including the requirement for approval by a research ethics committee, apply to both quantitative and qualitative studies. These are described in Chapters 23 and 24.

13.3 Qualitative Interviewing Methods

In-depth interviews of individuals use open-ended questions to explore viewpoints. They usually involve in-person conversations between one interviewer and one participant. Sometimes two researchers meet with one participant for safety or cultural reasons, or so that one researcher can ask questions while the other takes notes. Interviews are often audio- or video-recorded and then transcribed so that the exact words (and sometimes also the nonverbal expressions) can be coded and interpreted. Interviews are sometimes supplemented by other methods, such as participant diaries or journals.

The interviewer may have a list of initial questions that will be asked of each participant (a **semi-structured interview**) or may simply have a list of topics to be covered during each interview. These are merely starting points for eliciting responses from participants. The researcher can probe for more details about any response in order to gain fuller understanding of participants' experiences and perspectives. Interviewers should be aware of how their word choices, tone of voice, and body language may be interpreted or misinterpreted by interviewees. Interviewers should also be careful not to ask leading questions and not to move on to a new set of questions before full responses have been gathered from the current line of inquiry. If the interviewer is not certain what a participant meant by a particular statement, clarification can be respectfully requested. A typical in-depth interview is 1 or 2 hours long. See Chapter 19 for more information about interviewing techniques.

Audio recordings should be transcribed as soon as possible after an interview and reviewed for accuracy. All parts of the interview, including fillers (like "um" and "you know"), laughs, and other sounds should be included in the typed transcript.

13.4 Focus Group Discussions

Focus groups usually include about 8 to 10 people (plus or minus a few individuals) who spend 1 or 2 hours participating in a moderated discussion. Focus groups can be used to understand the norms of a group as well as to identify the diversity of perspectives that exist within a population.

Focus group participants are recruited through **purposive sampling** because they are able to provide insights about the study question. Research projects using focus groups often hold discussions with several different sets of informants. Membership in each group is designed to minimize power differentials and allow for the open sharing of perspectives. For example, a study of workplace safety issues might include separate groups for factory workers who use heavy equipment, their supervisors, and safety engineers at the factory. If supervisors and safety engineers were included in the discussions with the floor workers, it might be difficult for the people operating the machinery to be honest about their concerns. They might feel pressured to provide the answers they thought the company wanted to hear rather than acknowledging the need to address hazards.

Most focus groups are hosted by two researchers. One serves as the moderator who sets the agenda, facilitates the discussion, and keeps the conversation on track. The other serves as a note-taker while providing other support such as assisting with welcoming participants, collecting consent forms, operating recording devices and backup recorders, and time-keeping. Focus groups should be audio- or video-recorded so that complete transcripts can be created. The note-taker can track the key messages and themes that emerge during the discussion while also documenting observations like emotions and gestures that may not show up in the transcript.

The session should begin with the moderator establishing rapport with the group and setting the ground rules for the session. Participants need to understand that their involvement in the study is voluntary (even if they have been offered an incentive to participate) and they can leave at any time. The importance of privacy and respect must be emphasized. Participants should be asked not to disclose to outsiders what others say during the group discussion. For sensitive topics, it may be helpful to assign pseudonyms to group members so that their true names are not disclosed to other participants.

Once everyone has agreed to the plan for the session, the facilitator will begin posing questions to the group, carefully keeping the conversation focused on the core discussion items and moving forward at an appropriate pace. Participants should be encouraged to interact with one another and to identify shared perspectives while not succumbing to groupthink. Follow-up questions posed by the moderator in a neutral manner can help clarify individual and shared perspectives. Times of silence are acceptable when participants need a few quiet moments to process their thoughts. The moderator must ensure that everyone has an opportunity to speak and that no one dominates the conversation or interrupts other participants' comments. Being a good moderator requires practice. Mock sessions can be helpful training for the moderator role, and mentoring from an experienced facilitator is valuable for improving performance.

After the focus group has concluded, the moderator and note-taker should hold a debriefing session to discuss what worked well and what should be improved in the next round. The transcript of the session should be typed up soon after the session and reviewed for accuracy by both facilitators.

13.5 Coding Qualitative Data

The analysis of qualitative data usually involves coding and classifying observations, sometimes using software designed for this purpose. The first step in this process is carefully reading each transcript (or other document) and **coding** it by using words or short phrases to briefly summarize each item. These words can reflect content, attitudes, processes, or other foci. Next, the codes are grouped into categories so that major and minor themes can be derived from the groups of observations. The process of categorizing may reveal new meanings that were not explored with the initial coding, so several rounds of recoding and reclassifying may be necessary. These cycles are a valuable part of the analysis process (**Figure 13-2**). An examination of the final set of categories will reveal the concepts and meanings that answer the study question. These concepts may point toward more abstract theories, but the development of a new theory is not a requirement of qualitative analysis.

The qualitative data analysis process is often informed by particular analytic frameworks. **Narrative analysis** may draw on established theories, such as those from feminist theory and cultural studies, to help with the interpretation of the personal stories that the analyst is examining. **Discourse analysis** uses the tools of linguistics to analyze the written, spoken, or nonverbal language used by participants. Other frameworks derive from grounded theory and other philosophical orientations.

FIGURE 13-2 Codes, Themes, and Concepts

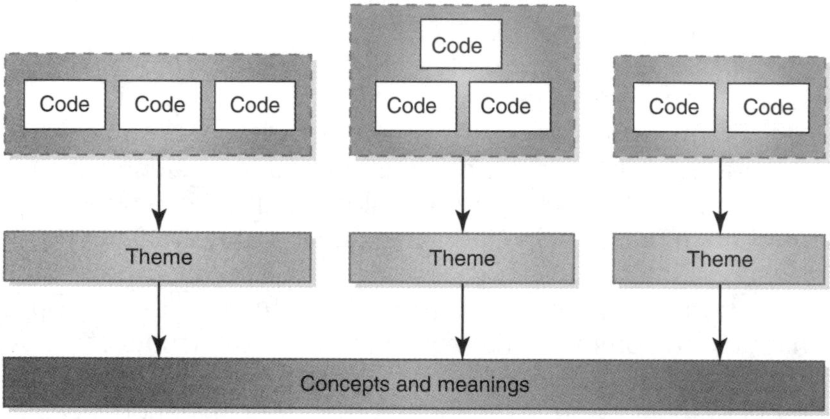

13.6 Mixed Methods Research

Qualitative research can stand alone, or it can be used in conjunction with quantitative surveys. **Mixed methods** studies draw on both quantitative and qualitative methods. Some mixed methods projects use a convergent parallel design to collect quantitative and qualitative data concurrently and then compare the results and interpret them. Some studies collect the data sequentially, completing one type of study first and then designing and implementing the other type of study. An explanatory study may collect quantitative data first, and then use a qualitative study to assist with interpretation of the results. An exploratory study may collect qualitative data first, and then use the insights from that study to design and implement a quantitative study. A qualitative study may be embedded within a quantitative study.

Integration of the two strands of a mixed methods study may occur at various times during the projects. Some research protocols do not consider the interface of the qualitative and quantitative results until the very end of the project when the findings are being interpreted. Other protocols weave both strands of the study together throughout the research process from the design stage through data collection, data analysis, and interpretation. Reports of the findings of qualitative and mixed methods studies often incorporate quotations that express participants' perspectives and experiences in their own words.

13.7 Monitoring and Evaluation

Monitoring and evaluation (M&E) are important management tools, and they both draw on a variety of qualitative and quantitative techniques. **Evaluation** includes a variety of approaches for examining the goals, processes, and/or outcomes of

projects (specific, time-limited activities), **programs** (ongoing groups of projects), and/or policies. The goal of these assessments is usually not to identify what is being done correctly or incorrectly, but to provide feedback about what is working well and what can and should be improved. **Monitoring** is ongoing assessment to ensure that projects and programs are staying on track.

In the health sciences, a typical **program evaluation** begins with a meeting at which stakeholders describe the purposes of the program being examined, how it was intended to function, how it is actually functioning, and what they themselves hope to learn from the assessment. Based on these conversations, an evaluation approach is selected. Evidence is gathered from a variety of sources, possibly including a review of existing program documents, surveys of stakeholders, interviews with key informants, and observations at program sites. All the evidence is then reviewed and categorized, perhaps using a framework like realist synthesis or SWOT. **Realist synthesis** uses a systematic process to find and analyze evidence for the complex reasons some programs succeed and others fail. **SWOT** identifies the strengths (internal organizational strengths), weaknesses (internal organizational limitations), opportunities (external strengths), and threats (external limitations, which might be political, economic, sociocultural, technological, environmental, or legal) of a program. Finally, practical suggestions are made based on the conclusions of the assessment.

A similar process can be used as a component of other forms of evaluative research, such as:

- Needs assessment
- Cost-effectiveness analysis
- Health services research, which examines factors related to the types of health services and providers available to a population, the organization and financing of those health services, and the impact of governments and policies on population health

13.8 Consensus Methods

The goal of some studies is to identify areas of consensus and areas of contention among individuals who are experts on a particular topic and/or a particular community or organization. The results of the deliberations are then used, for example, to select research priorities, to identify best practices, and to agree on plans of action.

Several techniques have been developed for shaping these conversations and the resulting conclusions. For example, the **Delphi method** is a structured decision-making and forecasting process in which participants engage in several rounds of:

- Completing individual questionnaires
- A facilitator summarizing and sharing the responses
- Panelists reconsidering their perspectives after reflecting on the opinions expressed by others

The goal is for each iteration to move the panel of experts closer to agreement.

CHAPTER 14

CORRELATIONAL STUDIES

A correlational, ecological, or aggregate study uses population-level data to examine the relationship between exposure rates and disease rates.

14.1 Overview

A **correlational study** uses population-level data to look for associations between two or more group characteristics (**Figure 14-1**). For example, a correlational study could answer questions like:

- Does the percentage of adults with multiple sclerosis tend to be higher in countries farther from the equator?
- Does the rate of asthma tend to be higher in cities with higher levels of air pollution?
- Does the prevalence of diabetes tend to be higher in provinces with a higher prevalence of obesity?

Correlational studies that explore an environmental exposure, such as distance from the equator or level of air pollution, may be called **ecological studies**. Correlational studies also are called **aggregate studies** because they only look at aggregate, or grouped, population-level data, and they do not include any individual-level data.

Because existing data sources are almost always used for correlational studies—that is, because nearly all correlational studies are secondary analyses—the key to success is identifying data sources that contain comparable information about the variables of interest. Information about all the variables of interest must be available for a suitable number of populations, which can be grouped by place or time. For example, place-based populations could consist of all member nations of the United Nations, all 50 states from the United States, the largest 20 metropolitan areas in the United Kingdom, all the counties in the U.S. state of Michigan, or a random sample of census tracts in Toronto. Time-based studies could use annual historical data for the past several decades from one or more place-based populations.

FIGURE 14-1 Key Characteristics of Correlational (Ecological) Studies

Objective	Compare average levels of exposure and disease in several populations
Primary study question	Do populations with a higher rate of exposure have a higher rate of disease?
Population	Existing population-level data are used; there are no individual participants.
When to use this approach	The aim is to explore possible associations between an exposure and a disease using population-level data.
Requirement	The topic has not been previously explored using individual-level data.
First steps	1. Select the sources of data that will be used. 2. Decide on the variables to include in the analysis.
What to watch out for	The ecological fallacy Limited publication venues
Key statistical measure	Correlation

14.2 Aggregate Data

For most correlational studies, at least one characteristic of the populations being examined is designated as an exposure, and at least one is designated as an outcome or disease. Most exposures and outcomes used in correlational studies are in the form of population-level statistics, such as the proportion of each population with a particular characteristic or the average value of the variable in the population. For example, the exposure may be the percentage of adults age 30 and older in the population who have not completed at least 12 years of education, the mean household income in the population, or the median age of the population. Alternatively, an exposure variable may represent an environmental measure that is likely to be fairly consistent across an entire population, such as the number of rainy days over a given year in each city being included in an ecological study or the average ultraviolet radiation index during midday in the hottest month of the year in those cities. The disease status of each population is also measured at the aggregate level. For example, an outcome metric might be the prevalence of obesity among adults in the countries being included in the analysis or the annual mortality rate from asthma in each province being included in the analysis.

FIGURE 14-2 Sample Data Table

Population	Exposure 1	Outcome 1
A	48.2	14.1
B	65.1	17.0
C	37.8	14.9

Before conducting a statistical analysis of aggregate data, the data from each population must be entered into a spreadsheet. Each population should be assigned to its own row in the spreadsheet. Each exposure and outcome should be assigned to its own column. The data should be filled into the cells in each column so that they line up with the correct population (see **Figure 14-2** for a sample data table). See Chapter 26 for more information about data management.

The analysis will be valid only if the data points are comparable. If multiple sources of data are used or if the data were collected over a lengthy period of time, then the definition of an exposure or a disease may differ from one population to another. For example, different countries might use very different definitions for what counts as access to clean drinking water or what constitutes literacy in an adult. The quality of the data may also vary when different sources are used. In some populations, exposures and diseases may be routinely undercounted or routinely over-diagnosed when compared to other populations. Because of the potential lack of comparability, researchers should interpret ecologic associations conservatively when multiple data sources are used.

14.3 Analysis: Correlation

On a scatterplot used to illustrate correlation, each point represents one population in the study. The exposure is plotted on the x-axis, and the outcome or disease is plotted on the y-axis (**Figure 14-3**). A trend line is fit to the data points, usually using a software program that calculates the line with the best fit.

- When all the points fall neatly along or very near a sloped line, the correlation is strong. A positive (upward) slope shows that higher levels of exposure are associated with higher rates of disease, as shown in Figure 14-3A. A negative (downward) slope shows that higher levels of exposure are associated with lower rates of disease.
- When the points are not exactly linear but a line for trend can be drawn through them, the correlation is mild or moderate, as shown in Figure 14-3B.
- When the points appear to be randomly placed and no obvious line can be drawn through them, or the best-fit line is horizontal, as shown in Figure 14-3C, then the correlation is weak or nonexistent.

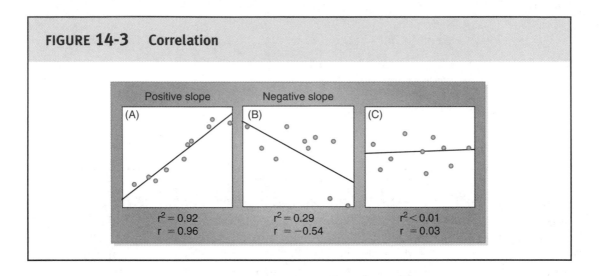

FIGURE 14-3 Correlation

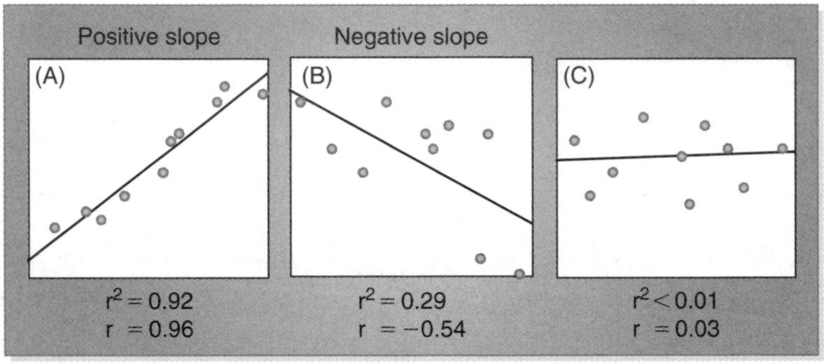

For continuous variables and other variables with responses that can be plotted on a number line, a **Pearson correlation coefficient (r)** can be calculated. For variables that assign a rank to responses or that have ordered categories, the **Spearman rank-order correlation** (designated by the letter r or the Greek letter ρ [rho] in most statistical programs) should be used. For both tests, the value of r (or ρ) ranges from −1, when all points lie perfectly on a line with a negative slope, to 1, when all points lie perfectly on a line with a positive slope. When $r = 0$, there is no association between the exposure and outcome. (Chapter 28 explains the difference between parametric tests like the Pearson correlation and nonparametric tests like the Spearman rank-order correlation and Kendall's rank correlation, which is often designated with the Greek letter τ [tau].)

The association between two or more variables can also be reported as the **coefficient of determination**, r^2, which shows how strong a correlation is without indicating the direction of the association. The value of r^2 ranges from 0 for no correlation to 1 for perfect correlation.

When more than two variables are being compared or the goal is to understand the relationship between two variables while controlling or adjusting for the effects of other variables, linear regression models are used to assess the associations (see Chapter 29).

14.4 Age Adjustment

Sometimes the populations being compared have very different age structures. For example, one or more populations might be considerably younger or older than the others. A younger population may have more favorable health statistics because fewer population members have developed the chronic diseases associated with aging. An older population may have less favorable health statistics simply because

FIGURE 14-4 Direct Age Adjustment

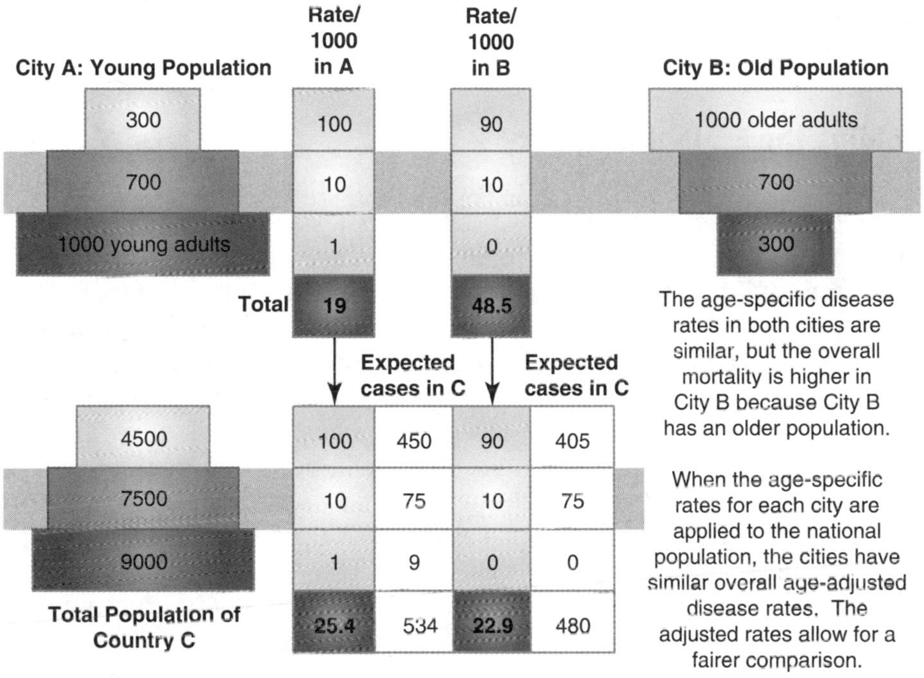

its members are more advanced in years. When the age distributions of populations being compared are known to be different, **age adjustment** can allow a researcher to make more accurate comparisons than are possible with **crude statistics** (raw or unadjusted statistics).

Direct age adjustment requires knowing the exposure or disease rates by age group in each population. To calculate an age-adjusted overall rate for each population, each population's age-specific rates are applied, one at a time, to a standardized population and then an all-ages rate in that standardized population is calculated. In **Figure 14-4**, two cities are compared. City A has a young population, and an overall disease rate of 19 cases per 1000 adults. City B has an older population, and an overall disease rate of 48.5 cases per 1000 adults. However, the age-specific rates in these cities are similar, with City B having slightly lower—not higher—rates in some age groups. If the rates from City A were the rates in the national adult population in Country C, the overall rate of disease nationally would be 25.4 per 1000. If the rates from City B were the rates in the national population, the overall rate of disease nationally would be 22.9 per 1000. These age-adjusted rates for the two cities show that the disease rates are similar, with City B having a slightly lower age-adjusted rate. These adjusted rates are directly comparable because they are based on the age distribution of the same standard population, and they allow for a fairer comparison of disease statue in the two cities.

Indirect age adjustment methods can be used to compare populations for which the population age distributions are known but age-specific rates of exposure and/or disease are not known.

14.5 Avoiding the Ecological Fallacy

Correlational studies compare groups rather than individuals. No individual-level data are included in the analysis, only population-level data. The incorrect attribution of population-level associations to individuals is called the **ecological fallacy**. Even when a population with a higher rate of exposure has a higher rate of disease than populations with lower exposure rates, individuals in that population who have a high level of exposure do not necessarily have the disease. The experience of an individual in a population may vary significantly from the population average. For example, it would be incorrect to assume that any one individual from a country with a high average body mass index (BMI) will be obese or that an individual from a country with a low average BMI will not be obese. However, it is appropriate to identify trends across populations and to use those observations to generate hypotheses for future individual-level studies that will test for relationships between the characteristics of interest in individuals. Correlational studies are a useful starting point for generating hypotheses about associations, but they are not the final word on risk factors for disease.

STEP

3

Designing the Study and Collecting Data

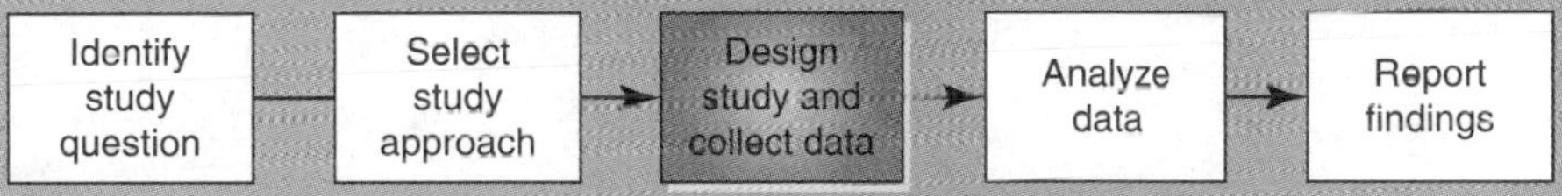

The third step in the research process is developing and implementing a detailed study plan. This section describes how to create a protocol and collect data for primary, secondary, and tertiary studies. The section also includes information about research ethics and about grant proposal writing.

- Research protocol development
- Primary studies that collect new data
  - Population sampling
  - Sample size estimation
  - Questionnaire development
  - Surveys and interviewing methods
  - Additional assessments
- Secondary analyses of existing data sets
- Tertiary analyses using systematic reviews and meta-analyses
- Ethical considerations, review, and approval
- Writing grant proposals

CHAPTER 15

Research Protocols

A research protocol is a detailed handbook describing all the actions that will be taken during the implementation of the research plan.

15.1 Overview of Research Plans by Study Approach

Once a study question and a study approach have been selected, the next step is to create a detailed research plan. A research **protocol** is a detailed written description of all the processes and procedures that will be used for data collection and analysis. The components of this plan will vary somewhat according to the study approach (**Figure 15-1**). For the collection of new data from individuals, the researcher needs to:

- Identify an appropriate way to sample and recruit participants
- Develop a questionnaire and other data collection tools
- Select methods for gathering and recording responses from participants
- Prepare an application for a research ethics review committee

If existing data will be analyzed, an appropriate data source must be identified and the data file and supporting materials acquired. If a systematic literature review will be conducted, the search strategy must be defined, eligible articles identified, and relevant information from each article extracted into a database. For all study plans, it is helpful to create a protocol that will guide each step of the data collection and management process.

15.2 Research Timelines

Most research protocols include a detailed schedule for the planned research project. It is therefore helpful to:

- Create a list of all the steps from planning the study through the dissemination of results.
- Create a calendar that shows when each of these steps is expected to be initiated and be completed.

FIGURE 15-1 Research Plans for Primary, Secondary, and Tertiary Data Collection

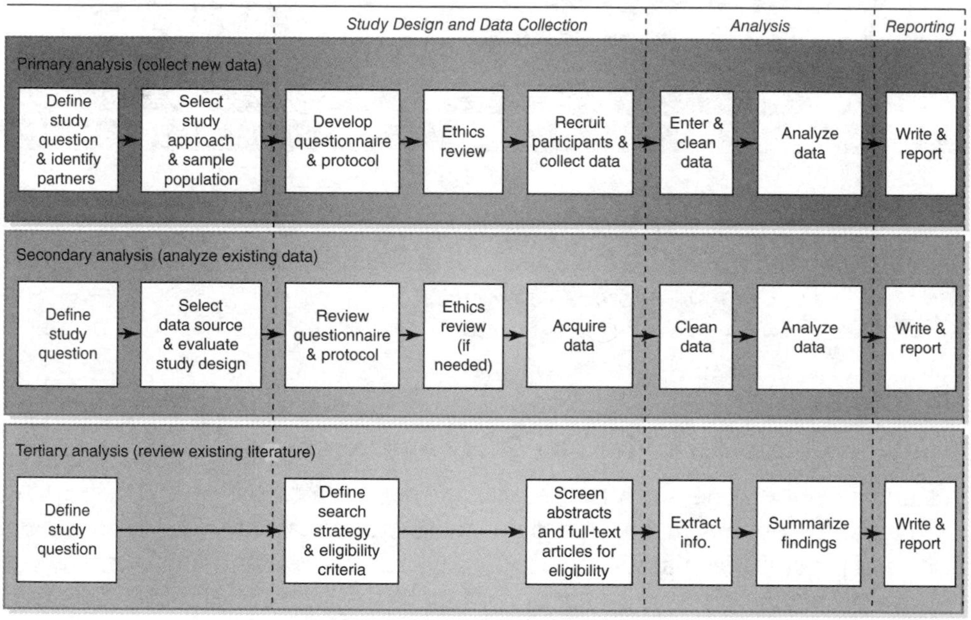

- Identify fixed deadlines that must be met, such as grant application deadlines and abstract submission dates for conferences where the work might be presented.
- Agree with collaborators on intermediate deadlines for research tasks that will help the project stay on track toward timely completion and will ensure that no important fixed deadlines are missed.
- Set up regular meeting times for the research team (whether in person, online, or via other communication modes).

A **Gantt chart** (**Figure 15-2**) can be very helpful for visually displaying the research timeline.

The internal due dates set by the research team will need to be somewhat flexible because predicting how long some steps will take can be difficult. For example, waiting for ethics approval or for the disbursement of funds from a granting agency might take several months instead of several weeks. Data collection might be completed far more slowly or more quickly than expected. Data entry or data cleaning might take much more time than originally anticipated. Additionally, relying on collaborators to complete some aspects of the work may result in delays. This is especially likely when the lead researcher is not in a position of authority. For example, a

FIGURE 15-2 Sample (and Simplified) Gantt Chart for a Year-Long Secondary Analysis Project

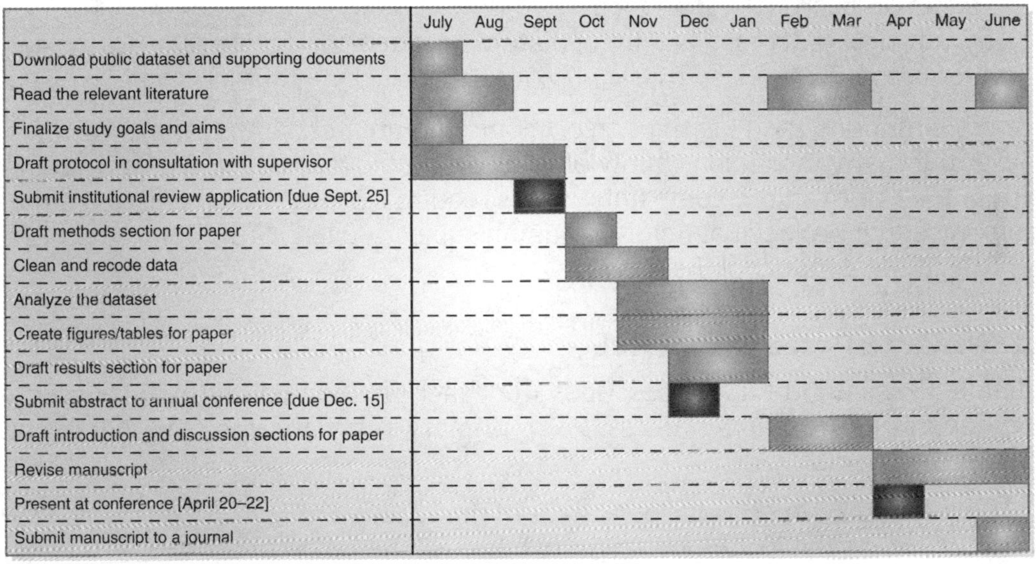

student researcher might not be able to push for a faster response when a supervisor is slow to provide feedback. Sometimes these holdups are not a major concern, but missed deadlines may be a serious problem when some collaborators have inflexible schedules or stringent degree requirements. Including a timeline in the protocol—even if it may need to be updated as the project is conducted—is a way to promote steady progress toward completion.

15.3 Researcher Responsibilities

Research projects tend to proceed most smoothly when all research team members have a shared understanding about each contributor's roles and responsibilities. The protocol should include the names of the people who have accepted responsibility for particular tasks, the dates they have agreed to work on those assignments, and the mechanisms that will be used to encourage careful and on-time completion of those items (such as emailed reminders sent by the lead researcher in advance of deadlines). It may also be helpful to identify a process for resolving conflicts. Sometimes one person, often a senior researcher, is designated as the adjudicator of delays in the submissions of agreed-upon deliverables, disagreements about the interpretation of the protocol or the nature of an assigned task, and other differences of opinion or awkward situations.

Universities, hospitals, and other institutions typically require one researcher to act as the **primary investigator (PI)** and to accept responsibility for guaranteeing that:

- The protocol is followed.
- The budget is properly managed.
- Any adverse outcomes are immediately reported to the institution's research ethics committee.

In some situations the PI is the person doing the greatest amount of work on the project, but many institutions allow only senior employees to serve as official institutional PIs. For example, some universities require a professor to be listed as the PI on any research project that involves human subjects, even if a student is taking the lead role in the conduct of the project.

15.4 Writing a Research Protocol

A detailed research protocol describes the exact procedures that will be used for every step of the research process. For a primary study, the protocol will explain, among other items:

- The main goal and specific objectives of the study
- The desired sample size and the steps that will be taken to acquire an adequate number of participants
- The specific processes that will be used for contacting and recruiting participants
- The precise procedures that will be used to obtain and document informed consent (or to document refusal to participate)
- The exact questions that participants will be asked and, if interviews will be used to gather information from participants, the instructions for how those questions will be asked
- The exact ways that responses to survey questions will be entered into a computer database, including the methods for recording missing responses
- The precise steps that will be taken to confirm the accuracy of the entered data
- The steps that will be taken to maintain the confidentiality of personal information that might be contained in the data set
- The plans for data analysis, including the particular statistical tests that will be used to answer the study questions
- If applicable, the precise laboratory procedures that will be used

For a systematic review, the protocol is quite different but equally detailed. It defines the exact criteria for an article's eligibility for inclusion in the review, and it spells out exactly how articles that cannot easily be classified according to the eligibility criteria will be handled. For all study designs, the protocol should anticipate likely dilemmas or areas of confusion and address them as completely as possible.

Ideally, a protocol should:

- Fully describe all the procedures that will be used for data collection and analysis
- List the anticipated dates of completion for each of the steps in the research process
- Provide details about the responsibilities of each member of the research team
- Describe the mechanism for updating any part of the research plan if revisions arise after approval of the initial protocol, noting that significant adjustments to the protocol may need to be approved by all relevant research ethics committees before they can be implemented

A strong protocol provides enough detail that another researcher could easily replicate the study. It should also be detailed enough that the entire methods section of any paper that will result from the project could be written before data collection begins.

15.5 Preparing for Data Collection

Before initiating data collection, make sure that all preparations have been finalized.

- Have all collaborators approved of their designated roles, responsibilities, and deadlines?
- Have all collaborators completed required ethics training?
- Are all supplies and equipment ready for use?
- Has the data management system been tested and found to be reliable?
- If applicable, have the final versions of all study documents (such as the informed consent statement and the questionnaire) been approved by all relevant research ethics committees?
- If applicable, are all participating laboratories ready to begin processing samples?

The following chapters provide information about some of the essential steps in preparing for primary data collection: identifying a sample population, developing a questionnaire and other forms of assessment, and ensuring that ethical standards are followed. Most of these steps must be completed before a proposal for grant funding can be finalized and submitted.

CHAPTER 16

POPULATION SAMPLING

An accessible and appropriate source of study participants for primary studies should be identified early in the research process.

16.1 Types of Research Populations

At least four different types of populations must be considered when preparing to collect data (**Figure 16-1**). Several different names are used to describe these four entities, but the concepts are the same for all health science fields.

- The broadest group is the **target population** to which the results of the study should be applicable.
- The **source population** is a well-defined subset of individuals from the target population.
- The **sample population** consists of the individuals from the source population who are invited to participate in the research project.
- The **study population** comprises the eligible members of the sample population who consent to participate in the study.

16.2 Target and Source Populations

A well-defined study question identifies a target population to which the results of the study should apply. A target population might be quite narrow. The goal might be to identify the cause of an outbreak of a drug-resistant bacterial strain in one wing of a long-term acute care hospital. Or the goal might be to measure the prevalence of binge drinking on one college campus. Alternatively, the target population might be relatively large: all adult males, a whole country, or all people with type 2 diabetes. Unless the target population is very small, it is usually not possible to invite all members of the target population to participate in the study.

FIGURE 16-1 The Study Population Is a Subset of Individuals Sampled from a Source Population

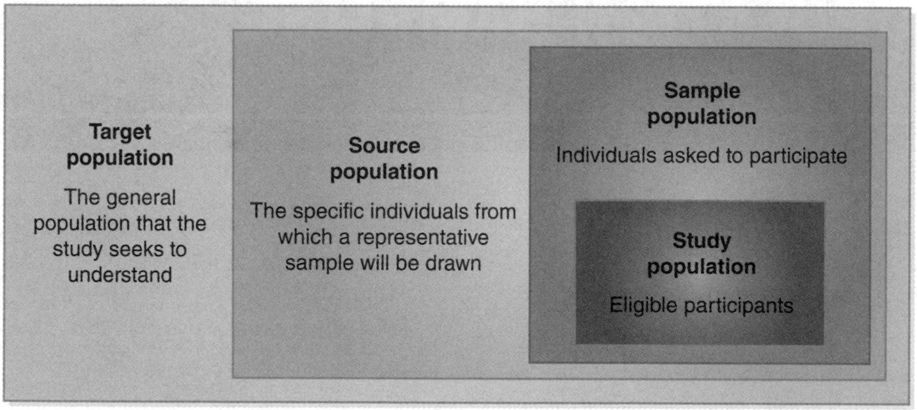

Instead, a more specific source population (sometimes called a **sampling frame**) should be identified. Ideally, the source population consists of an enumerated list of population members. For example:

- A list of the registry identification numbers for all women with a breast cancer diagnosis in the past 2 years who are indexed in a particular cancer registry
- A list of the names of all members of a professional sports league
- A list of the addresses for all households within 2 miles of a particular nuclear power plant

In each of these examples, it would be possible for a researcher to acquire or generate a list of all members of the source population. That means that the number of individuals (or households) in the source population can be counted. The count can then be used in the determination of an appropriate sampling method—one that might include the entire source population or a randomly sampled subset of it—and the calculation of participation rates.

16.3 Sample Populations

When the source population is small, every person who is listed as a member of the source population can be asked to participate in the study. In this situation, the source population is the same as the sample population. However, a source population is often much larger than the sample size required for a study. When the source population is very large, a portion of the source population may serve as a sample population.

A **population-based study** uses a random sampling method to generate a sample population that is representative of some well-defined larger population (which is usually a population that is not defined by a disease or exposure status). A variety of methods can be used to generate a sample population that is a representative subset of a source population. **Probability-based sampling** is usually the preferred option for producing a sample population that is similar to the source population as a whole. If a list of every individual in the source population is available, a computer program can be used to select at random the individuals who will be invited to participate. If the sample will be drawn from an entire city, then cluster sampling can be used to identify at random whole city blocks for inclusion in the sample population. Alternatively, the sample population might consist of all residents in the city living on every tenth street that runs north to south, starting with a randomly sampled street. Examples of these types of probability-based samples are shown in **Figure 16-2**.

Sometimes a non-probability-based **convenience population** can be selected based on the ease of access to those individuals, schools, workplaces, organizations, or communities. Convenience sampling must always be used with caution, since convenient sample populations are often systematically different from the target and source populations they are intended to represent. When possible, researchers should seek to confirm that the selected sample population has demographic and socioeconomic characteristics similar to those of the broader community the participants are intended to represent.

No matter which sampling method is used, the goal is to end up with a sample population that is representative of the source population and, ideally, of the target population, too. Researchers attempting to generate a random sample from the source population need to avoid the **non-random sampling bias** that could occur if each individual in the source population does not have an equal chance of being selected for the sample population. Researchers using a convenience sample must avoid the **ascertainment bias** that can occur if the convenience sample is not

FIGURE 16-2 Examples of Types of Probability Sampling

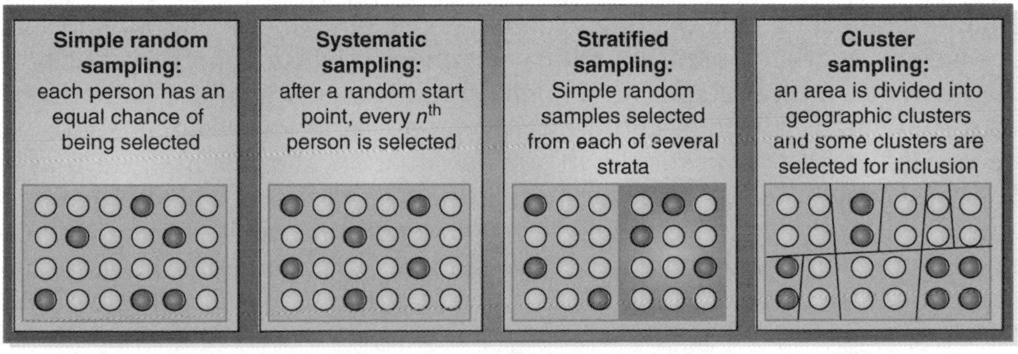
Simple random sampling:
each person has an equal chance of being selected
Systematic sampling:
after a random start point, every n^{th} person is selected
Stratified sampling:
Simple random samples selected from each of several strata
Cluster sampling:
an area is divided into geographic clusters and some clusters are selected for inclusion

representative of the source population as a whole. These and many other potential sources of bias can be eliminated or minimized with careful planning.

16.4 Study Populations

The individuals identified as the sample population will later be asked to participate in the study. The study population will consist of the members of the sample population who can be located, who consent to participation, and who meet all eligibility criteria. A 100% participation rate is extremely rare. At least some of the individuals in the sample population will ignore an invitation to participate. Some who respond to the invitation will choose not to participate. Others will turn out to be ineligible because they do not meet the inclusion criteria. A low response rate may result in **nonresponse bias** if the members of the sample population who agree to be in the study are systematically different from nonparticipants. However, a less than 100% participation rate is usually not a problem as long as the researcher:

- Uses acceptable and carefully explained sampling methods.
- Takes appropriate steps to maximize the participation rate.
- Recruits an adequately large sample size. (Chapter 17 explains how to estimate the sample size required.)
- Reports the number of potential participants at each stage.

16.5 Populations for Cross-Sectional Surveys

In a cross-sectional survey, the source population must be representative of the target population, and the sample population must be representative of the source population. The goal of most cross-sectional surveys is to describe a specific target population accurately. The results of these surveys are often used to make important resource and policy decisions.

Convenience samples rarely result in a study population that is representative of the target population. For example, suppose that the goal of a study is to quantify the prevalence of tobacco use among high school students in a county. The county's 15 high schools together serve as the target population and the source population. Selecting only one high school as the sample population is probably not sufficient. Working intensely with one school might maximize participation rates. However, the selected school might enroll students who are different from county students as a whole—more rural or urban, more or less diverse, or from more or less wealthy households. In such a situation, the results from that one high school would not be an accurate reflection of adolescent health across the county. A better option is to sample some students from each of the 15 schools, such as by randomly sampling 20% of the students in each high school based on the classroom they are in during the first period of the school day (**Figure 16-3**). Similarly, recruiting participants for a general population survey from among the spectators at a football game, the shoppers in a particular grocery store, or the

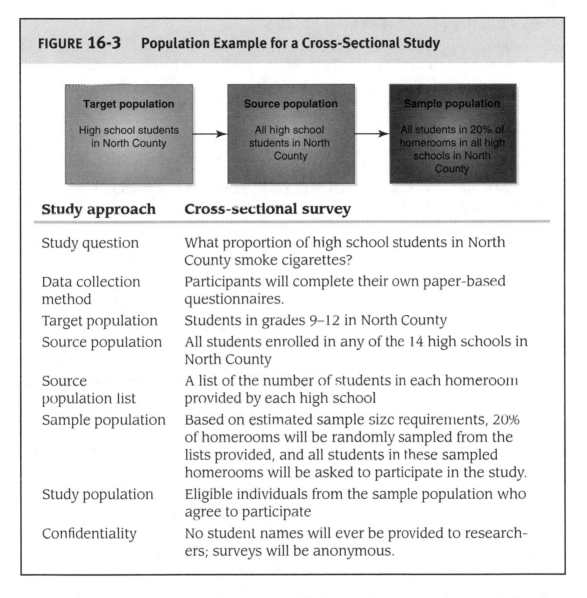

FIGURE 16-3 Population Example for a Cross-Sectional Study

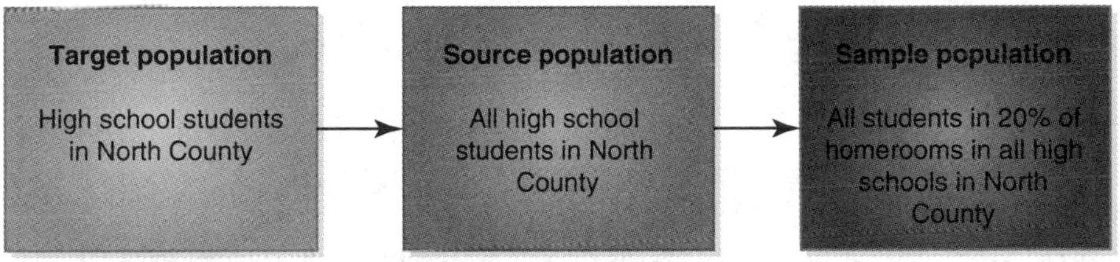

Study approach	Cross-sectional survey
Study question	What proportion of high school students in North County smoke cigarettes?
Data collection method	Participants will complete their own paper-based questionnaires.
Target population	Students in grades 9–12 in North County
Source population	All students enrolled in any of the 14 high schools in North County
Source population list	A list of the number of students in each homeroom provided by each high school
Sample population	Based on estimated sample size requirements, 20% of homerooms will be randomly sampled from the lists provided, and all students in these sampled homerooms will be asked to participate in the study.
Study population	Eligible individuals from the sample population who agree to participate
Confidentiality	No student names will ever be provided to researchers; surveys will be anonymous.

donors at a volunteer blood drive would likely result in a sample population that did not represent the target population.

Ideally, the researcher will identify a way to confirm that the source population is similar to the target population and that the sample population is similar to the source population. For example, the sample population for the survey in Figure 16-3 can be checked to verify that it yields a proportion of students by grade that is similar to the distribution of these characteristics for the total student populations of participating high schools. Similarly, the sample population for a survey of the general public should reflect the demographics of the target population in the most recent population census.

16.6 Populations for Case-Control Studies

When identifying possible participants for a case-control study, the first step is to find an appropriate and available source of cases. All cases must have the same disease, disability, or other health-related condition. The study's case definition should be very clear about the characteristics, signs, and symptoms that must be present or absent for an individual to be categorized as a case. For example, a researcher may want to select only candidates with advanced disease or, alternatively, may prefer to study only cases whose symptoms began recently. The case definition should specify both the inclusion and the exclusion criteria.

Hospitals, specialty clinics, public health offices, disease support groups, and advocacy organizations may be helpful resources for locating individuals or groups of individuals who are likely to meet the study's case definition. However, care must be taken to ensure that the sample population is not healthier, sicker, or more or less socially connected than the typical person who meets the case definition. (Another option may be to use the participants of a large longitudinal cohort study as the source population for both cases and controls. This kind of **nested case-control study** design minimizes recall bias because information about past exposures was collected at the time of the exposure and is not based on participants' memories. However, a cohort study will only yield a sufficient number of cases when the disease being studied is common.)

Once a source of cases is identified, a valid control group must be selected. This is a critical decision. The controls must be similar to the cases in every way except for their disease status. For example, it would be inappropriate to compare older adult women to teenage boys, to compare people with chronic heart disease to marathon runners, or to compare big-city businessmen to men who are subsistence farmers in remote areas. All cases and all controls must meet the same **eligibility criteria** except for the ones relating to disease status. (Having both a case definition and a control definition is helpful so that borderline cases are excluded from serving as either cases or controls.) Thus, a study that targets septuagenarian women should require both cases and controls to be women in their 70s (**Figure 16-4**). A study examining chronic disease should choose a control population representative of the general public, not a population that is unusually physically active. And cases and controls for any one study should be drawn from similar geographic and sociodemographic populations.

Controls can be drawn from many different types of source populations. For some hospital-based studies, it may be appropriate to use as controls individuals hospitalized with a condition other than the one being studied. For some population-based studies, random-digit telephone dialing may yield a representative population—or, because many people will refuse to answer personal questions over the telephone, this strategy may result in a very unrepresentative population. In some situations, friends or family members of the cases may be the best controls because they are likely to have backgrounds similar to the cases. When making this important decision, the researcher should consult a reference that specifically addresses the selection of appropriate participants for case-control studies, including the possibilities for matching cases to controls.

FIGURE 16-4 **Population Example for a Case-Control Study**

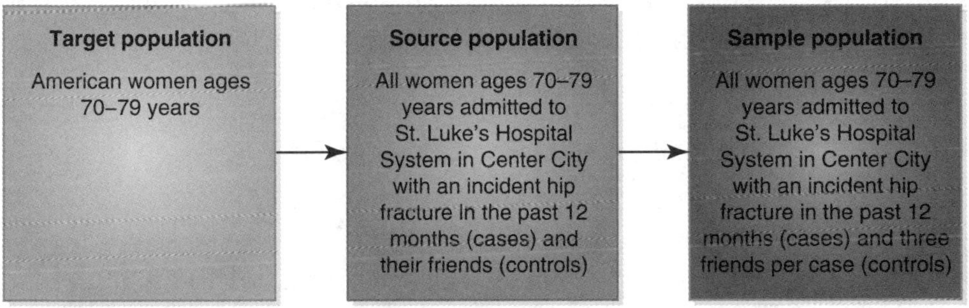
Target population
American women ages 70–79 years
Source population
All women ages 70–79 years admitted to St. Luke's Hospital System in Center City with an incident hip fracture in the past 12 months (cases) and their friends (controls)
Sample population
All women ages 70–79 years admitted to St. Luke's Hospital System in Center City with an incident hip fracture in the past 12 months (cases) and three friends per case (controls)

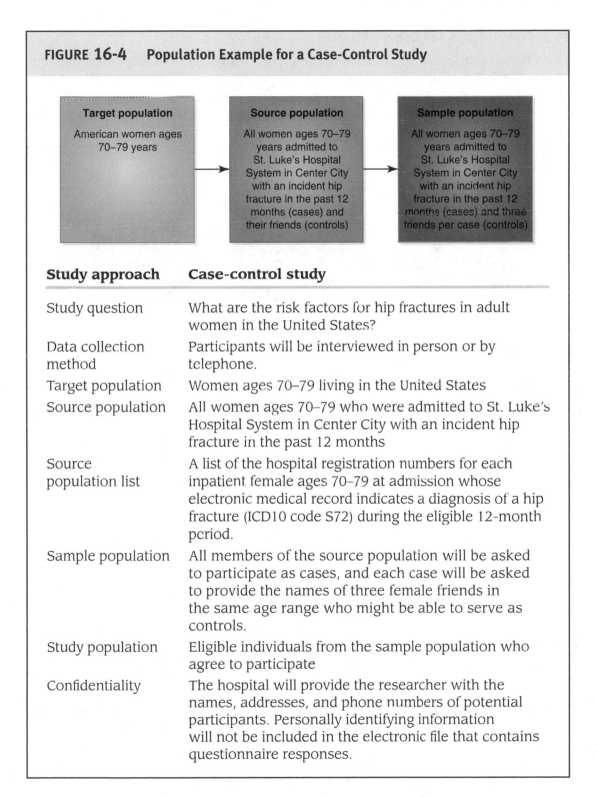

Study approach	**Case-control study**
Study question	What are the risk factors for hip fractures in adult women in the United States?
Data collection method	Participants will be interviewed in person or by telephone.
Target population	Women ages 70–79 living in the United States
Source population	All women ages 70–79 who were admitted to St. Luke's Hospital System in Center City with an incident hip fracture in the past 12 months
Source population list	A list of the hospital registration numbers for each inpatient female ages 70–79 at admission whose electronic medical record indicates a diagnosis of a hip fracture (ICD10 code S72) during the eligible 12-month period.
Sample population	All members of the source population will be asked to participate as cases, and each case will be asked to provide the names of three female friends in the same age range who might be able to serve as controls.
Study population	Eligible individuals from the sample population who agree to participate
Confidentiality	The hospital will provide the researcher with the names, addresses, and phone numbers of potential participants. Personally identifying information will not be included in the electronic file that contains questionnaire responses.

16.7 Populations for Cohort Studies

Identifying source and sample populations for a longitudinal cohort study is similar to the process for identifying these populations for a cross-sectional survey (**Figure 16-5**). There are some added concerns about needing to recruit a stable study population in order to retain as many participants as possible for

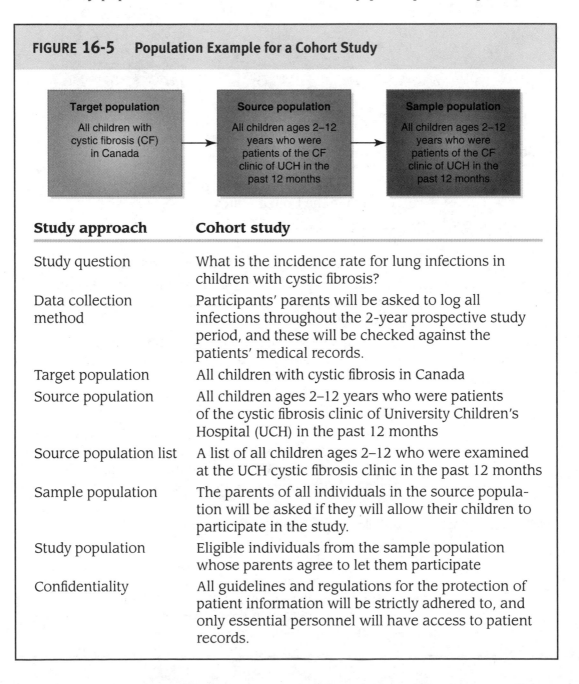

FIGURE 16-5 Population Example for a Cohort Study

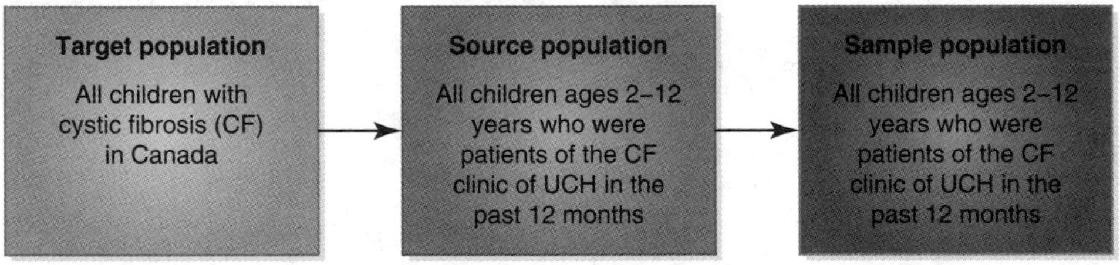
Target population
All children with cystic fibrosis (CF) in Canada
Source population
All children ages 2–12 years who were patients of the CF clinic of UCH in the past 12 months
Sample population
All children ages 2–12 years who were patients of the CF clinic of UCH in the past 12 months

Study approach	Cohort study
Study question	What is the incidence rate for lung infections in children with cystic fibrosis?
Data collection method	Participants' parents will be asked to log all infections throughout the 2-year prospective study period, and these will be checked against the patients' medical records.
Target population	All children with cystic fibrosis in Canada
Source population	All children ages 2–12 years who were patients of the cystic fibrosis clinic of University Children's Hospital (UCH) in the past 12 months
Source population list	A list of all children ages 2–12 who were examined at the UCH cystic fibrosis clinic in the past 12 months
Sample population	The parents of all individuals in the source population will be asked if they will allow their children to participate in the study.
Study population	Eligible individuals from the sample population whose parents agree to let them participate
Confidentiality	All guidelines and regulations for the protection of patient information will be strictly adhered to, and only essential personnel will have access to patient records.

the duration of the study. For cohort studies that seek to compare exposed and unexposed populations, identifying exposed and unexposed participants is similar to the steps for identifying cases and controls for a case-control study. For example, studies of the aftereffects of occupational exposures often recruit individuals exposed to on-the-job hazards (similar to cases for a case-control study) through employers, and ask those exposed persons to help recruit unexposed friends and family members to serve as a members of a comparison population (similar to the controls for a case-control study).

16.8 Populations for Experimental Studies

As is true for cross-sectional surveys, experimental studies require a source population that is reasonably representative of the target population. For example, suppose the goal of an experimental study is to test whether nutritional counseling during the first semester at a residential college prevents weight gain during the first year of college. For this intervention study to be valid, the researcher needs to recruit a reasonable cross-section of the first-year student population (**Figure 16-6**). Some sampling approaches would likely result in a study population that was much more concerned about weight than the average first-year student. Suppose the researcher asked for volunteers, recruited students majoring in nutrition, or sampled from among student athletes. Members of all three of these populations—volunteers for a wellness study, nutrition majors, and varsity athletes—are likely more attuned to their nutritional status than is typical for a first-year college student. These individuals are therefore less likely than the typical student to gain significant weight during the observation period. Minimal changes in weight would be observed during the year both in the intervention group receiving nutritional counseling and in the control group not being offered dietary advice as part of the study. Because there would be no significant difference in weight gain in the intervention and control groups, the intervention would be deemed unsuccessful. If a more representative study population had been recruited, the intervention might have been deemed a success.

Some experimental studies require participants to be exposed to potentially risky substances or activities. In such studies, the risk of harm can be reduced by selecting an appropriate source population and defining strict inclusion and exclusion criteria. For example, studies that involve exercise must target potential participants likely to be healthy enough to engage in physical activity. Studies of new drugs for advanced forms of cancer are often open only to extremely ill patients for whom standard therapies have not been effective.

Safety should always be the top priority when designing and implementing an experimental study. Precautions must be taken to protect participants from injury. For example, suppose all volunteers for an experiment will be injected with a solution. The researchers must ensure that potential participants have no known allergies to any of the ingredients in either the experimental substance or the placebo. An allergy to any ingredient must be listed as one of the exclusion criteria.

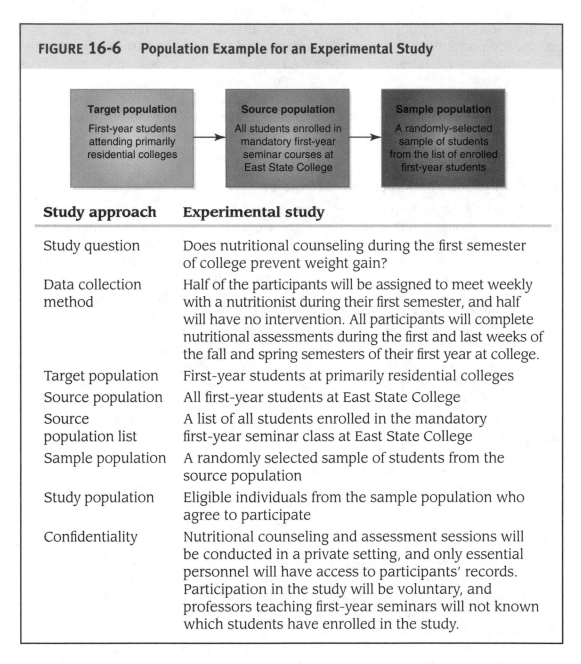

FIGURE 16-6 Population Example for an Experimental Study

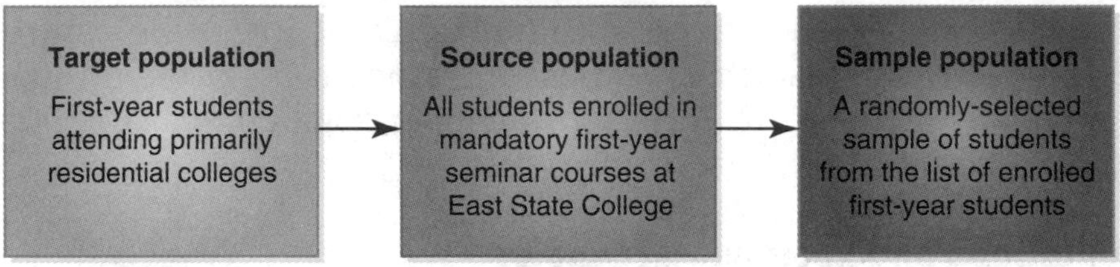
Target population
First-year students attending primarily residential colleges
Source population
All students enrolled in mandatory first-year seminar courses at East State College
Sample population
A randomly-selected sample of students from the list of enrolled first-year students

Study approach	Experimental study
Study question	Does nutritional counseling during the first semester of college prevent weight gain?
Data collection method	Half of the participants will be assigned to meet weekly with a nutritionist during their first semester, and half will have no intervention. All participants will complete nutritional assessments during the first and last weeks of the fall and spring semesters of their first year at college.
Target population	First-year students at primarily residential colleges
Source population	All first-year students at East State College
Source population list	A list of all students enrolled in the mandatory first-year seminar class at East State College
Sample population	A randomly selected sample of students from the source population
Study population	Eligible individuals from the sample population who agree to participate
Confidentiality	Nutritional counseling and assessment sessions will be conducted in a private setting, and only essential personnel will have access to participants' records. Participation in the study will be voluntary, and professors teaching first-year seminars will not known which students have enrolled in the study.

16.9 Vulnerable Populations

Vulnerable populations in health research include young children, some individuals with serious health issues, people in prison and some other socially marginalized populations, and others who might have limited ability to make an informed, autonomous decision about volunteering to participate in a research study. These populations should not be selected as the source population for studies that do not require their participation. At the same time, it is problematic when members of vulnerable populations are systematically excluded from research. In particular, the only way to study health issues of special importance to potentially vulnerable populations is to allow for their participation in relevant research projects. Pregnant women and children must be included in tests of the safety of pharmaceutical agents before they can be approved for wider use. Individuals with severe mental health disorders must be included in studies of psychiatric diseases. New therapies for life-threatening diseases must be tested in people with advanced illnesses. The critical health concerns of prisoners can be identified only by conducting research in prisons. The impact of interpersonal violence on health can be understood only by asking survivors about their experiences.

Research studies including members of vulnerable populations require extra consideration of the potential risks of research to participants. The study must be sufficiently important to justify gathering new data from members of a vulnerable population. The ability of every participant—or, for young children and those with significantly diminished cognitive abilities, a legally recognized representative—to provide informed consent free from coercion must be assured. Concerns about the increased risks of adverse effects from study participation must be addressed. For example, people with fragile health may have an elevated risk of injury from physical tests. Those with histories of abuse or mental illness may have a heightened risk of psychological damage from answering questions about sensitive topics. Chapter 23 provides additional information about the requirements of research involving vulnerable populations.

16.10 Community Involvement

Some studies benefit from or require the participation and support of whole geographic, cultural, or social communities and their leaders. The approval of community leaders does not negate the requirement to obtain individual informed consent from participants whose individual data will be collected. However, community buy-in for a project often improves participation rates, enhances the cultural competence of the research team, and ensures that the study's outcomes are valuable to the community.

A cross-sectional survey that will collect information from students may require the permission of school authorities in addition to the consent of the students and/or their parents and the approval of a research ethics committee. A clinical study that seeks to enroll participants with a rare disease may benefit greatly by partnering with an active disease support and advocacy network. A longitudinal study that intends to recruit and monitor whole villages will be most successful if formal and informal community leaders and other local representatives are actively involved in planning, recruitment, and retention. These connections with community representatives should be established early in the research planning process and maintained throughout the data collection and dissemination period.

Community-based studies often work best when they use research methods such as those developed for **Community-Based Participatory Research (CBPR)**. CBPR partnerships link academicians with community representatives who together identify research priorities for the community, design and implement appropriate data gathering and analysis activities, and then apply those findings to the development of new policies and programs in the community. Under a CBPR model, community participants are partners rather than study subjects, and all partners are involved in decision making throughout the entire research process.

CHAPTER 17

Sample Size Estimation

An adequate number of study participants is required to achieve valid and significant results.

17.1 Importance of Sample Size

When determining how many participants are needed for a study to be meaningful, the goal is to recruit just the right number of participants, not too many and not too few. The correct number is based on statistical estimations about how many people are required to answer the study question with a specified level of certainty. If more participants are recruited than are statistically required, resources are wasted, including the time of both the researcher and the superfluous participants. If too few participants are recruited, the whole study will be almost worthless because the sample will not have enough statistical power to answer the study question. Few researchers ever have the luxury of worrying about a surplus of participants, but many struggle to recruit a sufficient study population. A shortage can make getting statistically significant results almost impossible.

17.2 Sample Size and Certainty Levels

There is value in having a large sample size. Large samples from a population are usually better than small ones at yielding a sample mean close to the true population value. For example, suppose that the mean age in a population consisting of 20 people is 39 years (**Figure 17-1**). If a sample of only 3 people is taken (15% of the total population), there is some possibility that the sample mean will be close to the population mean of 39 years. But there is also a possibility that the sample mean will be distant from the population mean. If a larger sample of 8 people (40% of the total population) is selected from the population, then the sample mean is likely to be fairly close to the population mean.

Figure 17-2 shows an alternative display of the sample means that combines the mean age with its 95% confidence interval. A **confidence interval** is a statistical

FIGURE 17-1 Sample Size and Means

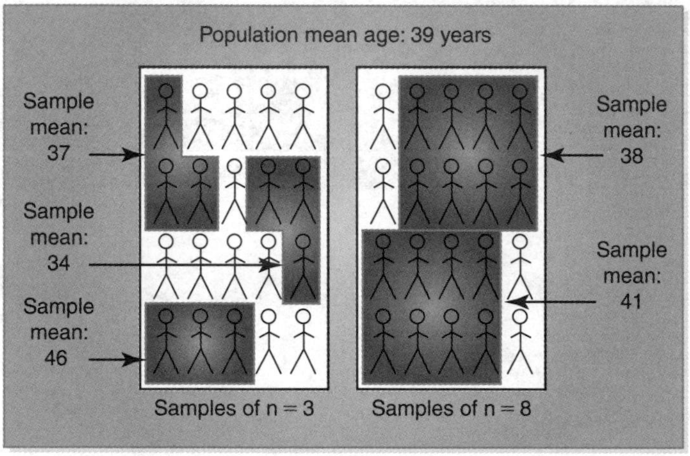

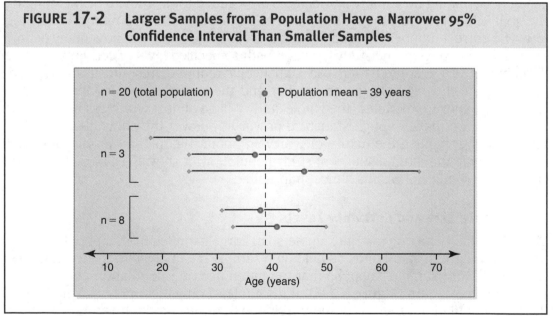

FIGURE 17-2 Larger Samples from a Population Have a Narrower 95% Confidence Interval Than Smaller Samples

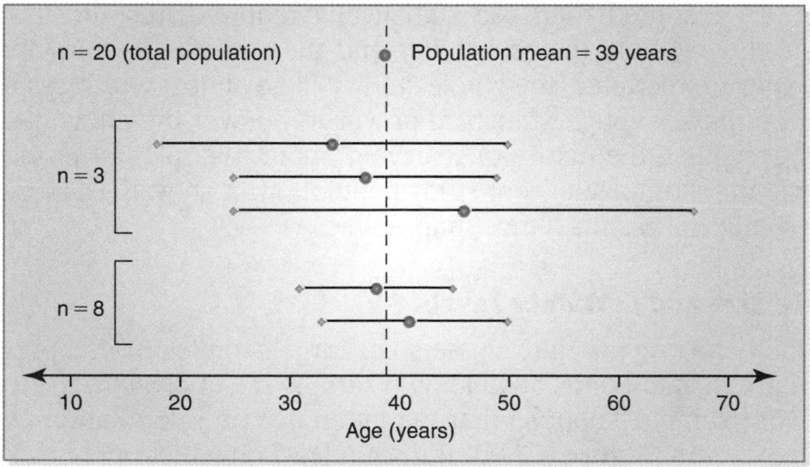

estimate of how close to the population value (in this case, the population mean age) a sample of a particular size is expected to be. When the sample size is small, the sample mean might be quite far from the mean in the total population. This is represented by a wide confidence interval that reaches far from the sample mean.

When a greater proportion of the total population is sampled for inclusion in the estimation of the mean age, the confidence interval for the mean age will be narrower because there is greater certainty about the sample mean being close to the population mean.

The black dots in the center of each of the five lines in Figure 17-2 represent the five sample means from Figure 17-1. The 95% confidence interval for each sample population is represented by the lines extending from the sample means. The 95% confidence interval is calculated for each sample based on the number of individuals included in the sample, the mean age of those individuals, and the standard deviation of their ages, which is a measure of how far apart the ages of the individuals in the sample are. For the top line in Figure 17-2, the sample mean is 34 years, and the confidence interval stretches from 18 to 50 years. Based on this sample, a researcher can be 95% confident that the mean in the total population is somewhere between 18 and 50 years. Indeed, the population mean of 39 years is captured in that range. If hundreds of random samples of 3 individuals are drawn from the total population of 20, about 95% of those samples will have a 95% confidence interval that overlaps the true population mean of 39 years. About 5% of the time, the random sample of 3 individuals will, by chance, include an unusually young or unusually old set of individuals, and the confidence interval will not overlap the population mean.

If all of the 20 people in the total population are included in the analysis, no confidence interval is required; the population mean age will be known exactly. If a sample of 18 of the 20 members of the population is drawn, the sample mean age will be very close to 39 years and the confidence interval will be so narrow that it will hardly extend beyond the dot representing the sample mean. Figure 17-2 shows that larger sample sizes generally result in sample means that are closer to the population mean. Larger sample sizes also have confidence intervals that are narrower than the confidence intervals generated by smaller sample sizes. More generally, larger sample sizes make it more likely that a study will yield statistically significant results.

17.3 Sample Size Estimation

A **sample size calculator** is more accurately called a **sample size estimator** because the range of suggested sample sizes is based on a series of assumptions about the expected characteristics of the sample population. This type of tool should be used early in the study design process to identify an appropriate goal for the number of participants who will need to be recruited for the study. Sample size calculators are available online, often at no cost, and are bundled with most statistical software programs.

Figure 17-3 shows examples of the kinds of inputs that must be provided for various study approaches in order to get a rough estimate of the required number of

FIGURE 17-3 Examples of Sample Size Calculation

Characteristic	Cross-Sectional Survey	Case-Control Study	Cohort Study	Experimental Study
Study question	What proportion of the population has the exposure or disease?	Are cases more likely than controls to have the exposure?	Are exposed people more likely than unexposed people to develop the outcome?	Are exposed people more likely than unexposed people to have a favorable outcome?
Population size	5000	—	—	—
Anticipated percentage with exposure or disease	15%	—	—	—
Confidence for anticipated exposure percentage	±3%	—	—	—
Ratio of controls to cases	—	2	—	—
Ratio of unexposed to exposed	—	—	1	1
Anticipated percentage of controls exposed	—	25%	—	—
Anticipated percentage of unexposed with disease or outcome	—	—	10%	70%
OR worth detecting	—	1.5	—	—
RR worth detecting	—	—	1.3	1.25
Confidence level $(1 - \alpha)$	95%	95%	95%	95%
Power $(1 - \beta)$	—	80%	80%	80%
Estimated sample size	~500	~350 cases and 700 controls	~1850 exposed and 1850 unexposed	~90 exposed and 90 unexposed

participants. A best guess must be used for most of these inputs because accurate information will not be available until after the study has been completed. The values for inputs can be informed by previous studies, but those prior publications will likely not allow a researcher to be certain about whether, for example, the proportion of cases with the exposure of interest will be the same 25% mentioned in the article or will instead be 20% or 30%. Trying a variety of values for the input variables in a sample size calculator will show that even slight changes in input values may result in a considerable difference in the estimated sample size required (**Figure 17-4**). When the level of certainty about inputs is low, it is wise to err on the side of a larger sample size.

17.4 Power Estimation

Another way to check for sample size requirements is to work backward from the number of participants likely to be recruited to see whether a study population of that size will provide adequate statistical power for the study design. **Power** is related to the ability of a statistical test to detect significant differences in a population when differences really do exist. For example, suppose that there really is a substantial difference in the mean weight of cases and controls in a case-control study or that an exposure in a cohort study is truly a risk factor for the disease outcome of interest. In such situations, a study needs adequate power to be able to detect those meaningful differences or associations. When two proportions are close to one another, very large sample sizes are required to detect a significant difference between those proportions. When an incidence rate ratio has a point estimate close to 1, a very large sample size will be required to yield a confidence interval that is statistically significant and does not overlap 1.

Figure 17-5 illustrates the definition of statistical power. Population-based studies aim to have study populations that reflect their source populations. Sometimes, however, either because of chance or because of a study design flaw (such as a sample size that is too small), the sample does not capture the true experience of the population. **Type 1 (type I) errors** occur when a study population yields a significant statistical test result even though a significant difference or association does not actually exist in the source population. The probability of a type 1 error is often noted by the Greek letter alpha (α). Most studies use $\alpha = 5\%$ as the value for statistical significance, which corresponds to statistical tests using a 95% confidence interval (and a *p*-value of $p = 0.05$). When $\alpha = 5\%$, about 1 in 20 statistical tests will result in a type 1 error. **Type 2 (type II) errors** occur when a statistical test of data from the study population finds no significant result even though a significant difference or association actually exists in the source population. The probability of a type 2 error is often referred to using the Greek letter beta (β). Power is defined as $1 - \beta$, so a 20% likelihood of a type 2 error (that is, $\beta = 20\%$) corresponds to a power = 80%.

FIGURE 17-4 Sample Size Estimates for a Case-Control Study

Situation	Ratio of Controls to Cases	Anticipated Percentage of Controls Exposed	Anticipated Percentage of Cases Exposed	Odds Ratio (OR) Worth Detecting	Estimated Sample Size Required	Estimated Number of Cases Required	Estimated Number of Controls Required
Base case (Figure 17-3)	2	25%	33%	1.5	1050	350	700
1:1 ratio	1	25%	33%	1.5	950	475	475
10:1 ratio	10	25%	33%	1.5	2750	250	2500
Lower % exposed	2	10%	14%	1.5	2025	675	1350
Higher % exposed	2	30%	39%	1.5	976	325	650
Lower OR	2	25%	29%	1.2	5400	1800	3600
Higher OR	2	25%	40%	2.0	345	115	230

FIGURE 17-5 Power and Errors

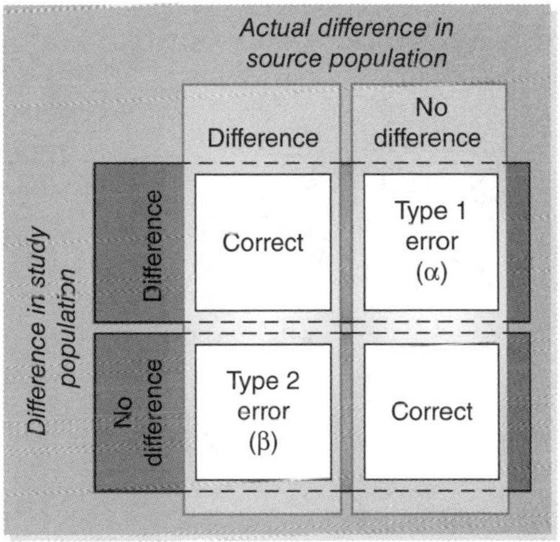

Examples of power estimation for various study approaches are shown in **Figure 17-6**. Like sample size estimates, power estimates require best guesses about the expected findings of the study. The standard expectation is that a study's analyses should have a power of 80% or greater. If the power estimates for a study are lower than desired, the easiest way to improve the power is to increase the sample size.

17.5 Refining the Study Approach

These sample size estimates refer to the study population (the actual number of participants) and not the sample population (the number of individuals invited to participate in the study). Because the participation rate is unlikely to be 100%, the sample population needs to be larger than the number suggested by sample size calculations in order to yield a study population of adequate size.

Be prepared to rethink the study approach if the power for the estimated number of available participants is not sufficient. For example, if a researcher expects to be able to recruit about 300 participants but the sample size estimates suggest that 870 participants will be required, then the intended study design will not work. In this situation, the study question, study approach, and/or the target and source populations must be modified. A new plan must be crafted that is suitable for the sample that the researcher can reasonably expect to recruit.

FIGURE 17-6 Examples of Power Calculation

Characteristic	Cross-Sectional Survey	Case-Control Study	Cohort Study	Experimental Study
Number of exposed	100	—	2500	70
Number of unexposed	250	—	1500	70
Number of cases	—	250	—	—
Number of controls	—	490	—	—
Percentage of exposed with disease or outcome	40%	—	13%	85.7%
Percentage of unexposed with disease or outcome	26%	—	9%	64.3%
Percentage of cases with exposure	—	32%	—	—
Percentage of controls with exposure	—	25.5%	—	—
Confidence level $(1 - \alpha)$	95%	95%	95%	95%
Estimated power $(1 - \beta)$	~70%	~45%	~97%	~80%

CHAPTER 18

QUESTIONNAIRE DEVELOPMENT

A questionnaire is a tool for systematically gathering information from study participants. Survey instruments can be designed for self-reporting or as scripts for interviews.

18.1 Questionnaire Design Overview

A **questionnaire** (or **survey instrument**) is a tool for systematically gathering information from study participants. A good questionnaire is carefully crafted for a specific purpose. Questionnaire design usually works best when it starts with the identification of the general and specific content to be covered by the survey instrument and then progresses to choosing the types of questions and answers for each topic to be assessed. In some situations, validated question banks are available and questions can be selected from them. Once a survey instrument is drafted, the wording of each question (and its associated response items, if applicable) should be checked carefully. The questions within each section and the sections themselves should be in logical order. The formatting of the document (or the computer file) should be visually appealing and easy to read. Prior to its use, the survey instrument should be pretested and revised as necessary (**Figure 18-1**). This chapter provides details about each of these steps in questionnaire development. The researcher should also consult specialty reference manuals for additional information about designing a valid and useful questionnaire for a particular study.

FIGURE 18-1 Questionnaire Design Plan

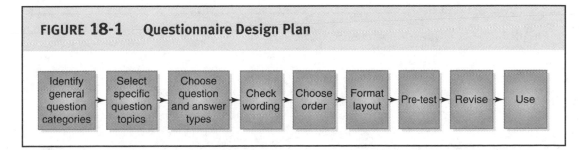

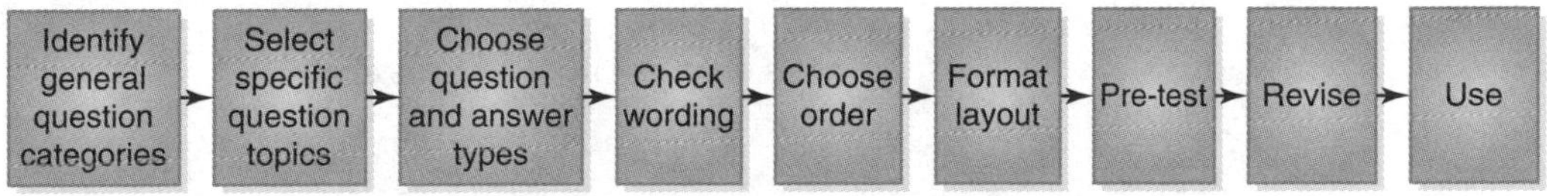

18.2 Questionnaire Content

The first step in designing a questionnaire is to list the topics that the survey instrument must cover. This list generally includes all of the exposure, disease, and population (demographic) areas that are the focus of the study question (**Figure 18-2**). The questionnaire may also include questions about factors that might influence the relationships between key exposures and outcomes; these factors are often called **potential confounders**. For example, adults who smoke tobacco products may be more likely than other adults to consume large volumes of alcohol. In a study of the relationship between smoking and liver disease, alcohol consumption could be a potential confounder. Because smokers are more likely than nonsmokers to drink, tobacco users may appear to be at a greater risk of liver disease than nonsmokers, even if the rate of liver disease is the same in smokers who drink as it is in nonsmokers who drink. Asking questions about both tobacco use and alcohol use enables the researcher to statistically adjust for different levels of alcohol use by smokers and nonsmokers and thus to more accurately examine the possible relationship between smoking and liver disease. A thorough search of the literature for studies on similar topics will help in identifying the range of question areas that should be included in the questionnaire.

It is often helpful to start with a list of the main categories of questions to be asked and then to add detail about the specific topics to be covered. For example, a survey of physical fitness might include sections on:

- Demographics
- Cardiorespiratory fitness
- Muscle strength
- Muscle endurance
- Flexibility
- Balance
- Body composition

These same categories could be used for a self-assessment tool or for a laboratory-based assessment tool. A survey about risk factors for breast cancer might have sections on:

- Sociodemographics (such as age, ethnicity, education level, and income)
- Family health history

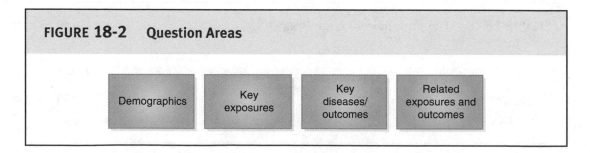

FIGURE 18-2 Question Areas

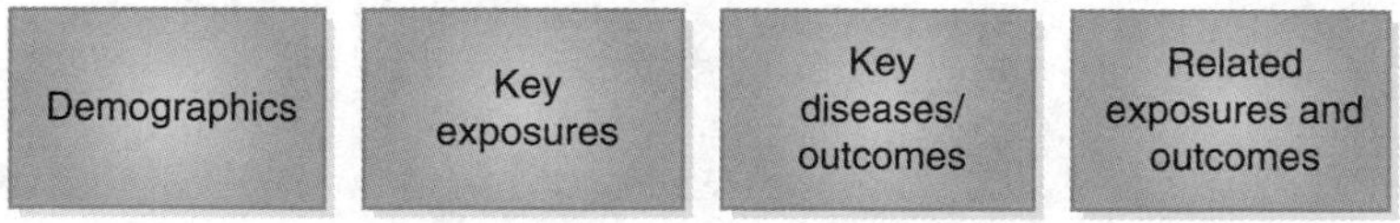

- Personal health history (such as previous diagnoses of benign breast diseases and the date of the last screening mammogram)
- Reproductive history (including questions about menstrual cycle characteristics, pregnancies, and use of hormones)
- Lifestyle factors (such as alcohol use, exercise history, and working night shifts)

The questionnaire must include questions confirming that participants meet the eligibility criteria for the study. For example, if only currently registered students are eligible to participate in a university-based cross-sectional survey, one of the first questions should be about school enrollment status. Participants who report that they are not students will be excluded from analysis based on their answer.

The questionnaire must also be able to accurately place participants into key categories. For example, in case-control studies, researchers need to ask questions that allow them to confirm that all cases meet the case definition and that all controls meet the control definition. Prospective cohort studies examining rates of incident disease require a series of questions about both exposure status and disease status. The answers to these questions must allow each participant to be classified as exposed or unexposed, and they must provide evidence that no participant had the disease of interest at the start of the observation period.

A final consideration is the length of the survey. A survey that is too short will miss potentially crucial information. A survey that is too long may yield a low response rate.

18.3 Types of Questions

After determining the broad categories of questions and the specific topics to be addressed in each section, the next step is to decide which types of questions are most appropriate. Each survey item should be assigned a specific question type, such as a date question or a yes/no question. Examples of various question types are shown in **Figure 18-3**. Decisions about the types of questions to ask must include considerations of which statistical tests the researcher wants to be able to run on the collected data. For example, the tests used with numeric data (such as *t*-tests, ANOVA, and linear regression) are different from the tests used with categorical data (such as Chi-square tests and logistic regression). Figure 27-2 provides additional information about variable types and statistical analysis. A consultation with a statistician early in the planning phase of a study can be invaluable for ensuring that the questionnaire and data analysis plan are strong and valid.

Closed-ended questions (alternatively called **close-ended questions**), which allow a limited number of possible answers, are usually easier to statistically analyze than **open-ended**, or **free response**, questions. The main limitation of closed-ended questions is that they may force respondents to select answers that do not truly express their status or opinions. Open-ended questions allow participants to explain their selections and qualify their responses, to give multiple answers, and to provide responses not anticipated by the researchers. However, open-ended questions take longer to ask and

FIGURE 18-3 **Examples of Types of Questions**

Type	Sample Question	Sample Response Option for the Sample Question
Date	What is your birth date?	__ __ - __ __ - __ __ __ __ m m - d d - y y y y
Numeric	What is your height without shoes (rounded to the nearest half inch)?	__ __ . __ inches
Yes/no	During your lifetime, have you smoked more than 100 cigarettes?	❑ Yes ❑ No
Categorical/ multiple-choice: nominal (no rank)	What is your sex?	❑ Female ❑ Male
	What is your favorite type of film?	❑ Action/drama ❑ Comedy/musical ❑ Documentary ❑ Other: ____________
Categorical/ multiple-choice: ordinal (ranked)	What is the highest level of education you have completed?	❑ Less than high school ❑ High school ❑ Some college but no degree ❑ College/university degree or advanced degree
	How much do you agree with this statement?: "No matter how much I exercise, I will not be able to lose weight."	❑ Strongly disagree ❑ Disagree ❑ Neutral ❑ Agree ❑ Strongly agree
	On a scale of 1 to 5, with 1 meaning poor and 5 meaning excellent, how would you rate your hearing (without the use of a hearing aid)?	Poor__________Excellent ❑ 1 ❑ 2 ❑ 3 ❑ 4 ❑ 5
Paired-comparisons	Do you prefer to drink coffee or tea?	❑ I prefer coffee ❑ I prefer tea ❑ I like coffee and tea equally ❑ I do not drink coffee or tea

FIGURE 18-3 (continued)

Type	Sample Question	Sample Response Option for the Sample Question
Rank-ordering	List the following four political issues in order from most important to you (1) to least important to you (4): crime/safety, environment/energy, foreign policy/defense, taxes/revenue	Number from 1 (most important) to 4 (least important): ___ Crime/safety ___ Environment/energy ___ Foreign policy/defense ___ Taxes/revenue
Open-ended/ free-response	What is your biggest personal health concern at present?	____________ ____________

answer, and they may result in irrelevant answers. Recoding free response answers into objective and meaningful categories for statistical analysis is often a time-consuming and imprecise process. Open-ended questions are often most useful when they are used to capture initial impressions or to clarify responses to closed-ended questions.

Closed-ended questions come in a variety of formats, including date and time variables (which can be used to calculate the length of time between events), numeric variables, and categorical variables. **Categorical** questions can have as few as two options (called **dichotomous** responses), like just having "yes" and "no" responses, or they can have dozens of possible answers. Categorical variables can also be ranked (**ordinal**) or unordered (**nominal**). Ordinal responses have an inherent order, and nominal responses do not have any built-in order. For example, a question about educational level is ordinal because some levels of education involve more years of school than other levels do. A question about occupational category is nominal because there is no obvious way to rank occupations as diverse as plumbing, farming, teaching, nursing, sales, and law. Less used question types include paired comparisons and rank-ordering questions.

18.4 Anonymity

For some study topics, researchers must ensure that the responses given by participants do not reveal their identities to researchers or to others who might access study materials. **Anonymity** protects participants and allows them to provide honest answers to sensitive questions. For example, clients of a community organization serving drug abusers should not be asked to complete a questionnaire about illegal activities if there is any risk that their identities could be ascertained from their questionnaire forms. Patients completing a satisfaction survey might not report genuine concerns about their physical therapists if they fear that their comments will allow their identities to be unmasked and their comments reported to their care providers. Community members sampled for participation in a telephone-based opinion survey might not feel comfortable expressing candid perspectives about health care policies when they are aware that an interviewer knows their telephone number and address and can therefore determine their name and identity.

Many questions can be asked in more than one valid way. The researcher must decide which question type and which level of precision for responses is most appropriate for the study goal and the study population. For example, participants' ages can be ascertained in a number of ways. One is by asking for the date of birth and calculating the number of years between the birthdate and the interview or survey date. However, asking for such specific personal information may raise concerns about anonymity because birthdates could be personal identifiers in a small population. Additionally, the fear of providing that individually identifying information may mean that many participants will skip the question entirely. Some may even drop out of the study rather than provide a birthdate. To protect participants and reduce fears about privacy, the researcher could ask for each participant's current age in years rather than asking for a birthdate. Even then, age in years could reveal the identity of some individuals in the study population. In surveys of residential college students, for example, most participants will fall into a fairly narrow age range, and much younger or older students will stand out. In such situations, it might be best simply to ask participants to indicate which age range they belong to (such as ≤ 20 years or ≥ 21 years).

Similar decisions must be made about each component of the questionnaire that could allow for the ascertainment of the identities of participants in a survey intended to be anonymous. If participants could be harmed by being identified as a member of a study population or by having their responses linked to their identities, or if identifiability might limit the truthfulness of survey responses, then there must be a solid plan in place for protecting the privacy of all participants and the confidentiality of the information they share.

18.5 Types of Responses

Once the types of questions have been selected, a decision must be made about the kinds of responses that are appropriate for each question.

- For numeric responses, the question should state exactly how specific the answers should be. Should height be reported to the nearest inch, to the nearest half-inch, or to the nearest centimeter? Should height be reported in feet and inches (like "5 feet 6 inches"), or should it be reported only in total inches (as "66 inches")?
- For categorical questions, the response categories should be listed. Sometimes an "Other" category should be included so that respondents can fill in their own answers if none of the listed responses is applicable. Consider all possible responses for each question, and include as many items as needed.

- For ranked questions, decisions must be made about how many entries to include on the scale and whether there will be a neutral option. Most scales with a neutral option list 5 to 7 categories; most scales without a neutral option list 4 or 6 categories. (These are sometimes called **Likert items** or **Likert scales**.) Sample response scales are shown in **Figure 18-4**.

For self-report surveys, a decision must also be made about whether to add a category for "not applicable" or "I do not know." For questionnaires to be used as scripts, a "refused to answer" category is needed. Other examples of these types of alternate responses are "no opinion," "not sure," "hard to say," "no answer," "I prefer not to answer," "I do not understand," and "I forget."

Some questions must be answered by all participants because they are essential for determining eligibility for the study. For example, all participants in a study comparing adults with and without tattoos must answer a question about their tattoo history. Most people can answer that question very easily, so an "I do not know" response is not required. Anyone who skips that question when completing the survey form will be deemed ineligible for inclusion in the analysis.

However, for a question like "When was the last time you had your blood sugar levels tested?" it may be important to know whether the respondent is uncertain about the answer. That uncertainty might be considered a valid and interesting response. Neglecting to list "I do not know" as a possible response would force many people to choose an answer they were not sure about. This might hide important information. It might also lead to systematic inaccuracies in the data. For example, information bias may occur if participants who do not know the answer to a question systematically default to providing the answer they assume the researcher wants to hear.

FIGURE 18-4 Examples of Five-Point Responses for Ranked Questions

Strongly disagree	Disagree	Neutral	Agree	Strongly agree
Dissatisfied	Somewhat dissatisfied	Neutral	Somewhat satisfied	Satisfied
Very negative	Somewhat negative	Neither negative nor positive	Somewhat positive	Very positive
Poor	Fair	Good	Very good	Excellent
None	Few	Some	Many	Very many
Never	Rarely	Sometimes	Often	Always
Not important	Slightly important	Somewhat important	Very important	Extremely important

18.6 Wording of Questions

After drafting the questionnaire, check each question for clarity.

- Does each question ask what it is intended to ask?
- Is the language of each question clear and neutral?
- Will members of the study population understand the language?
- Do questions about sensitive topics use language acceptable to the source population?

Also check to be sure that the responses are carefully worded.

- Are the response options clearly presented?
- For scaled questions, is the rank order clear? (For example, is it obvious that 1 is "strongly disagree" and 5 is "strongly agree"? Or, alternatively, that 1 is "excellent" and 7 is "poor"?)
- For questions with unranked categories, is the order of possible responses alphabetical or otherwise neutral?

Figure 18-5 lists examples of questionnaire problems that should be avoided, including problems related to language, content, and response items.

18.7 Order of Questions

Many questionnaires start with easy or at least general questions before moving to more difficult or sensitive questions. The questions should be in an order that flows naturally from one topic to another, and similar questions should be grouped. Sometimes similar questions with similar response types can be best asked consecutively. Other times, it is better to mix up such questions to prevent habituation. **Habituation** occurs when respondents have given the same answer to so many questions in a row ("agree... agree... agree...") that they continue to reply with the same response, even one that does not reflect their true perspectives, because that response has become routine. Think carefully about how previous questions could taint the answers to later ones. For example, once a participant has considered a variety of opinions about a topic, he or she can no longer provide an unbiased first impression. Thus, the researcher may want to order questions about impressions this way:

- First, an open-ended question to garner a first impression from participants: "What do you do most often when _____?"
- Second, a series of yes/no questions to clarify beliefs, perceptions, and practices: "Do you ever _____?"
- Last, a concluding, open-ended question to allow participants to express final impressions: "Now that you have considered the possibilities, what would you say you do most often when _____?"

FIGURE 18-5 Problems to Avoid

Problem	Example	Problem with the Example
Big words/ jargon	Have you ever had a myocardial infarction?	Participants may not know that a "myocardial infarction" is a technical term for a heart attack.
Undefined abbreviations	Have you ever been told that you have BPH?	Participants may not know that BPH is short for benign prostatic hypertrophy or that BPH means an enlarged prostate.
Ambiguous meanings	What kind of house do you live in?	Without seeing a list of appropriate responses, it is not clear if the answer should be "an apartment," "a rental," "a split-level duplex," or "a single-family home."
Vagueness	Do you exercise regularly?	"Regularly" is not defined. A person who exercises most days of each week might assume that "regularly" means daily and say "no." Another person who exercises once a month may consider that regular. It would be better to ask "In a typical week, how many days do you exercise for at least 30 minutes?"
Double negatives	I did not find this visit with my doctor to be unpleasant. ❑ Disagree ❑ Neutral ❑ Agree	The wording of this question makes it hard to figure out whether a person who was satisfied with a visit should agree or disagree.
Faulty assumptions	Do your gums bleed during regular dental cleanings? ❑ Yes ❑ No	The question assumes that everyone has routine dental cleanings. If "I do not visit the dentist" is not an answer option, a person who does not have dental cleanings is forced to answer no.

FIGURE 18-5 Problems to Avoid (continued)

Problem	Example	Problem with the Example
Two-in-one	Do you exercise at least 3 times a week and eat a healthy diet? ❑ Yes ❑ No	Combines two separate questions: one for exercise and one for diet.
Impossible to recall accurately	How many servings of carrots did you eat most weeks when you were a child?	Adults will not be able to remember this level of detail about their childhood diets.
Too much detail	List any prescription medications you have taken for 1 month or longer in the past 10 years.	Unless the respondent has had very few prescriptions, answering this question is impossible without looking up medical records.
Sensitive questions	Have you ever hit, scratched, bruised, or otherwise physically injured an intimate partner?	This question is unlikely to be answered truthfully if the response should be yes,and it may raise concerns about confidentiality and potential legal requirements for reporting abuse.
Hypothetical questions	Have you ever thought that you would like to lose 10 or more pounds?	Anyone could have felt this at some point in time, but the question does not clarify whether this is a long-term longing or a thought that crossed the respondent's mind for the first time upon reading the question.
Leading questions	What is your impression of the quality of work done by the dedicated public servants who work at the county health department?	This question clearly intends to lead respondents toward a positive answer (and may unintentionally have the opposite effect).

FIGURE 18-5 (continued)

Problem	Example	Problem with the Example
Leading answers	What is your impression about the quality of services provided by Center City Hospital? ❑ Fair ❑ Good ❑ Great ❑ Excellent	This question's response options clearly are intended to lead to a positive response; there is no "poor" option.
Answers with a poor scale	How many hours a week do you watch television? ❑ 0 ❑ 1–3 ❑ 4–7 ❑ 8 or more	Even though most people watch more than 1 hour of television daily, which would put them in the "8 or more" response category, they may not want to choose an "extreme" answer. Their inaccurate responses will lead to a false report. Alternatively, these response options may cause respondents to misread the question as how many hours a *day* they watch television.
Lack of specificity	What is your income?	It is not clear if income refers to earnings per hour, week, month, or year, or whether it refers to pre- or post-tax income.
Missing answer options	What color are your eyes? ❑ Brown ❑ Blue	Many possible eye colors are missing.
Overlapping answer options	In a typical week, how many days do you eat fish? ❑ 0 ❑ 1–3 ❑ 3–5 ❑ 5–7	Participants who eat fish 3 days a week or 5 days a week will not know which response to select.

18.8 Layout and Formatting

The next step in questionnaire design is formatting the document so that it is organized, easy to read, and easy to record answers on. The layout of the survey instrument will vary depending on the mechanism of data collection used.

For a written survey (sometimes called a paper-and-pencil survey) that respondents complete on their own, the answer sheet should clearly indicate where and how responses should be marked (**Figure 18-6**). Use a readable and large font. **White space** (blank areas) on the page is helpful for separating sections and making the page visually appealing. If necessary, very clear instructions for **skips** should direct interviewers or respondents to jump over sets of non-applicable questions. A cover letter or list of instructions should tell respondents how to record their answers, such as:

- "Select the one answer that best describes you."
- "Fill in the oval in front of your answer completely using blue or black ink."
- "Circle all options that apply to you."
- "Write your answer in block capital letters, as shown in the example below."
- "If you answered 'NO' to Question 4, then skip to Question 8. If you answered 'YES' to Question 4, then please answer Questions 5, 6, and 7 before moving on to Question 8."

An Internet-based or computer-based survey has the benefit of allowing the researcher to build skips into the program so that irrelevant questions do not even

FIGURE 18-6 Example of a Self-Response Questionnaire

Basic Information

1. What is today's date?	__ __ - __ __ - __ __ __ __ m m d d y y y y		
2. What is your date of birth?	__ __ - __ __ - __ __ __ __ m m d d y y y y		
3. What is your sex?	☐ Female	☐ Male	☐ ______

Health History (*Check one answer box for each question.*)

4. Have you ever been diagnosed with breast cancer?	☐ Yes	☐ No	→ *If **No**, then skip to Question 8.*
5. Have you had a mastectomy (either partial or complete)?	☐ Yes	☐ No	

appear on the screen. Questions can be presented over several webpages, and this design strategy can be used to force participants to provide an answer to one or more questions before the next set of questions is revealed. However, making some fields required may create problems. Required fields force a person who does not want to provide an answer to one required question to quit the survey and leave all subsequent items unanswered. As with paper-based surveys, attention must be paid to layout, font, color, and spacing.

When survey data are collected though interviews (**Figure 18-7**), the interviewer reads the questions aloud and records the respondent's spoken answers. In addition to the questions, the script must include an opening statement, transitions between sections of the survey, and closing sentences. The questionnaire must clearly indicate the sections to be read aloud, the procedures for recording responses on paper or in a computer file, and other instructions.

After formatting, survey documents should be carefully checked for grammatical errors, misspellings, missing questions, gaps in logic, unclear instructions, formatting errors, and other organizational issues. If the questionnaire appears to be too long, it may be helpful to identify less-important questions and remove them.

18.9 Reliability and Validity

A reliable and valid questionnaire (or other assessment tool) measures what it was intended to measure in the population being assessed. **Reliability** (or **precision**) is

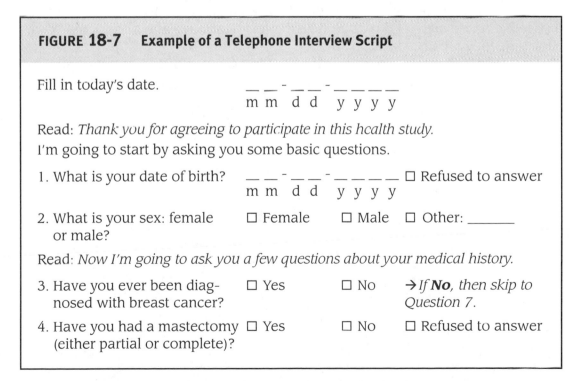

FIGURE 18-7 Example of a Telephone Interview Script

Fill in today's date. __ __ - __ __ - __ __ __ __
mm dd yyyy

Read: *Thank you for agreeing to participate in this health study.*
I'm going to start by asking you some basic questions.

1. What is your date of birth?	__ __ - __ __ - __ __ __ __ (mm dd yyyy)		☐ Refused to answer
2. What is your sex: female or male?	☐ Female	☐ Male	☐ Other: ______

Read: *Now I'm going to ask you a few questions about your medical history.*

3. Have you ever been diagnosed with breast cancer?	☐ Yes	☐ No	→ *If* ***No****, then skip to Question 7.*
4. Have you had a mastectomy (either partial or complete)?	☐ Yes	☐ No	☐ Refused to answer

demonstrated when consistent answers are given to similar questions and when an assessment yields the same outcome when repeated several times. **Validity** (or **accuracy**) is established when the responses or measurements are shown to be correct. **Figure 18-8** illustrates the differences between these concepts. A dart-thrower who hits the same spot on a target consistently is reliable, but if that cluster is not centered at the bull's-eye then the thrower lacks accuracy.

One aspect of reliability is **internal consistency**. Some survey instruments ask the same question several different ways, or ask a series of similar questions, in order to confirm the stability of participants' responses. For example, a questionnaire might include two questions that are opposites of one another, like "I enjoy eating most fruits" and "In general, I do not like to eat fruit." The expectation is that all respondents who say the first item is true will say that the second item is false, and vice versa. If a very high proportion of respondents' answers meet this expectation, then that is evidence that the responses are reliable. Internal consistency in a data set can be confirmed with tests of **intercorrelation** that assess whether two or more related items in a survey instrument measure various aspects of the same concept. **Cronbach's alpha** and the **Kuder-Richardson Formula 20 (KR-20)** are both measures of internal consistency among questionnaire items. Both of these metrics are expressed as a number between 0 and 1, and scores near 1 indicate an assessment tool with minimal random error and high reliability. (Tests of intercorrelation used to examine the reliability of survey instruments are not the same as tests of correlation that compare two or more independent variables.) Another facet of reliability is **test-retest reliability**, which is demonstrated when people who take a baseline assessment and then re-take the test later have about the same scores each time they are tested.

Several approaches are used to evaluate the accuracy of assessment tools that rely on self-reporting, such as psychometric tests and surveys about attitudes and

FIGURE 18-8 Reliability and Validity

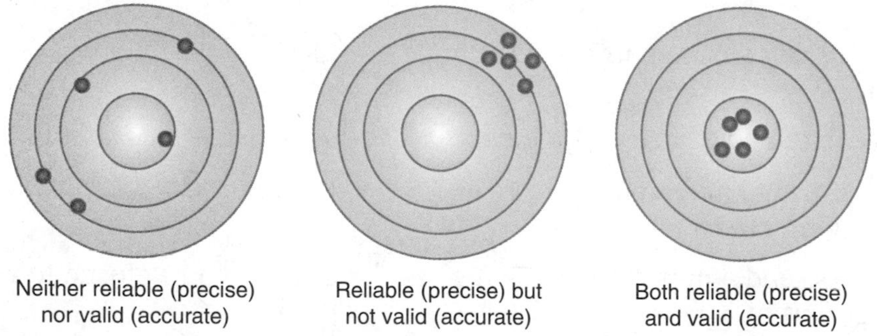

perceptions. These tools are often considered to be proxy measures for an underlying theoretical construct that cannot be directly measured. For example, happiness and intelligence cannot be directly measured with physical or chemical tests, but survey instruments can be designed to measure them indirectly. Some researchers use the word **concept** to describe theories informed by observations and use the term **construct** to describe theories informed from more complex abstractions. For example, there is no particular threshold at which an object becomes "heavy" or a person becomes "rich," because those definitions will vary for different individuals, but measurements of weight and income can guide the evaluation of these concepts. In contrast, notions like "trust" and "leadership" are more difficult to quantify. Other researchers consider a concept to be a general abstraction and a construct to be a multidimensional concept that has been carefully defined and crafted for research purposes. In practice, the terms concept and construct are often used interchangeably.

Content validity, sometimes called **logical validity**, is present when subject matter experts agree that a set of survey items captures the most relevant information about the study domain. Content validity requires consideration of the technical quality of the survey items as well as their representativeness of all the dimensions of the theoretical construct being measured by the survey instrument. Some statistical methods, such as **principal component analysis (PCA)**, can provide information about which items in an assessment tool might be redundant or unnecessary and can be removed. **Face validity** is present when content experts and users agree that a survey instrument will be easy for study participants to understand and correctly complete.

Construct validity is present when a test (such as a set of questions in a survey instrument) measures the theoretical construct the test is intended to assess. Construct validity requires the development of an explicit theoretical construct and a rigorous examination of how well an assessment tool represents that construct. Ideally, empirical tests can be used as part of the examination of construct validity. **Factor analysis**, structural equation modeling, and various measures of correlation are often used for this process of identifying interrelationships among variables measuring different aspects of the same theme. **Convergent validity** is present when two indicators that the underlying theory says should be related are shown to be correlated. **Discriminant validity** is present when two indicators that the construct says should not be related are shown not to be associated.

Criterion validity, sometimes called **concrete validity**, uses an established test as a standard (or criterion) for validating a new test that examines a similar theoretical construct. For example, a new test of intelligence can be validated against standard IQ tests, and a shorter version of a widely used assessment tool can be validated against the longer original version. There are two main approaches to examining criterion validity. **Concurrent validity** is evaluated when participants in a pilot study complete both the existing and new tests and the correlation between the test results is calculated. **Predictive validity** is appraised when the new test is correlated with subsequent measures of performance in related domains. Suppose researchers create a new test intended to predict success in medical school. Concurrent validity could be demonstrated by comparing scores on the new test with scores on the MCAT, which is the current standard test for medical college admission in the United States. Predictive validity could be demonstrated by administering the test to incoming medical students and comparing their results on the new test with their performance on the initial licensing exam (USMLE Step 1) taken 2 years later.

18.10 Commercial Research Tools

One way to improve validity is to include survey questions or modules that are identical to the ones used in previous research projects. Unfortunately, access to survey questions is often not possible in the health sciences. Copies of questionnaires from some disciplines are almost never included in published papers and are only rarely posted on researchers' websites. As a result, new research projects usually require the development and testing of a completely new survey instrument. However, several widely used and validated tests are available to researchers, such as:

- The Beck Depression Inventory and the General Health Questionnaire (GHQ), which assesses psychological status
- The Mini-Mental State Examination (MMSE), which evaluates cognitive function
- The SF-36 and SF-12, which both measure health-related quality of life **(HRQOL)**

The Buros Institute's *Mental Measurements Yearbook* provides reviews of thousands of available tools used in psychological and educational assessment. Some of these tools are free of charge, but most are commercial products that require payment for use. For some instruments provided at no charge, researchers must pay to have the results scored and validated against previous users of the survey instrument.

18.11 Translation

Translation of the survey instrument into one or more additional languages may be necessary if the source population contains speakers of more than one language. (Translation may also be required when an ethics review committee requires materials to be presented in the committee's preferred language as well as in the language of the sample population.) Researchers using multiple languages must be certain that the translated version expresses the same meaning as the original survey. Accuracy may require the rephrasing of whole sentences, not just direct word-for-word translations.

One way to ensure that the correct meaning is being conveyed is to use **back translation**, or **double translation**. One person translates the questionnaire from the original language to a new language; a second person then translates the survey instrument in the new language back into the original language. A comparison of the original version of the survey with the back-translated version will reveal where the second-language translation does not match the intended meaning of the original version. A second approach is to have two translators independently translate the survey instrument from the original to the new language. Then the two translations are compared to see which words and phrases best convey the precise meaning and complexity of the original questionnaire.

18.12 Pilot Testing

A **pilot test**, or **pretest**, of the questionnaire is helpful for checking, among other issues:

- The wording and clarity of the questions
- The order of the questions
- The ability and willingness of participants to answer the questions
- The responses given, and whether the responses match the intended types of responses
- The amount of time it takes to complete the survey

The researcher should ask several volunteers to help with the pilot test. These volunteers should be from the target population and meet the eligibility criteria for the study (in terms of age, disease status, and/or other key factors), but they should not be members of the sample population. They should be asked to complete the preliminary survey and then provide feedback about content, clarity, layout, timing, and other factors. Feedback may be provided individually or as part of a focus group. The survey instrument should be revised based on these observations. Several rounds of pilot testing may be required to develop a sound survey instrument.

CHAPTER 19

Surveys and Interviews

Most primary studies collect data from individual participants using an interview method or a self-administered questionnaire. Self-reported surveys are usually the least costly and least time-consuming way to gather information. However, interviews may allow for more detailed information to be gathered and can be accompanied by laboratory and other tests.

19.1 Interviews Versus Self-Administered Surveys

The first decision to make about data collection is whether to have a member of the research team interview participants or to have participants record their own answers (**Figure 19-1**). **Interviews** may be conducted in person or via telephone. A key advantage of using interviews to gather data is that trained interviewers record the responses, and they can ensure the accuracy and completeness of each questionnaire. A major benefit of **self-administered surveys** is that it allows for the cost-effective collection of data from a large number of

FIGURE 19-1 Examples of Methods for Collecting Data

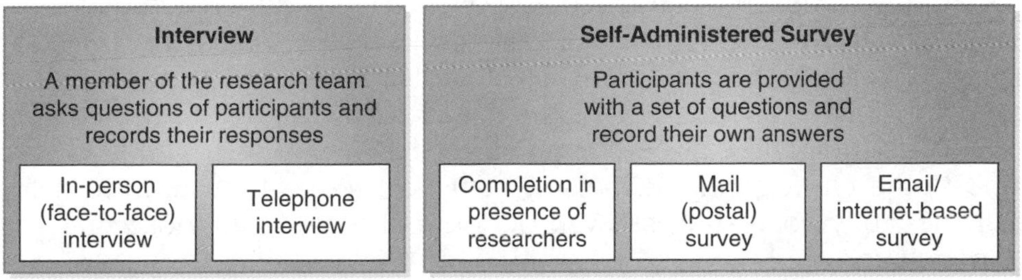
Interview
A member of the research team asks questions of participants and records their responses
In-person (face-to-face) interview
Telephone interview
Self-Administered Survey
Participants are provided with a set of questions and record their own answers
Completion in presence of researchers
Mail (postal) survey
Email/ internet-based survey

participants. Self-administered surveys may also be the best way to get honest answers to sensitive questions. Self-administered questionnaires can be completed at a specific study site, such as a workplace or school or hospital, or they can be delivered by mail or the Internet.

The most important considerations when deciding which approach to use are the goals of the study and the expectations of the sample population members. Additional considerations are cost, time, and potential barriers to participation. For example, in terms of financial and time costs:

- Interviews may require major time commitments from study personnel.
- Mailed surveys incur direct costs related to photocopying, postage, and data entry.
- Internet-based surveys may have relatively low costs if a free or low-cost survey-hosting website is used.

In estimating the cost per participant, consider the likely participation rate. Mailing out 10 surveys may be necessary to receive one completed questionnaire, and the budget and sample size estimates should reflect this expectation.

Time is another consideration. Asking participants to complete their self-administered questionnaires at the same place and time can generate a lot of data quickly. For example, a school-based survey could gather data from hundreds of students during one 20-minute period. One-on-one interviews may take a considerable amount of time per participant, and it may take months to schedule all of the needed interviews. Mail surveys may trickle in over an extended period of time and make it challenging for a researcher to know when to stop waiting for additional responses to arrive.

The barriers to participation also vary according to the data collection method. Transportation to the interview site may be difficult for some interviewees. Discomfort with the telephone or computer may be a challenge for others.

19.2 Recruiting Methods

Once a data collection method has been selected, the next step is to decide on an effective method for recruiting members of the sample population to be participants in the study. The goal of recruiting is to maximize the participation rate among members of the sample population so as to yield a study population that is reasonably representative of the source population. Ideally, the researcher should try to find a way to compare the characteristics of participants to the demographics of the source population as a whole. For example, in a school-based study the proportion of participants by grade can be compared to the overall distribution of students by grade in the participating schools. A statistical test can be used to determine whether the study population skewed old or young or was a close match to the source population.

The best method for initiating contact with potential participants is often related to the intended data collection method (**Figure 19-2**).

- If the plan is to interview people in person, the best recruiting method may be to visit potential recruits at work, at school, at home, at a public venue, or at another appropriate location. Alternatively, if the contact information for sampled individuals is available, which would be true if recruiting patients from a collaborating clinic or recruiting employees from a cooperating corporation, then interviews could be set up by sending a letter or an email of invitation and then following up with calls to all of the sampled individuals.
- If the plan is to interview by telephone, it may be possible to recruit some participants with cold calls. However, the participation rate will likely be higher if a letter of invitation is sent first. Sending a letter will also allow for the acquisition of signed informed consent forms prior to the interview, if they are required.
- If the plan is to collect data via the Internet, then contacting potential participants via email or a website may be the most effective method.

FIGURE 19-2 Examples of Methods for Contacting Members of the Sample Population

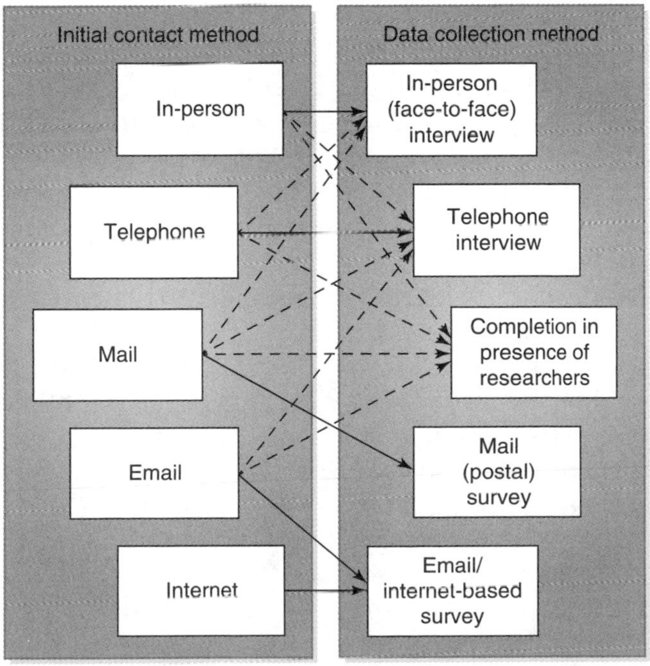

Participation rates will likely be higher if recruits understand the importance and value of the research project. For example, suppose that the plan is to interview members of a selected organization by phone. The response rate is likely to be highest if interviewers start each phone conversation with potential participants by explaining why the participants are being contacted, how their contact information was acquired, and how completing an interview will assist the organization. The participation rate may be quite high, even for unscheduled telephone calls, because the importance and relevance of the study are addressed at the start of the call. Support for the study may be even higher if the study plans are shared ahead of time in an organizational newsletter or via an email to all members.

In contrast, only a few out of every hundred calls made by **random-digit dialing**—calls to a computer-generated list of unscreened telephone numbers—may yield one person willing to participate in a survey. Even then, many willing participants may turn out to be ineligible for the study. Additionally, a growing problem with using random-digit dialing is that mobile phone numbers are often unlisted and are not necessarily indicative of the user's geographic location. These issues may further reduce the representativeness of study populations recruited by random-digit dialing. Nevertheless, using the first minute of a phone call to explain why a particular study will make a difference in the world or to a particular community may increase the willingness of randomly dialed individuals to participate.

Other ways to increase the participation rate are to provide multiple invitations and opportunities to participate and to make participation as easy as possible. Mailed survey packets should include a concise cover letter that explains the purpose and importance of the survey and discloses any necessary information such as financial sponsorship and contact information for the research team. The mailed packet should also include the survey instrument and a preaddressed stamped envelope so that the completed survey can easily be returned to the researcher. A few weeks after the initial mailing, a reminder postcard or a second copy of the questionnaire should be sent to those who have not yet responded. The follow-up mailing should reaffirm the study's importance and express gratitude to those who have already returned a completed survey as well as those who intend to do so. Similarly, multiple phone calls on different days of the week and at different times of the day may have to be made to reach potential participants by telephone. Multiple email invitations to complete a computer-based survey may be required to get recruits to fill out an online questionnaire. Including a step-by-step guide for using the survey website may make participation more accessible to those who are willing to participate but uncomfortable with new technologies.

Incentives such as small gifts or the opportunity to be entered into a drawing to win a prize may be an effective means of encouraging participation among those invited to be in the study. Any inducements, gifts, or compensation must be approved by an ethics review committee prior to being offered.

19.3 Data Recording Methods

A decision must also be made about how responses will be recorded and when they will be entered into a computer database. There are two basic options (**Figure 19-3**). One is to record the responses on paper and to enter or scan them into a computer database later. The other is to have interviewers or participants enter responses directly into a database.

Paper questionnaires have several benefits. In some environments, they are required for the collection of data from a large number of participants at one time, as would be the situation when all students attending a school are asked to complete a questionnaire during the same 20-minute period. Paper instruments allow for the easy collection of signatures on informed consent statements, and some researchers value having paper records as a backup to electronic files. But paper-based surveys have a serious disadvantage: Unless somewhat expensive optical scan forms are used, all responses have to be manually entered into a computer at a later time. Data entry is often a very time-consuming process, and that can become costly.

The major advantage of computer-assisted surveys is that they eliminate the need for later data entry. They may also simplify the questionnaire by automatically removing any questions not relevant to a particular study participant. For example, they may skip questions specific to females for participants who identify themselves as being male. The main limitation of computer-assisted surveys is that some populations are uncomfortable with computer technology. Discomfort with technology may be expressed in several ways. Older adults who have limited access to the Internet or do not routinely use computers may systematically choose not to participate

FIGURE 19-3 Methods for Collecting and Recording Survey Data

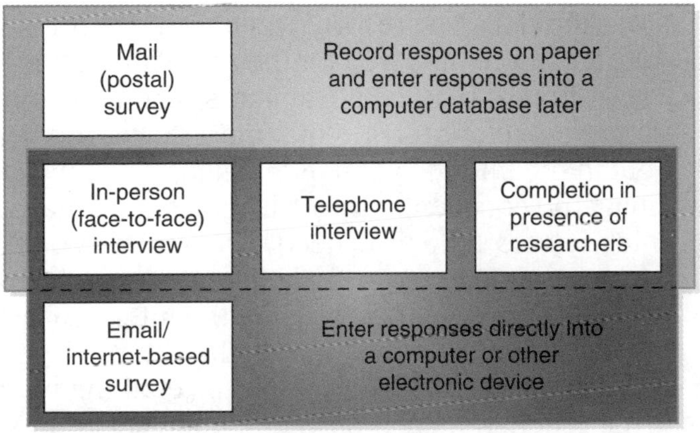
Mail (postal) survey
Record responses on paper and enter responses into a computer database later
In-person (face-to-face) interview
Telephone interview
Completion in presence of researchers
Email/ internet-based survey
Enter responses directly into a computer or other electronic device

in an Internet-based survey. Some interviewees will be distracted by an interviewer entering responses into a computer as they give their responses. These individuals might not be similarly bothered by an interviewer with a clipboard who is jotting down their comments on a piece of paper. Additionally, having a limited number of computer terminals or portable electronic devices available for participant use may become a barrier to project success. For example, suppose that health fair attendees are being asked to complete an exit survey using handheld computers. Most people in the process of leaving a venue will not choose to wait 15 or more minutes for a tablet computer to become available to them (unless there is a very desirable reward for participation). The participation rate may be very low, and the study population may not be representative of health fair attendees as a whole because only the most patient people will be have recorded their answers.

19.4 Training Interviewers

The interview process should be the same for all participants in a study. Uniformity is easiest to accomplish when all interviewers are provided with the tools they need to follow a standardized set of procedures. All interviewers should undergo role-specific training and have an opportunity to practice their interview skills. Each interviewer should be given a comprehensive interviewer handbook that provides information about the purpose of the study, details about interview logistics, an annotated script for the in-person or electronic interview, and annotated copies of all study forms. The training and handbook should:

- Explain the interview process step-by-step
- Specify exactly how to ask questions and record responses
- Identify any prompts or follow-up questions that the interviewer must use or is allowed to use
- Emphasize any restrictions against asking for clarification about particular items
- Provide checklists for handling problems that might arise during an interview, such as interruptions

All of this information should also be recorded in the study protocol.

Interviewers usually feel more prepared for their role after attending one or more training sessions. Facilitators often begin training sessions by explaining the purpose of the research project, emphasizing the importance of strictly following the procedures spelled out in the interviewer handbook, and making clear the absolute necessity of maintaining the confidentiality of all information that study participants share with them. Interviewers may also need to complete additional institution-mandated research ethics training sessions. The remainder of the training session is usually dedicated to understanding and practicing the interview process.

The questionnaire should be examined in detail so that all interviewers understand what each question is asking, how to pronounce all the words in each question, how to phrase the reading of each question, and how to present the possible answers for questions that are not open-ended. All paper response forms and/or computer-assisted data entry programs should be closely examined so that every interviewer understands exactly how to record participant responses.

Each interviewer should have the opportunity to participate in several mock interviews from start to finish, including the informed consent process. Clear guidelines and lots of practice will help to create skilled, confident, and reliable interviewers (**Figure 19-4**). Well-trained interviewers will know how to make participants comfortable, how not to intentionally or unintentionally guide participants toward particular answers rather than letting participants provide candid responses, and how to complete all survey forms consistently and completely.

FIGURE 19-4 Characteristics of Well-Trained Interviewers

Characteristic	Actions That Demonstrate the Characteristic
Respectful	• Communicates pleasantly and professionally with all study participants and members of the research team • Has practiced interviewing enough to be comfortable with both the script and the interview process • Asks supervisors for assistance when it is needed
Organized	• Begins each scheduled interview session on time • Has all necessary materials on hand prior to the start of each interview session • Maintains meticulous records and completes all files and paperwork promptly
Considerate	• Dresses and grooms appropriately for in-person interviews • Is alert to modifiable conditions that may make interviewees uncomfortable, such as loud background noises or dim lighting • Allows adequate time for participants to respond to each question
Articulate	• Speaks at an appropriate pace and volume • Enunciates clearly • Uses an appropriate tone of voice (and, for in-person interviews, appropriate facial expressions and gestures) • Rereads questions and/or the list of closed-ended responses when a participant does not understand the question or the acceptable responses

FIGURE 19-4 Characteristics of Well-Trained Interviewers (continued)

Characteristic	Actions That Demonstrate the Characteristic
Consistent	• Reads the script exactly as it is written • Probes for answers only when the script indicates that probing is approved • Does not provide explanations for any question unless an explanation is provided in the script or approved in the interviewer handbook
Impartial	• Avoids verbal and nonverbal expressions of approval or disapproval • Does not express personal opinions • Avoids leading interviewees toward a particular answer (for example, by placing special emphasis on particular words in a question or by probing until receiving a particular desired response)
Honest	• Does not fabricate or falsify reports • Records responses to open-ended questions verbatim, without rephrasing, paraphrasing, "correcting," or interpreting them
Careful	• Completes all steps of the interview process in the correct order, as prescribed by the interviewer handbook • Documents informed consent prior to conducting an interview • Does not skip any component of the interview • Completes all response forms correctly

CHAPTER 20

Additional Assessments

Surveys and interviews are the most common sources of health data, but other measurements are often important supplements to self-reported information.

20.1 Supplementing Self-Reported Information

Self-reports, such as those made during interviews and the completion of questionnaires, are essential data sources, but they have significant limitations. Respondents may not tell the truth, either because they do not accurately remember the answers or because they want to provide "correct" answers. Also, they may not know some of their health measures, such as their current weight or blood pressure. Laboratory tests and other objective measures can be used to supplement and validate self-reported data and to quantify attributes that require independent assessment. This information is usually collected in person by a member of the research team. This chapter presents some of these additional types of data along with examples of the ethical considerations associated with them.

20.2 Anthropometric Measures

Anthropometry is the measurement of the human body, and anthropometric measurements are often important in health research, especially in studies of nutritional status. Some of the most common body measurements are:

- Height (stature)
- Weight
- Waist circumference
- Hip circumference
- Mid-upper-arm circumference (MUAC)
- Skinfold measurements that estimate the body fat percentage

Standard methods should be used to take all anthropometric measurements. Any tools used for the measurements should be carefully calibrated to ensure accuracy and reliability.

The individuals taking the measurements should be trained to use all equipment properly and to record results to the appropriate level of precision. They should also ensure privacy for participants while the measurements are being taken, such as by conducting assessments in a designated examination room or behind a screen or room divider. It is often best for two members of the research team to be present when measurements are being taken. When a child is being measured, it may be necessary for a parent or guardian to be present with the child. Research ethics committees may be able to offer guidance on legal and safety requirements related to physical examinations.

20.3 Vital Signs

Basic **vital signs** are physiological measurements that can be quantified accurately after minimal instruction. These include:

- Body temperature
- Blood pressure
- Pulse (heart rate)
- Respiratory rate (breathing frequency)

A thermometer is used to measure body temperature. A manual or electronic sphygmomanometer (a blood pressure cuff) is used to measure systolic and diastolic blood pressure. Resting pulse and respiratory rate do not require any instruments other than timekeeping devices.

All assessors should be trained to use the same techniques. For example, guidelines for measuring blood pressure should specify the appropriate sitting position or other posture for the person being assessed as well as the way the back and arm should be supported, perhaps by resting the arm on a surface. The measurement protocol should spell out the instructions that should be given to the participant about removing clothing from the arm, sitting back in the chair and putting his or her feet on the floor without crossing the legs, and not talking or moving during the measurement of the blood pressure. The research handbook should also state whether blood pressure should be measured in a particular arm or both arms as well as indicating whether the blood pressure should be measured once or several times. Deviation from any of these procedures may cause a recorded blood pressure to be higher or lower than it would be if the protocol had been followed. Standardization increases the precision and validity of the measurements. Additionally, tests of inter-rater reliability can be used to confirm that all assessors generate similar or identical results when they measure the same person.

20.4 Clinical Examination

A well-trained clinician can make accurate and reliable assessments of many health states that machines are unable to assess well. For example, a clinician can examine:

- Heart sounds
- Breath sounds and other respiratory functions

- Bowel sounds and the condition of the abdomen
- The range of motion (ROM) and the condition of the joints
- The condition of the skin, hair, and nails
- The health of the eyes, ears, nose, and mouth
- Mental status
- The ability to conduct activities of daily living
- Other signs of health or disease

When a clinical examination is part of the data collection process, an assessment form should carefully describe each component of the examination, including the exact procedures to be used and the specific diagnostic criteria for each item on the assessment form, as well as the order in which these elements should be examined. Care should be taken to ensure the comfort, privacy, and safety of each person being assessed.

20.5 Tests of Physiological Function

Tests of physiological function can provide helpful information about health status. For example, spirometry measures lung function, electrocardiography (ECG) measures heart function, electroencephalography (EEG) measures brain function, and audiometry measures hearing acuity. The costs associated with these tests must be considered when designing primary data collection protocols. Although some medically necessary tests may be covered by patient insurance plans, tests conducted primarily for the benefit of researchers must be paid for by the research team. Because of cost considerations, secondary analyses of existing medical records may be the best option for researchers whose study questions require the use of expensive equipment. When tests are conducted as part of a primary research protocol for research purposes rather than clinical purposes, the research team must decide ahead of time, in consultation with specialists in medical ethics, whether the results of the studies will or will not be shared with patients and/or their health care providers. This decision must be disclosed to participants during the informed consent process prior to any measurements being taken.

20.6 Laboratory Analysis of Biological Specimens

Tests of blood, urine, stool, saliva, and/or other biological specimens may be helpful for identifying the presence of a disease or markers for a disease, the characteristics associated with having a disease, and the risk factors for a disease. Some immunologic, genetic, and other studies require the collection of new body fluids or tissue biopsies, either as part of routine clinical practice or specifically for the purposes of the research project. Before new specimens are collected, a research ethics committee must verify that the potential physical risks to participants caused by the collection of the sample will be minimized. Some studies may be able to make use of existing specimen banks. These samples may be fully anonymous, or they may be linked to other information about the donor. The use of existing samples also requires ethics committee review and approval. Participants may have a right to the results of the laboratory tests conducted on their own biological specimens, and the protocol should discuss how notification will occur.

20.7 Medical Imaging

Medical imaging techniques are sometimes used to visualize parts of the human body. Examples are radiography (X-rays), computed tomography (CT) scans, magnetic resonance imaging (MRI), and ultrasound. The resulting images may be useful to researchers for purposes of diagnosis and/or for the assessment of responses to therapies.

20.8 Tests of Physical Fitness

Many different tests can be used to measure physical fitness levels:

- Cardiorespiratory fitness can be assessed using a 1-mile walking test, a 1.5-mile run test, or some other test of aerobic fitness.
- Measures of muscle strength and endurance include timed curl-ups, push-ups, pull-ups, flexed arm hangs, bench presses, leg presses, and grip tests (using a handgrip dynamometer).
- Flexibility can be measured using a sit-and-reach test (often measured with a flexometer) and other activities that stretch the lower back, hamstrings, or other muscle groups.
- Additional tests of fitness may assess agility, balance, coordination, speed, power, and reaction time.

Researchers must make the safety of participants their top priority. Appropriate precautions must be taken to ensure a safe environment. Participants walking or running on a treadmill must be given clear instructions about how to step on and off the belt; they must wear appropriate footwear; they must use any automatic-stop safety clips and other devices recommended by the manufacturer; and they must be monitored throughout the test. The treadmill must be situated away from walls or other objects that could cause harm to someone falling off the treadmill. The use of a harness might be required for participants with poor balance. Study participants walking or running on an outdoor track must be alerted to any bumps, dips, or other hazards on the track and must not be allowed to be tested in conditions of extreme heat, humidity, or precipitation. Participants who have an existing injury or other impairment or condition that might make movements dangerous should not be allowed to participate without medical authorization, legal approval, and close supervision.

20.9 Environmental Assessment

Both the natural and built environments can have an impact on human health. Consider just a few of the many environmental factors that may affect the safety of the home:

- Is the entrance to the home accessible, or are there stairs or other barriers to access for people with mobility limitations? Are any stairs in the home loose or uneven? Do all stairs have handrails? Is any carpeting in a stairway firmly affixed to each step? Are all stairways free of clutter? Do exterior and interior stairs have adequate lighting?

- Does the home have adequate temperature control to prevent extreme heat and extreme cold?
- Do residents have reliable access to clean drinking water?
- Is the kitchen free of pests and rubbish?
- Does the bathtub or shower have a nonslip surface to prevent falls? Is the water heater set to prevent scalding and burns? Is the bathroom free of water damage, moisture, and mold?
- Has the home been tested for toxic substances such as lead paint and asbestos? Is the home ventilated to prevent the buildup of radon gas? Are household chemicals, such as cleaning supplies, safely stored?
- Is the home equipped with working smoke alarms and carbon monoxide detectors?
- Are there sidewalks that facilitate safe walking near the home? Is the home located near a park, a playground, or another place where residents can safely engage in physical activity and recreation?

Similar lists of questions could be developed for schools, healthcare facilities, workplaces, and other locations.

Some of these questions can be answered by trained observers. These assessors may describe findings qualitatively, assigning ratings like "high" or "low" to observed conditions based on predefined lists of rating criteria. Other assessments require quantitative measurement of environmental contaminants, such as tests of paint chips for lead or tests of basement radon levels. For some types of hazards, the exposure dose, frequency, and duration must be ascertained. Risk assessments may be conducted at one point in time or at several time points. Researchers must have the permission of owners and/or residents before they enter a building or conduct environmental assessments of a structure.

20.10 GIS (Geographic Information Systems)

Sometimes a map and/or spatial analysis of important features in the study area helps answer the study question. If so, a **GPS (global positioning system)** receiver can be used to acquire the geographic coordinates (in latitude, longitude, and altitude) for relevant locations, such as the homes of participants, nearby hospitals and other health care facilities, roads, schools, religious and social organizations, grocery stores, recreation facilities, water sources, and industrial sites. The coordinates for public locations can be collected by anyone, but permission from the owners or residents of private land may be needed before entering their property to take a GPS reading. The GPS coordinates for the homes of participants is individually identifying information, so precautions must be taken to protect geographically linked personal data.

20.11 Inter-Rater Reliability

Statistical tests can be used to determine the extent of agreement between two assessors who are evaluating the same study participants. For example, a measurement known as the **kappa statistic** can indicate whether two radiologists examining the same set of X-rays reach the same conclusion about the presence or absence of a fracture more or less often than expected by chance. If the two radiologists agree as often as expected by chance, $\kappa = 0$. If they agree on the interpretation of 100% of the X-rays shown to both of them, $\kappa = 1$. If they agree more often than expected by chance, kappa will have a positive value somewhere between 0 and 1. Although complete agreement is rare, a valid study will have a value of kappa that is close to 1. Other measurements of **inter-observer agreement** or **inter-rater agreement** (also called **concordance**) can also be used to assess the validity and consistency of other assessment tools and procedures (**Figure 20-1**). More detailed information about quality control techniques is available in reference books.

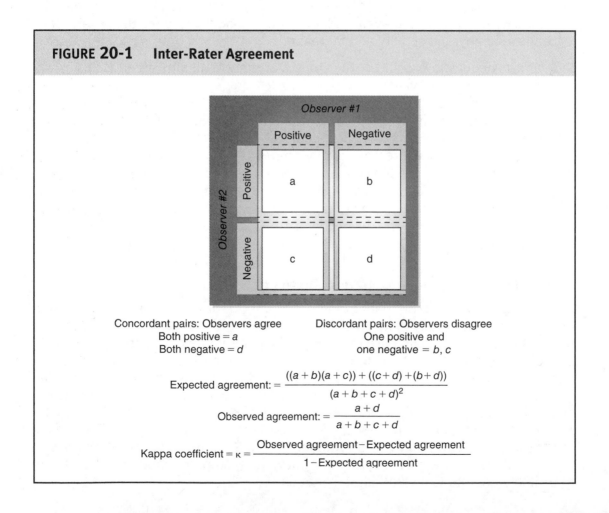

FIGURE 20-1 Inter-Rater Agreement

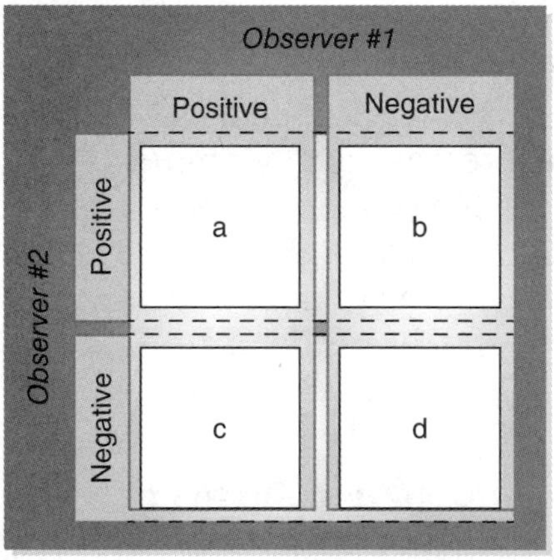

Concordant pairs: Observers agree
Both positive = *a*
Both negative = *d*

Discordant pairs: Observers disagree
One positive and
one negative = *b*, *c*

$$\text{Expected agreement: } = \frac{((a+b)(a+c)) + ((c+d)+(b+d))}{(a+b+c+d)^2}$$

$$\text{Observed agreement: } = \frac{a+d}{a+b+c+d}$$

$$\text{Kappa coefficient} = \kappa = \frac{\text{Observed agreement} - \text{Expected agreement}}{1 - \text{Expected agreement}}$$

CHAPTER 21

Secondary Analyses

Some health research studies analyze existing clinical records, survey data, or population data rather than collecting new information.

21.1 Overview of Secondary Analysis

For some studies, the data collection stage of the 5-stage research process is the step of acquiring existing data sets for secondary analysis. These data files may be publicly available individual-level or population-level data, privately held survey data, or electronic or paper health records. Whatever the data source, what makes a project a **secondary analysis** is that the researcher conducting the statistical analysis has not had (and does not have) any contact with the individuals whose data are being examined.

A researcher conducting a secondary analysis contributes to scientific knowledge by analyzing and interpreting accumulated data that might otherwise remain untapped. Sometimes a researcher can download an entire data set from an Internet website or have it sent by email. Such files often contain already cleaned data that are ready to analyze within minutes of receipt. At other times, the data are available only as paper records or electronic files from which the relevant information must be extracted and entered into a new computer database prior to analysis.

21.2 Publicly Available Data Sets

A growing number of governmental agencies allow researchers access to their **anonymized data sets** (also called **deidentified data sets**) that have had all potentially identifying information removed from the files. These organizations are experts at collecting data but often do not have the resources to conduct a thorough statistical analysis of an entire data set before it becomes relatively obsolete. Sharing data with external researchers is therefore a cost-efficient way to extract as much information as possible out of data sets, especially when the data were expensive to collect. Some research teams supported by federal funding agencies and some private organizations are also required to make their data available to researchers upon request, and others voluntarily share their data.

Available data sets are often listed on the websites of government health agencies. For example, the U.S. Centers for Disease Control and Prevention (CDC) website provides data from several nationwide cross-sectional studies, including the National Health and Nutrition Examination Survey (NHANES), the National Health Interview Survey (NHIS), the National Health Care Surveys, and the Behavioral Risk Factor Surveillance System (BRFSS). Other agencies within the U.S. Department of Health and Human Services (HHS) also make data sets available to researchers, including the Administration for Community Living (ACL), the Agency for Healthcare Research and Quality (AHRQ), the Centers for Medicare and Medicaid Services (CMS), the Health Resources and Services Administration (HRSA), the Indian Health Service (IHS), the National Institutes of Health (NIH), and the Substance Abuse and Mental Health Services Administration (SAMHSA). The U.S. Environmental Protection Agency (EPA), the U.S. Department of Veterans Affairs, the U.S. Census Bureau (which sponsors the American Community Survey), USAID (which sponsors the Demographic and Health Surveys in DHS-participating countries across the globe), and other agencies also participate in data sharing.

Additional data sets are available from other national, state, and provincial governments in addition to United Nations agencies like the World Health Organization. For example, Statistics Canada provides access to data sets such as the Canadian Community Health Survey (CCHS) via the Research Data Centres Program, and the United Kingdom's Medical Research Council (MRC) Research Gateway links researchers to available population health data. Other data sets are available from compilation sites such as the Global Health Data Exchange (GHDx), which is hosted by the Institute for Health Metrics and Evaluation (IHME).

Some sponsoring organizations that have made their data sets available to the public at no cost to the user allow those files to be downloaded on demand from their websites. Sometimes there is a screening process. The researcher may be required to submit a formal request and to have a research plan approved by an oversight committee before the requestor can be provided with a copy of the data by email or via a link to a password-protected download site. Although these data files are often provided at no cost to the researcher, sometimes they must be purchased. Additionally, access to some data files is limited to citizens or residents of the country in which the data were collected.

A researcher conducting secondary analysis needs to understand all the methods that were used for data collection and to become familiar with all the variables in the data files. In addition to downloading the data files, the researcher should download and read all supporting documents, such as the project overview, protocol, or handbook; the questionnaire; the codebook; and any published articles that describe the origins of the data set and previous analyses of the variables in it.

Investigators who make their data available to the public often do not expect to be coauthors on papers written by independent analysts. However, they may expect their contributions to be recognized and/or the sources of funding and technical support to be acknowledged. The supporting documents should state the expectations; if they do not, the researcher should ask a contact person for clarification. Also, sometimes the analysis requires assistance from the individuals involved in designing the study and/or collecting and processing the data. If so, those individuals may qualify for coauthorship even if the supporting documentation does not say that this is necessary; those individuals should be asked about their expectations.

There are some major limitations associated with using already available data. One is that the analyst is limited to exploring only the topics and specific questions included in the original survey. A related concern is that the analyst has to trust that the data were collected using valid and standardized methods and that the supporting documentation accurately describes the actual procedures used for data collection. Another challenge arises when the analyst has questions about the data collection and management procedures that are not spelled out in the supporting documents. Finding someone who can answer those questions might be difficult. Some download websites do not list the name of a contact person, and some of the listed contacts may not have been integrally involved in the study design and data collection process. A final issue is the risk of duplicating the analysis that someone else has done or is doing. A literature search may uncover related works that have been published or are in press, but it will not identify analyses in progress or papers under review by journals. The contact person for the data set may not know whether other researchers are conducting an analysis of the data or what topics other researchers are focusing on. Even with these potential difficulties, secondary analysis is often an excellent option for researchers with strong statistical skills but limited time and/or data collection resources.

21.3 Private Data Sets

Individual researchers and small research teams may have data available that have not yet been analyzed. The researchers may have computerized data files that have not yet been fully explored, or paper records may have been set aside because they are not a current priority of the research team. Sometimes the original researcher or research team may have published the results of some portion of the data set, but left unanalyzed some of the other potentially significant, interesting, and novel aspects of the data set. In these situations, the original researchers may be open to a new researcher taking the lead on analyzing an underexplored portion of the data set and writing up the results for possible publication.

A request for access to a private data set is most likely to be granted when the new researcher has some existing connection to the original researcher. Students are most likely to have success asking their own professors for data sets to analyze. If students are interested in the work of a research group at another university or hospital, they may find it helpful to ask their professors to reach out to friends at the other institution. The ethics review committees of both institutions may need to approve the data sharing plan, especially if identifiable information might be included in the data file.

When privately held data are shared with a new investigator, the original researchers usually expect to be coauthors on any resulting publication. The roles and responsibilities of each party should be agreed on as early as possible in the research process, preferably before the data files are shared.

21.4 Clinical Records

Clinical records are a common source of data for case series. Individuals working in clinical settings often can apply to gain access to patient records for research purposes. Most clinical sites require researchers to submit an application form to an oversight committee for review and approval prior to being authorized to access the data. The application must explain the goals of the study, the process that will be used to identify eligible patient records, the specific information that will be extracted from each patient's files, the steps that will be taken to protect the confidentiality of the data file, and the analysis plan. Applicants must also provide evidence of having successfully completed both research ethics training and specific instruction about patient privacy laws and policies. For example, researchers working with patient records in the United States must be prepared to comply with the **Health Insurance Portability and Accountability Act (HIPAA)** Privacy Rule.

Sometimes the relevant information can be extracted from an electronic database. When electronic records are not available, a data extraction form can be created and used to compile the relevant information from each patient file. The extracted information can be entered directly into a computer database or recorded on paper for later data entry. Whenever possible, the data files should not contain any individually identifying information.

A major limitation of using existing clinical records is that patient records are often incomplete. Researchers cannot make any assumptions about the missing information. For example, researchers cannot assume that the absence of information about a symptom means that the patient did not experience the symptom. The patient might have had the symptom but failed to mention it to the clinician. Perhaps the clinician did not specifically ask whether the symptom was occurring. Maybe the patient did mention the symptom but the clinician did not record it, perhaps because the symptom did not seem especially relevant. Similarly, researchers cannot assume that the information in the medical records of one health care provider tells a complete story about those patients' health status. Consider medication use. Researchers cannot assume that a patient is not taking a particular medication just because that patient's records at one clinical site do not mention that the patient has been prescribed that drug. The patient might have been prescribed the medication by a clinician at some other site. And, even if the patient's records show that a prescription was written for a particular medication, that does not mean that the patient filled the prescription and took the drug. If the research question requires complete information about symptoms or medication usage or other details, a primary study design may be necessary.

21.5 Health Informatics, Big Data, and Data Mining

Health informatics applies advanced techniques from information science and computer science to the compilation and analysis of health data. **Bioinformatics** typically focuses on analysis of molecular-level data (or, less often, tissue-level data). Clinical informatics and public health informatics usually focus on patient or population-level data. The tools of health informatics can be used to create novel data sets for research purposes.

Big data refers to the analysis of data sets that are so large and complex that they require access to powerful hardware and special statistical software applications. These data sets may include data for many thousands or even millions of individuals from:

- **Electronic health records (EHRs)** or **electronic medical records (EMRs)**, some of which use SNOMED CT (Systematized Nomenclature of Medicine Clinical Terms) as a standard terminology
- Billing records, which often use ICD codes (International Classification of Diseases codes) based on diagnoses or **CPT codes** (Current Procedural Terminology codes) based on procedures
- Laboratory records, which often use **LOINC codes** (Logical Observation Identifiers Names and Codes)
- Medication records, which often use NDC codes (National Drug Code identifiers)
- Social media posts and other sources of information derived from the Internet
- A diversity of other sources

Text mining and other forms of **data mining** can be used to extract particular phrases from large sets of records. Clinical informatics projects might use data mining techniques to explore hospital records. Public health informatics projects might use data mining and computational linguistics to explore social media events. Big data approaches have the power to reveal patterns and trends that are not apparent in smaller data sets analyzed with traditional statistical methods. Specialized training is usually required before researchers are prepared to implement data mining and other big data methods.

21.6 Ethics Committee Review

Use of hospital records for research purposes always requires review by one or more research ethics committees. If the data for a secondary analysis come from a private source, then, prior to even looking at the data set, the analyst usually must obtain clearance from his or her own institution and perhaps also from the institution that houses the data. The application for permission to analyze existing data is often shorter than the application required for primary studies, and review is usually able to be expedited. It is better to err on the side of submitting an unnecessary proposal than to erroneously presume that a project is exempt from review without confirming the validity of this assumption. Chapter 24 provides information about the ethics review process.

Most publicly available data, especially those collected by government agencies or federally sponsored researchers, were collected under protocols approved by one or several research ethics committees and then stripped of all personal identifiers prior to being shared. Additional approval by an ethics committee at the institution where the secondary analysis will be conducted is often not required when several conditions are met:

- The data were collected after approval by a trusted organization's research ethics committee.
- The data set contains no individually identifying information.
- The data to be analyzed are publicly available.

However, researchers are responsible for becoming familiar with the requirements of their host institutions and ensuring that their work is compliant with all institutional policies. When there is any doubt about whether review is required, the Institutional Review Board should be consulted.

CHAPTER 22

Systematic Reviews and Meta-Analyses

Tertiary analyses gather all prior publications on a specific topic and summarize them. A systematic review is the careful compilation and summary of all publications relevant to a particular research topic. A meta-analysis creates a summary statistic for the results of systematically identified articles.

22.1 Overview

Although much scientific research is about the identification of new results in a single study population, the goal of a review article is to engage in the scholarship of integration: to synthesize what is already known about a topic by connecting previous studies and offering new interpretations of their contributions to scientific knowledge. A review article in the health sciences requires:

- An extensive search of the literature
- The extraction of key information from relevant articles
- The clear and concise presentation of this information

Writing a review article—whether a narrative review, systematic review, or meta-analysis (**Figure 22-1**)—is a way to become an expert in the literature on a well-defined topic. This knowledge is a good outcome in and of itself, and a tertiary analysis can also be a helpful step in preparing for future primary or secondary analyses. Well-written and comprehensive review articles often become foundational for new research in the field because they summarize what is known about an area of inquiry. Because reviews provide a concise summary of the literature, published review articles may be cited more frequently than the typical article reporting on an individual field study.

However, review articles have limitations. Not all journals publish review articles, especially reviews that the editors do not solicit, so their likelihood of publication might be lower than that of other study approaches. Also, reviews are sometimes regarded as exhibiting less originality than other types of scholarship. A good review requires meticulous library work followed by the careful compilation and interpretation of information, yet reviews are sometimes perceived to be a less rigorous form of research than projects collecting new data and/or involving statistical analysis.

22.2 Selecting a Topic

When starting a tertiary analysis, the most important decision is the selection of a topic that is narrow enough that all the relevant publications can be acquired. The topic may need to be modified after a preliminary search, depending on the number of articles available. If an initial search of an abstract database yields only

FIGURE 22-1 Key Characteristics of Reviews and Meta-Analyses

Approach	Narrative Review	Systematic Review	Meta-Analysis
Objective	Synthesize existing knowledge	Synthesize existing knowledge	Synthesize existing knowledge
Primary study question	What conclusions about this topic are supported by previous studies?	When all previously published studies on this topic are examined, what conclusions can be drawn?	When the results of all previously published studies on this topic are merged, what is the summary statistic?
Population	Published literature	Published literature	Published literature
When to use the approach	The goal is to describe a new perspective on a topic that can be supported by the existing literature.	The goal is to compare the findings of previous studies on a well-defined topic.	The goal is to summarize previous findings using pooled statistics.
Requirements	The researcher has excellent library access.	The researcher has excellent library access.	The researcher has excellent library access.
	The researcher has a unique perspective on the topic.	The researcher can obtain every relevant article.	The researcher has strong quantitative skills.

FIGURE 22-1 (continued)

Approach	Narrative Review	Systematic Review	Meta-Analysis
First steps	1. Decide what story the article will tell.	1. Decide on the specific objectives of the review. 2. Select the search methods that will be used to find potentially relevant articles. 3. Select inclusion and exclusion criteria for articles.	1. Decide on the specific objectives of the review. 2. Select the search methods that will be used to find potentially relevant articles. 3. Select the inclusion and exclusion criteria for the articles. 4. Decide how to assess the quality of the studies. 5. Decide how the results of the studies will be combined into one summary statistic.
What to watch out for	Limited publication venues	Publication bias	Studies that cannot be fairly compared
Key statistical measure	No statistics are required.	No statistics are required, but providing some results from included studies may be helpful.	Summary measures for included studies must be reported.

8 possibly relevant articles, the topic probably needs to be expanded; if a search produces 352 articles, the topic needs to be narrowed to a more specific disease condition, to a smaller geographic area, or to a reduced scope. For example, a review of risk factors for cardiovascular disease would be cumbersome. A very long book would be required in order to cover all the identified risk factors, and an article-length summary would provide such a superficial level of information that it would not be useful. There is a greater likelihood of success for a review article with a narrower scope—one that limits the types of risk factors, the particular cardiovascular diseases, and the population groups included in the analysis.

22.3 Library Access

No review article can be written without excellent library access because *every* relevant article must be identified and obtained during a systematic review. This usually requires access to a university library that allows patrons to make numerous interlibrary loan requests. Before starting a review project, a researcher should check with a university librarian regarding the library's journal access policies and the fees that patrons may have to pay to acquire articles that are not part of the library's collections or subscription services. The researcher must also prepare to maintain a meticulous system for tracking articles that have already been acquired, those that have been requested but not yet received, and those that need to be requested.

22.4 Narrative Reviews

Narrative reviews tell a story about a topic using evidence from the literature to support the "plot." A narrative review might summarize important clinical aspects of a disease or summarize the epidemiological profile for a well-defined population. Because they are intended to convey a perspective and not merely compile facts, narrative reviews must be carefully organized by theme, methodology, chronology, or some other guiding principle. A narrative may also be appropriate when the researcher has developed a unique conceptual framework or theory that can be illustrated with examples from the literature. However, narrative reviews are becoming less common as editors and reviewers push for the use of systematic methods. Researchers must be prepared to justify their selection of a narrative approach. A narrative review works best when the researcher has a unique perspective on a topic and/or a particular expertise in the field that can be drawn on without using a systematic search strategy.

22.5 Systematic Reviews

Systematic reviews use a predetermined and comprehensive searching and screening method to identify relevant articles. This process is designed to minimize the bias that might occur when researchers handpick the articles they want to highlight. Therefore, after the identification of a focused study question, the most important decisions in a systematic review are the selection of keywords and inclusion criteria.

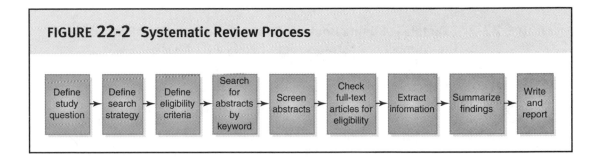

FIGURE 22-2 Systematic Review Process

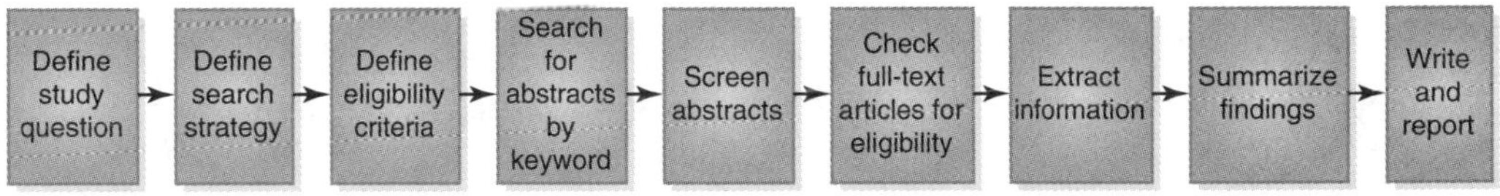

The goal is to craft a search strategy that identifies all the articles ever published on the narrow, well-defined area covered by the review. Once potentially relevant articles have been identified from a search of one or several abstract databases, each candidate article is screened to see whether it meets all of the inclusion criteria. Relevant information is extracted from all eligible articles and presented in a summary table, then the trends and key observations are summarized. In sum, the systematic review process requires:

- Identification of an appropriately narrow study question
- Selection of a well-defined and valid search strategy
- Screening of all potentially relevant articles to determine whether they meet the predefined eligibility criteria
- Extraction of relevant information from all eligible articles
- Summarization of the findings of these articles

Figure 22-2 presents the systematic review process. In some situations, it is appropriate to create a summary statistic by pooling data from the included studies, but this type of meta-analysis is not required.

22.6 Search Strings

After selecting a well-defined study question, the next step in a systematic review or meta-analysis is to compose appropriate search strings. A helpful first task is an exploration of the MeSH dictionary (available through the PubMed website) in order to identify the definitions of key terms as well as synonyms and related terms. For example, a search for "health care costs" shows that synonyms for this term include "treatment cost" and "medical care costs." Subheaders (sometimes called child terms) for "health care costs" include "direct service costs," "drug costs," "employer health costs," and "hospital costs." And "health care costs" fall under the headers (sometimes called parent terms) of "health care economics and organizations," "health care quality, access, and evaluation," and "delivery of health care."

A next step is to begin building candidate search phrases using keywords or MeSH terms along with **Boolean operators** such as AND, OR, and NOT (**Figure 22-3**). The exact search string(s) used for a systematic review should be presented in the

FIGURE 22-3 Examples of Using Boolean Operators to Expand or Restrict the Number of Abstracts Identified in a Database

Search String	Approximate Number of "Hits" in PubMed
cancer	3.5 million
bladder cancer	70,000
schistosomiasis	25,000
"schistosomiasis"[Mesh]	21,000
Schistosomiasis mansoni	10,000
cancer AND schistosomiasis	1500
bladder cancer AND schistosomiasis	650
bladder cancer AND *Schistosomiasis mansoni*	40
bladder cancer OR schistosomiasis	90,000
bladder cancer NOT schistosomiasis	65,000
colorectal cancer	200,000
colorectal cancer AND schistosomiasis	150
bladder cancer AND colorectal cancer AND schistosomiasis	20
(bladder cancer OR colorectal cancer) AND schistosomiasis	800

Note: Because the PubMed database is constantly adding new abstracts, the numbers in this table will not exactly match the results of a new search.

methods section of the resulting research report (or, if a variety of lengthy search options—such as the names of all countries in the world region of interest—were applied to various databases, in an appendix). Square brackets or other notation can be used in the text to indicate the start and end of each search string. A search for [a OR b] will find any abstract that includes "a" or "b" or both. A search for [a AND b] will yield only those abstracts that include both terms. More complex search strings may use parentheses, such as [a AND (b OR c)], which will find any abstract that includes both "a" and "b" or includes both "a" and "c."

Understanding the language used by MEDLINE and by other databases allows for the design of a database-appropriate search string. For example, in MeSH language a "child" is defined as a person who is 6 to 12 years old. Individuals who are 2 to 5 years old are classified as "preschool children" and those who are 13 to 18 years old are "adolescents." A keyword search of [child]—that is, a search for the word "child" in all of the titles and abstracts of articles indexed in PubMed—will yield hundreds of thousands more hits than a search for ["child"[Mesh]] that only searches for articles indexed with "child" as a MeSH keyword. The particular term or terms used in the search must be selected carefully.

To check the appropriateness of search terms, identify a handful of articles known to be relevant to the study question, then confirm that the search string captures all of these articles. If the search misses one or more of those key references, then the search strategy needs to be modified. However, this process must not be used to exclude disliked articles, which would cause the inclusion bias that systematic reviews seek to minimize.

Once a validated system for identifying eligible articles is in place, the selected abstract databases are systematically searched for articles that might meet the inclusion criteria. If the topic is appropriately narrow, then keyword searches can often reduce the number of abstracts and/or articles that must be screened for eligibility to a reasonable number, often fewer than 100 articles.

22.7 Search Limiters

Researchers must be cautious about artificially limiting the number of articles that will be identified during a literature search. Any limiters must be justified. For example, researchers must be able to answer the following types of questions:

- Why was the search restricted to articles indexed in MEDLINE rather than using a more diverse set of databases (such as CINAHL, PsycINFO, and SciELO in addition to MEDLINE)? If no justification is obvious, then the search should include multiple databases.
- Why was the search restricted to English-language papers rather than including a more comprehensive set of articles? This question is especially important for reviews covering the global population and not just English-speaking countries. A researcher's lack of fluency in other languages is not an acceptable justification for including only English-language articles. Online translation programs can assist with multilingual searches. For studies focused on countries with rich literatures in non-English languages, a collaborator who is fluent in those languages can be recruited.
- Does the use of a broad search term like "adult" or "United States" help or hurt a search, given that many papers reporting on these populations do not include these descriptors as keywords or even mention them in their abstracts?

Researchers should be especially cautious about using the built-in filters available in some abstract databases. For example, PubMed allows researchers to use filters to restrict results to particular types of articles (such as clinical trials or reviews), particular species (such as human-only studies), and even particular age groups (such as infants or adults age 65+ years). These limiters only work if an article was indexed appropriately by the submitting journal. Because many articles about humans do not add "human" as a keyword, and many studies do not include keywords for the ages of participants or even the study design, the built-in limiters often exclude many studies that would otherwise be eligible for the review. It is usually better to use study-specific exclusion checklists to remove abstracts that are ineligible rather than to artificially limit the number of abstracts using filters.

22.8 Eligibility Criteria

As the database searches are being conducted, each identified article's title and abstract are reviewed to determine whether the article is likely to be eligible for inclusion in the systematic review. When an abstract is not available or the abstract does not allow a determination about ineligibility to be made, the full text of the article must be read.

The decision about eligibility is based on pre-determined lists of inclusion and exclusion criteria. For example, suppose that an analysis of the connections between tobacco use and lung cancer included as some of its inclusion criteria:

- The study used a case-control or cohort study design
- The article reported an odds ratio or rate ratio for the relationship between cigar smoking and lung cancer
- The study included at least 50 participants with lung cancer

This study would then have as some of its exclusion criteria:

- The study used a cross-sectional design, an experimental design, or any design other than a case-control or cohort study
- The article did not include information about cigar use
- The article did not report a statistic for the association between cigar smoking and lung cancer
- The study included fewer than 50 participants with lung cancer

Researchers must be able to justify each of the inclusion and exclusion criteria they select for a systematic review. This means that they must be able to satisfactorily answer questions like:

- Why were only randomized controlled trials included rather than also considering case-control, cohort, and other observational studies? Studies of causality are often appropriately limited to reviews of experimental studies, but reviews that are not focused on causation generally do not need to exclude observational studies.
- Why were articles published before the year 2005 excluded? In many situations, older papers will still be relevant to the study question and they should not be excluded based solely on presumed obsolescence. For example, a study seeking to characterize current prevalence rates or examining a recently implemented public health law might safely exclude studies that are more than 10 years old, but a study examining risk factors might not be justified in excluding older papers. (Note that when the year can be justified as an important inclusion

criterion, the year of data collection should usually be used for determining eligibility rather than the year of publication. It would be inappropriate to include a study that collected data in 1995 and published the results in 2005 while excluding a study that collected data in 2003 because it published the findings in 2004.)

- If a quality assessment was part of the inclusion criteria, what evaluation tools were used to assess the quality of the studies and the risk of bias in their results? (A variety of quality assessment scales, checklists, and other approaches are available to guide these processes.) Was this a fair mechanism to use to decide which studies merit inclusion in the review?

Most systematic reviews end up with about 15 to 25 included articles after screening, although some have many more than that. The full text of each of these articles must be read to confirm eligibility. Ideally, each article should be assessed by at least two independent reviewers. **Figure 22-4** summarizes this process. The count of articles at each step—identification, screening, checks of eligibility, and inclusion in the analysis—should be included in the research report.

FIGURE 22-4 Systematic Search Strategy and Counts to Report

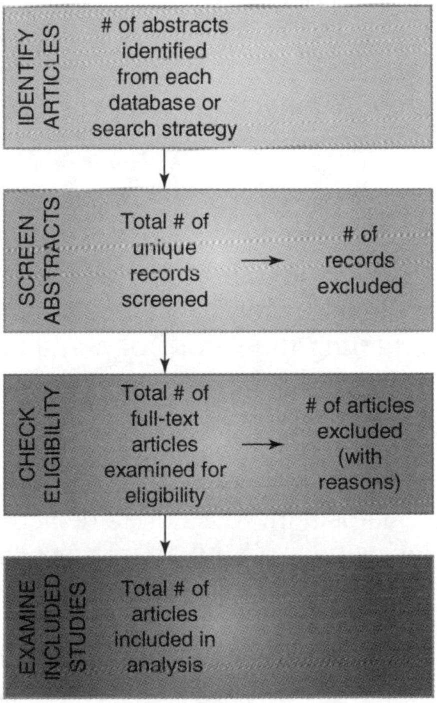

Three additional strategies may be considered to complement database searches. One is "**snowballing**," looking up every article cited by eligible articles in order to identify other articles that might be relevant but not indexed in the selected databases. Another is searching the **gray literature**, research reports that are available to the researchers but have not been externally reviewed and formally published. A third option is to conduct **hand searching** in which all articles in the tables of contents of selected volumes of relevant journals are scanned for reports on the topic of interest. The methods used for these expanded searches must be disclosed in the research report, and any documents found through these supplemental search methods must meet all of the inclusion criteria.

22.9 Data Extraction

Once all eligible articles are identified, the content of these articles is summarized in data extraction tables that list descriptive characteristics such as:

- The study location
- The years of data collection
- The study design
- The study population and sample size
- The definitions used for key exposures and outcomes
- The key findings of interest, including both quantitative (numeric) results and qualitative conclusions
- An evaluation of the quality of the study

A data extraction table allows for easy compilation and comparison of observations relevant to the study question. A condensed version of the table is usually included in the research report.

22.10 Systematic Review Results

The researcher should record and report both statistically significant findings ($p < 0.05$) and statistically insignificant findings ($p \geq 0.05$) that are related to the main study question. When interpreting the results of a systematic review, studies that find no statistically significant results for an item of interest are just as valuable as those that find a significant association. A report may state, for example, "Five of 40 published studies of the association between exposure A and disease B found an increased rate of disease B among those exposed to A; the remaining 35 studies found no association." That is a more accurate depiction of the literature than a report that merely says, "Five studies found an increased risk of disease B in those exposed to A." The latter statement incorrectly implies a consensus that exposure A is significantly associated with disease B. One of the primary contributions of systematic reviews to the health science literature is the ability to identify both areas of consensus and areas of disagreement and uncertainty that need to be further examined.

Systematic review reports also need to address the possible influence of publication bias on the findings. **Publication bias** occurs when articles with statistically significant results are more likely to be published that those with null results. If 10 studies look at the association between the same exposure and disease, the one study that finds the exposure to be risky is much more likely to be published than the 9 null result studies. Even if the other 9 studies are published, they are likely to highlight some other statistically significant aspect of their research and to downplay the lack of a positive or negative association between that exposure and disease. Proving that publication bias has occurred may not be possible, but the presence of consensus should be conservatively interpreted when only a limited number of studies have been published on a topic or the results are mixed.

22.11 Meta-Analysis

The goal of a **meta-analysis** is to combine into one summary statistic the results of several high-quality quantitative studies that used similar methods to collect and analyze their data. After the study question has been defined, meta-analysis usually begins with a comprehensive systematic review of the literature to identify every possibly relevant article. Each of these articles is read to ensure that it meets the inclusion criteria, which are usually more restrictive than they are for general systematic reviews. These restrictions are important because a summary statistic is only meaningful when every study included in the meta-analysis has very similar definitions for exposures and outcomes, similar study designs and methods, and similar populations. Trying to combine dissimilar studies could hide real and meaningful differences among the study populations.

The steps of a meta-analysis are:

- Use a systematic search strategy to identify relevant articles
- Carefully read each study
- Assess the quality and comparability of each study
- Extract statistical results from each of the studies that meet all of the inclusion criteria for the meta-analysis
- Combine comparable statistical results into one summary statistic

The summary statistic should usually adjust for the confidence intervals of the contributing statistical measures.

22.12 Pooled Analysis

A meta-analysis creates one summary statistic by pooling the results of studies identified during a systematic review. Only comparable statistics from similar studies can be pooled. For example, a summary estimate of efficacy can be estimated from several high-quality randomized controlled trials with the same active intervention, the same type of control, and similar population groups. However, the results from studies that use different study designs, different interventions, or dissimilar population groups should not be pooled.

Before pooling the data, the researcher must show that the results of the studies are comparable. **Homogeneous** (similar) studies can be combined into a summary statistic, but caution should be used if the studies are **heterogeneous** (dissimilar). The amount of variability in the measure across studies can be examined using a **Cochran's Q** statistic for homogeneity and the **I^2 statistic** that adjusts the Q statistic based on the number of studies being pooled. I^2 is reported as a percentage from 0% to 100%, where higher percentages indicate a greater presence of heterogeneity. When there are a large number of included studies or a very small number of included studies, other statistical tests may be more appropriate.

If a summary statistic appears to be appropriate given the variability among the studies, the next step is to select a model that will be used for creating a pooled estimate of the **effect size**, which is the estimated value of a measure like an odds ratio, rate ratio, efficacy, correlation coefficient, or difference in means. There are two main choices: a fixed effects model or a random effects model.

- A **fixed effects model** can be used to create a pooled estimate when the studies are fairly homogenous.
- A **random effects model** is required when the tests of heterogeneity show that the included studies are dissimilar.

The point estimate for the summary measure will be similar for both model types. However, a random effects model will result in a wider 95% confidence interval for the summary statistic because the random effects model will adjust for the variability between the included studies.

Once a model is selected, a specialized computer software program can be used to estimate the value of the pooled statistic (such as a pooled Mantel-Haenszel adjusted odds ratio) and its confidence interval. The contribution of each study to the pooled estimate is usually weighted based on the sample size of the included studies, although other approaches to **weighting** can be used. Step-by-step guides to meta-analysis techniques are available from The Cochrane Collaboration and other groups.

22.13 Forest Plots and Funnel Plots

The contributing studies and the summary measure for a meta-analysis are often displayed using a **forest plot** (**Figure 22-5**). A forest plot usually has:

- A horizontal axis showing effect size.
- A vertical line showing the effect size that indicates no effect (such as an odds ratio of 1).
- A row for information from each included study that uses a square or other marker to indicate the point estimate for the effect size and uses a horizontal line to show the 95% confidence interval. Markers for the point estimate are

FIGURE 22-5 Example of a Forest Plot

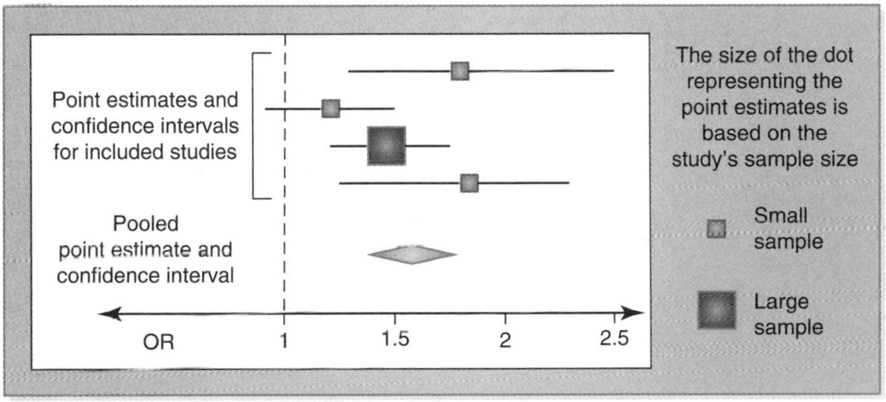

FIGURE 22-6 Example of a Funnel Plot

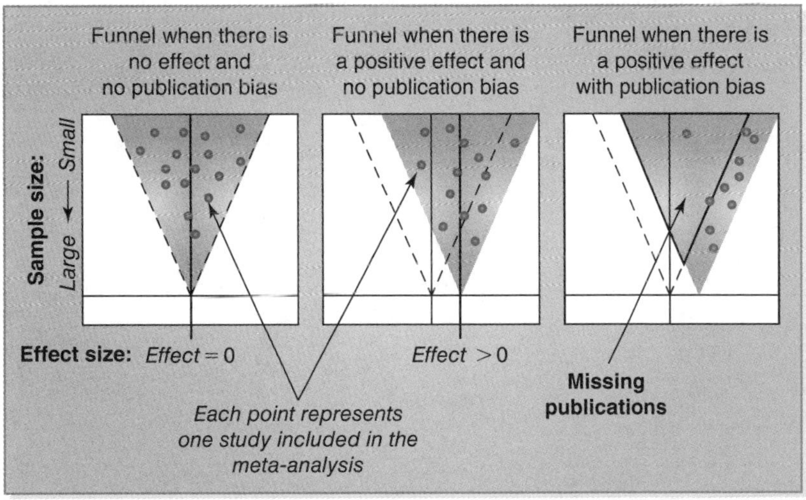

often presented in different sizes that show how each study was weighted in the meta-analysis. Small markers usually indicate studies with small sample sizes, and large markers usually indicate studies with large sample sizes.

- A representation of the summary measure and its confidence interval, often shown using a diamond shape.

There are two main threats to the validity of a meta-analysis: poor quality of included studies and publication bias. The selection criteria used during the systematic review process can eliminate studies of questionable validity. The possibility of the preferential publication of studies that report a statistically significant and/or favorable outcome can be examined using a **funnel plot**. A point for each study included in the meta-analysis is graphed on a plot that shows the effect size on the *x*-axis and the number of participants on the *y*-axis (**Figure 22-6**). If no publication bias has occurred, the points for the included studies will form a triangle. If publication bias has reduced the number of publications with statistically insignificant results, a part of the cone will be missing. In that situation, the pooled estimate is likely to have overestimated the true effect size.

CHAPTER 23

ETHICAL CONSIDERATIONS

Researchers have an ethical obligation to minimize the risks that research may pose to participants.

23.1 Foundations of Research Ethics

The ethical standards for human health research have evolved quickly over the past several decades. One of the first standards was the **Nuremburg Code**, which in 1947 mandated voluntary consent for experimental studies of humans. The **Declaration of Helsinki** was written by the World Medical Association in 1964 to provide guidelines for physicians conducting clinical trials. The ***Belmont Report***, published by the U.S. National Commission for the Protection of Human Subjects of Biomedical and Behavioral Research in 1979, defined key research principles. The Belmont Report is a foundational document for the current U.S. federal policy for protecting human research participants, which is often simply called the **Common Rule**. All of these documents have influenced research laws, policies, and regulations in countries across the globe.

Experimental studies have traditionally raised the greatest ethical concerns because the researcher assigns participants to try a new product, take a new drug or supplement, adopt a new behavior, or otherwise engage in an activity they would not normally do. Research ethics require that adequate, but not coercive, benefits be offered to participants. An appropriate control must be selected. Safety must be monitored. The ability of participants to continue to have access to the new product or service after the conclusion of the research project must be considered prior to the study's implementation.

Observational studies have traditionally been considered less risky because the research team is not imposing changes on the participants. However, observational studies usually still require informed consent from participants, and the researcher must still take care to maintain the confidentiality of all data and to minimize the physical, psychological, or other potential harms to participants. All patient protection regulations, such as the Health Insurance Portability and Accountability Act (HIPAA) Privacy Rule in the United States, must be strictly adhered to for observational as well as experimental studies.

23.2 Respect, Beneficence, and Justice

The three core principles of biomedical research ethics are now usually considered to be respect for persons, beneficence, and distributive justice. Each protocol for a primary research project in the health sciences (and most secondary research projects) should be carefully inspected to ensure its compliance with these principles. This level of scrutiny is required by research ethics review committees and by professional standards.

Respect for persons is a broad concept that emphasizes voluntariness. The principle of **autonomy** requires that only the individual (or his or her legal guardian) is authorized to make the decision about whether to volunteer to participate in a research study. For almost all research projects that involve interaction with individual participants and/or their personally identifiable data, each potential participant must be fully informed about the benefits and burdens of the study, the procedures involved, and the plans for use of the data collected. Recruits must make an autonomous choice to participate or not to participate. Respect for persons also requires many other considerations, including:

- Choosing an appropriate source population for the research question or, if conducting community-based participatory research, selecting an appropriate research question for the source population
- Developing a scientifically valid and rigorous study protocol that will answer the research question
- Making research procedures as minimally invasive as possible
- Using a nondiscriminatory process to sample and recruit participants
- Recruiting the correct number of participants required to have adequate statistical power for the study
- Confirming that all participants understand the informed consent materials and process
- Maintaining the confidentiality of all shared information

Beneficence means that the study should do good. Beneficence is often paired with **nonmaleficence**, which means that the study should do no harm. To meet the requirement of beneficence, a research proposal must have a high likelihood of benefiting individual participants and/or the communities from which they are drawn. For most studies, the opportunity to contribute to scientific knowledge is considered an adequate benefit to participants, although in some cases more specific individual and community benefits are offered. Researchers conducting beneficent research should be able to justify the necessity for and the importance of the research project.

Nonmaleficence requires the research team to minimize potential physical, psychological, financial, social, or other harms to participants, as well as to ensure an acceptable balance between risks and benefits. For example, the principle of "do no harm" means that experimental studies must identify ahead of time what events would lead to early termination of the study. Discontinuation might be appropriate when the intervention appears to be dangerous or when it appears to be so beneficial that it would be unethical not to immediately offer the intervention to the individuals assigned to the control group. Another way to minimize harm is to provide participants in studies that might cause emotional distress with information about local counseling services.

Distributive justice seeks to ensure that the benefits and burdens of research are equitable. Vulnerable populations should not be selected as the source population for research studies targeting the general population, because that might unfairly burden a disadvantaged population group. At the same time, members of understudied populations who happen to be sampled at random for a study of the general population should not be excluded from participation unless there is a defensible reason for why exclusion is necessary. Also, to be just and not exploitative, the source population must have access to the results of the research study. For example, if an experimental pharmaceutical therapy proves to be effective and safe, participants in the clinical trial usually should have the continued opportunity to access the drug after the trial is over. Justice is about the long-term impact of the study, and not just the immediate benefit to the individual participants and the community from which they were drawn.

Figure 23-1 highlights some of the many questions that researchers should ask and answer about their own protocols prior to formal review by an ethics committee. **Figure 23-2** illustrates the kinds of questions that can be asked for community-based projects to complement key questions for individual-focused projects. International health research guidelines, such as those developed by the Council for International Organizations of Medical Sciences (CIOMS), and national and disciplinary research guidelines may identify additional areas of concern that need to be considered as protocols are developed.

23.3 Incentives and Coercion

Researchers need to consider the ethical implications of offering an inducement to potential participants to encourage them to enroll in a study, offering reimbursement for the direct or indirect costs of participation, or compensating participants for their efforts. The principle of beneficence does not require monetary compensation to be offered. For many research projects in the health sciences, the innate reward of contributing to science is a sufficient benefit of participation. At the same time, the principle of nonmaleficence requires that participation in a research project should not be an undue burden to participants. In some situations, reimbursing participants for their travel and other expenses and/or compensating them for their time may be appropriate.

Incentives are sometimes offered to research recruits and participants. To increase the participation rate, researchers may reasonably offer a small gift to

FIGURE 23-1 Eight Central Considerations ("8 Cs") in Research Ethics

Category	Examples of Questions to Ask
Contribution	• Why is the proposed project important? • How will individuals and/or communities benefit from this study?
Compensation	• Will individuals or communities that participate in the study be offered any form of inducement, reimbursement, or compensation? If so, what will be offered, and is it appropriate? Is the offer so high that it could be seen as coercive or so low that the study could be seen as exploitative? • Are the risks of participation minimal? • How will study-related injuries be handled? • Are the risks and benefits balanced?
Consent	• How will potential participants be informed about the study? • How will consent to participate be documented? • Will a test of comprehension of the informed consent statement be required? • If applicable, how will consent (and possibly assent) be acquired for children and other members of potentially vulnerable populations? • If applicable, will community meetings be held prior to beginning the study?
Confidentiality	• How will the privacy and confidentiality of participants and their personal information be maintained?
Community	• Why is research in the selected population important? • Is the source population appropriate for the goals of the research study? • Will the selection process be fair? • Will the sample size be adequate? • Are potentially vulnerable participants adequately protected? • Has the protocol been adapted to address the cultural expectations of the source population? • If applicable, has the community agreed to participate in this project?
Conflicts of interest	• Who is contributing to the project's finances and/or logistics? • Might potential conflicts of interest inhibit the ability of a researcher to conduct ethical and unbiased research?

FIGURE 23-1 (continued)

Category	Examples of Questions to Ask
Collaborators	• Are all members of the research team adequately trained to conduct ethical research? • What steps will be taken during data collection and analysis to ensure that the protocol and all ethical standards are adhered to by all members of the research team?
Committees	• Which research ethics committee(s) needs to review the project? • If applicable, what community organizations have been consulted about the proposed project?

FIGURE 23-2 Sample Ethical Considerations for Individual- and Community-Based Research Projects

	Individual Participants	Community Participants
Respect	• What steps have been taken to protect individual rights? • Has the risk of coercion in recruitment been considered and minimized? • Is the informed consent process more than just signing a piece of paper? • Do participants in sensitive studies have privacy? Will their participation be kept secret? • Will data shared with the researchers be kept confidential? Will it be locked in a protected place and not shared unless individually identifiable information is removed?	• What steps have been taken to ensure that a community's values are respected? • Are appropriate community-based research methods being used? • Have community representatives and a local oversight committee been consulted about the project?

FIGURE 23-2 Sample Ethical Considerations for Individual- and Community-Based Research Projects (continued)

	Individual Participants	Community Participants
Beneficence	• How will individuals benefit from participation? Free services, supplies, or medicines? Free health education? Gifts or money? Contribution to knowledge?	• How will a participating community benefit from the research project?
Nonmaleficence	• What steps have been taken to minimize physical, psychological, financial, social, and other risks to participants? • Is counseling available for participants in sensitive studies? • Is appropriate reimbursement for travel costs and other expenses being offered?	• What steps have been taken to ensure that a community is not burdened by research participation?
Justice	• What are the long-term benefits for individual participants? For example, will they gain increased knowledge about their health status? • What will happen to participants after the study is completed? Will the results of the study be shared with them?	• What are the long-term benefits of participation to the community? • Will the researchers have an ongoing relationship with the community?

all participants or enter everyone who completes a questionnaire into a drawing for a more substantial gift that one randomly selected participant will receive. It may also be appropriate to provide free treatment for some types of conditions examined by the study, such as iron pills for participants found to have anemia after a blood test or de-worming medication for participants found to have intestinal parasites. These medical treatments must be provided with appropriate clinical supervision, and health education must also be provided to the recipients of these treatments to ensure that they complete the therapy correctly and safely. For some clinical trials, covering all medical expenses directly related to participation in the study may be expected and appropriate. The tests and procedures that will be covered and those that will not be provided and paid for by the research team must be fully disclosed to participants prior to their enrollment.

However, the desire to reward or thank participants with gifts must be balanced with the need for participation in any research project to be voluntary. When an individual feels coerced into participation, the principle of **voluntariness** is violated. **Coercion** could include social pressure or requests from authority figures that make it difficult for an individual not to agree to enroll in a study. For example:

- Employees asked by their supervisors to enroll in an occupational health study may fear losing their jobs if they do not agree to participate.
- Patients asked by their own physicians to register for a clinical trial may fear that their medical care will suffer if they do not comply with the request.
- People in jail or prison may believe that participation in a research study is mandated or will yield unspecified rewards, even if they are told that participation is voluntary and there will be no direct benefits to participants.

Coercion can also be instigated by generous incentives, such as free medical care and monetary compensation, which could significantly impair the ability of an individual to make an informed decision about the risks as well as the benefits of participation. To minimize the risk of coercion, researchers have to be very transparent about what participants will gain from participation in a research study and what they will not gain.

23.4 Informed Consent Statements

Informed consent statements provide essential information about research projects to potential research participants so that they can make a thoughtful decision about whether to enroll in a study. The key components of an informed consent statement are summarized in **Figure 23-3**. The statement must use clear, simple language to describe the study aims, the procedures and expectations of participants, and the benefits and the possible risks of participation. The statements should emphasize that participation is voluntary and that any participant can withdraw from the study at any time without penalty. Many research institutes provide informed consent statement templates that recommend particular language approved by ethics experts and the institution's legal advisors. The template might need to be modified to ensure that the language in the consent statement is accessible to the members of a particular study's source population.

23.5 Informed Consent Process

Informed consent is intended to be a process, not merely a piece of paper. The principle of autonomy dictates that potential participants in a research study have the right to make their own decisions about whether to participate and that they must

FIGURE 23-3 Content for the Informed Consent Statement

Content Area	Description
Research	A definition of "research" and a statement that the study involves research
Purpose	An explanation of the purpose and aims of the research process (except in the rare situations in which that interferes with the research goals)
Participants	A description of how and why certain individuals or communities were invited to participate in the research project and an estimate of the total number of individuals who will be recruited
Procedures	A description of the study procedures (including any physical exams, collection of biological specimens, randomization or blinding processes, interventions, or other procedures that are part of the study protocol) and the expected duration of the individual participant's involvement in the study
Benefits	A description of benefits to participants and/or to society, including a clear explanation of the compensation to be offered or a clear statement that the participant will receive no direct benefits
Risks	A description of the possible risks, discomforts, and costs associated with participation, a statement that involvement in the project may involve unforeseeable risks, and a description of how study-related injuries will be handled
Confidentiality	A description of the steps that will be taken to maintain confidentiality
Voluntariness	A statement that participation is voluntary and that the participant may withdraw from the study at any time with no penalty, along with a description for the process of withdrawing from the study
Contact information	Contact information for the researchers
Signature	Space for the participant's signature

be provided with information that will allow them to make informed choices. The goal is not to acquire signatures from potential participants, but to ensure that participants truly understand the research process.

The informed consent process consists of the following steps:

- Reading the informed consent statement aloud to a potential participant or allowing the individual to read a copy of the statement
- Allowing adequate time for the potential participant to consider whether he or she wants to participate
- Answering any questions
- Asking whether the individual wants to participate in the study and is willing to sign an informed consent form

Acquiring a signature is not the end of the process. The lines of communication between researchers and participants must remain open during and even after the data collection process. All participants must be given a copy of the informed consent statement that includes contact information so that they can contact the researchers if they have concerns about the study or desire to withdraw.

The researcher should ensure that participants understand the research process and the consent document. A brief test of comprehension may be helpful. For example, recruits for an intervention study may be asked to say in their own words what "randomization" means. A correct answer will demonstrate an understanding that each participant may be assigned to a control group rather than to the active intervention group and that participants do not have a choice in the matter. An incorrect or incomplete answer may require additional explanation of the research process prior to acquisition of a signature on a consent document. The goal is not merely informed consent, but **understood consent**.

23.6 Informed Consent Documentation

For most research studies, the expectation is that each study participant will sign a printed copy of the informed consent statement. This written record provides legal protection for the institution sponsoring the research project because it shows that participants agreed to the terms of the study. For telephone interviews, informed consent documents may be mailed to potential participants, signed, and mailed back to researchers prior to the interview. For computer-based surveys, an electronic signature can be provided.

In a limited number of observational studies, the full process of acquiring and documenting individual informed consent may not be required. For example, if researchers will observe groups of individuals in public places, where participants have no reasonable expectation of privacy and will not interact with the researchers, consent is not required. Some anonymous questionnaires do not require an intensive informed consent process when:

- The responses cannot be linked to individuals.
- The survey instrument does not ask sensitive questions.

- The researchers will not physically examine individuals or collect biological specimens.
- The questionnaire is so short that describing the study would take longer than completing the questionnaire form.
- There are no foreseeable risks to participants.

In these situations, the completion of the survey form can sometimes be considered adequate proof of willingness to participate. Any request not to require the full consent process must be approved by a research ethics committee.

In some situations, documentation of informed consent is important but written documentation of consent is not acceptable. For example, written consent may not be appropriate when the source population has a low literacy rate. When few potential participants are able to read or write, participants might provide a thumbprint or some other mark to indicate consent. Alternatively, if it is deemed inappropriate to ask people who cannot read a document to sign it, oral consent may be preferable. **Oral consent**, also called **verbal consent**, must usually be witnessed by an independent third person (someone other than the researcher or the participant), and in some cases a declaration of consent is also audio-recorded.

23.7 Confidentiality and Privacy

Privacy is the assurance that individuals get to choose what information they reveal about themselves. The right to privacy means that:

- Individuals have the right to refuse to allow their personal information to be shared with researchers.
- Individuals who agree to participate in a study involving face-to-face interviews should have the option of meeting with researchers in a place where no one outside the research team will be able to observe or overhear the interview.
- The identities of participants in a research study should not be disclosed to unauthorized persons.

Confidentiality is the protection of personal information provided to researchers. One way to guarantee confidentiality is not to collect any personally identifiable information, such as names, addresses, government-issued identification numbers, birthdates, or other data that can easily be linked to an individual. This is often an option for cross-sectional surveys, but it is not possible for prospective or longitudinal studies in which baseline data about individuals must be linked to their own follow-up data. When individually identifying information must be collected, many steps throughout the research process can be taken to protect the information.

- All paper records should be stored in a locked file box in a locked room, and all computerized data files should be password-protected.
- Names and other personal identifiers should not be included in data files that contain sensitive personal information. Instead, two separate files should be

created, one for identifying information and one for all other data. These should be linked only by a unique study identification number.
- Only essential research personnel should have access to the file containing personally identifying information.
- At some point after the end of the study, and in compliance with the rules of the relevant research ethics committees about how long documentation of informed consent must be stored, individually identifying records should be destroyed.

23.8 Sensitive Issues

Researchers asking questions about sensitive issues must decide ahead of time how to handle disclosures. Sensitive issues may include questions concerning:

- Drug or alcohol abuse
- Sexual practices and preferences
- Psychiatric illnesses
- Immigration status
- Participation in illegal activities
- Genetic disorders
- Other information that could materially damage a participant if it was made known to the public

When written documentation of consent is not acceptable because participants could be harmed by being linked to the study, a **waiver** of the need to document consent can be requested. This is not a request for waiver of the consent process, only for permission not to collect written documentation of consent. The research team can also apply for a **certificate of confidentiality** (or the equivalent in the study country) that protects the identity of participants from being subject to court orders and other legal demands for information. When working with vulnerable populations or sensitive information, the relevant research ethics committees should be consulted about what alternative methods for documenting consent they will consider acceptable.

In some situations, guaranteeing confidentiality may be impossible because withholding critical information from authorities would violate the law. For example, legal mandates may obligate researchers to alert the police about child abuse, intimate partner violence, or suicidal ideation and planning, and to inform public health authorities about diagnoses of infections designated as notifiable conditions. The decision about whether or how to collect data related to these issues may require consultation with a legal expert and local authorities.

Participants in studies of serious genetic diseases should be offered genetic counseling and given the opportunity to decide whether they want to know the results of tests. A qualified genetic counselor can assist with development of appropriate protocols.

23.9 Cultural Considerations

A research protocol must be appropriate to the culture or cultures of the expected study participants. For example, culturally appropriate recruiting may take different forms. In some cultures, a small gift may be expected as a token of goodwill before an individual is asked to participate in a study. In other parts of the world, this would be considered coercive because it would create a perceived debt owed to the researcher. In some cultures, participants may expect a small gift upon completion of the study. In other cultures, such a gesture of appreciation might make volunteers feel that the gift somehow devalues their donation to science. Participants from some cultures expect to share tea or coffee or a light meal with researchers before any questions are asked. People from some cultures may expect that all health research will be conducted in an impersonal clinical setting. In some parts of the world, prospective participants might need to know that community leaders, such as government officials, religious leaders, or tribal leaders, have approved of the project and are monitoring it. In other cultures, the association of authorities with a research project may raise concerns about voluntariness, confidentiality, and the potential misuse of data.

The informed consent process may also need to be adapted to local custom. Although individual participants are always required to provide consent for their own participation, potential participants may need time to consult with their spouses, parents, or other family members prior to giving consent. For some community-based studies, a meeting of the whole community should be held so that everyone is confident that they are all hearing the same story from the research team. It may be helpful to have a local advisory board facilitate communication between the community and the research team. The informed consent statement and study materials may need to be available in multiple languages.

The survey instruments and data collection processes must also be culturally appropriate, and researchers must be trained in culturally respectful interview techniques. Topics that are openly discussed in one culture may be sensitive in another. Tests that are only mildly uncomfortable in one culture may be extremely distressing in another. For example, although people in some cultures are sensitive about the measurement of body weight, other cultures may not care about weight but may be uncomfortable with the measurement of height. There may be formal or informal restrictions on who can conduct an interview or a physical examination. Female participants may be unwilling to be examined by a male, or older participants may be uncomfortable being interviewed by a much younger person. Some participants may expect to be alone with just a researcher, and others will expect to have a family member present for the entire process.

If the research team does not include members of the target population, it is important to work with representatives of the source community when developing and revising the protocol. Additionally, some research ethics committees require a cultural expert to examine the protocol as part of the review process.

23.10 Vulnerable Populations

Vulnerable research populations may be considered to include children, prisoners, comatose patients, or some other groups of people who have restricted autonomy or might be at elevated risk of harm from research participation. Additionally, special considerations may be required for research involving fetuses, women who are pregnant or may become pregnant, adolescents, some cognitively impaired persons, traumatized patients with altered mental status, terminally ill people, older adults, members of racial and ethnic minority groups, students, employees, healthy volunteers who cannot therapeutically benefit from clinical research projects but may be at risk of harm, and international populations.

In addition to defending why a particular research project must focus on a potentially vulnerable population, extra care must be taken to ensure that the selection process is fair, potential participants understand that participation is voluntary, and participants (and/or their legal representatives) are fully informed about the possible benefits and risks of the study as well as about the requirements of participation.

Although most members of vulnerable populations can make their own choices about whether to participate in a research project, children and some adults with cognitive impairments may not be considered competent to make an informed decision. In this situation, a legally approved guardian is allowed to grant consent on behalf of the study participant. Whenever possible, in addition to having the legal representative's consent, potential participants should **assent** to their own participation.

23.11 Ethics Training and Certification

Research ethics committees usually require everyone who will be in direct contact with research participants and/or their personal data to complete formal research ethics training. Many institutions offer their own courses, either in-person or online, and several funding agencies and nonprofit organizations also offer training that is publicly available. In addition to providing guidance on the protection of human subjects, the training modules may cover more general principles for the **responsible conduct of research (RCR)**. RCR training programs typically spell out expectations and procedures for disclosing conflicts of interest, avoiding research misconduct, reporting research ethics or personnel violations, and otherwise exhibiting professionalism.

After completing modules on various aspects of research ethics and passing an exam, a certificate of completion (usually valid for 1 to 3 years) is issued as evidence that the investigator has been appropriately trained in research ethics. Copies of these certificates should be saved because research ethics committees often require proof of ethics training for all members of the research team.

CHAPTER 24

Ethical Review and Approval

Research ethics committees protect study participants, researchers, and host institutions by carefully reviewing research protocols prior to their implementation.

24.1 Ethics Committee Responsibilities

The three primary goals of **research ethics committees (RECs)**, often called **Institutional Review Boards (IRBs)**, are to:

- Protect the "human subjects" who will participate in observational or experimental studies or whose personal information will be examined by researchers
- Protect researchers by preventing them from engaging in activities that could cause harm
- Legally protect the researcher's institution from the liability that could occur as a result of research activities

(Separate **Institutional Animal Care and Use Committees (IACUCs)** oversee research with animals.)

The major functions of ethics review boards are to:

- Review new and revised research protocols
- Approve or disapprove of those protocols
- Ensure that informed consent is documented (if required)
- Conduct continuing review of long-term research projects

To verify the achievement of these goals, IRBs maintain careful records of their procedures and membership; all proposals, consent statements, and supporting documents; all correspondence; and minutes of all meetings that chronicle the decisions made to exempt, approve, or disapprove proposals and the justifications for these decisions. Researchers must provide all documents requested by the review committee, including all requested status reports.

IRBs overseeing research funded by the U.S. federal government must be certified by the U.S. government as having **federalwide assurance** (FWA). IRBs with FWA agree to adhere to U.S. research laws, regulations, and policies (that is, the "Common Rule") and to release their written operational procedures to the U.S. government if requested to do so. Both IRBs in the United States and in other countries can apply for FWA status and FWA renewal.

24.2 Ethics Committee Composition

Research ethics committees are usually composed of at least five members, preferably from diverse backgrounds, including both scientists and nonscientists. Each member reviews the proposal and then meets with the others to discuss it and to determine whether it meets the requirements of the institution. An outside scientific expert and/or community representative may also be consulted about the research plan.

Because of the number of individuals involved in protocol review, even the most efficient ethics review committees may need a month or longer to issue an exemption or an approval or to make a request for a revision to be made to the protocol, which must then be reconsidered by the committee before final approval. For complicated proposals, the review may take several months. Examples are studies involving:

- Invasive procedures
- Sensitive questions
- Potentially harmful interventions
- Deception about the study aims
- Waiver of written informed consent
- Multiple sites
- International research

A research timeline should assume a lengthy review period. The application should be submitted to the ethics committee as early as possible in the planning process in order to minimize the risk that delays in the approval process will complicate the timing of data collection and other research activities.

24.3 Application Materials

Some research ethics committees ask applicants to provide a narrative research statement that addresses a list of possible ethical concerns. Others mandate the completion of dozens of pages of forms that require answers to a long series of questions about the project (even when most questions warrant an answer of "not applicable"). **Figure 24-1** summarizes the questions that research ethics committees commonly examine during the review process. A research protocol or narrative statement about a planned project should address each of these points and any others required by the committees evaluating the proposal.

FIGURE 24-1 Examples of Information Requested and Examined by Ethics Review Committees

Category	Considerations
Participants	• What is the anticipated composition and size of the study population? • How will participants be recruited? Does the recruitment method raise any concerns about coercion? • What are the inclusion and exclusion criteria? Are they reasonable? • Is the source population appropriate for the study question? • Are potentially vulnerable subjects protected, if applicable?
Risks and benefits	• Why is the study important and necessary? How will the proposed study benefit participants and/or their communities? • How will data be collected? Will existing data, documents, records, or specimens be used? Will individuals or groups be examined using surveys, interviews, focus groups, oral histories, program evaluations, or other methods? Will interviews be audio or video recorded? Will noninvasive clinical measures be taken? Will participants be asked to engage in exercise or tests of endurance, strength, or flexibility? What machines will be used to collect data, and will collection involve radiation exposure? Will blood, hair, nail clippings, sweat, saliva, sputum, skin cells, or other biological specimens be collected noninvasively? Will drugs or devices be tested? • What are the potential physical, psychological, financial, or other risks to participants? • Are the risks minimal (or at least minimized)? • Are the risks reasonable compared to the anticipated benefits?

FIGURE 24-1 Examples of Information Requested and Examined by Ethics Review Committees (continued)

Category	Considerations
Informed consent	• Does the informed consent statement adhere to institutional guidelines? • How will informed consent be sought? • How will informed consent be documented? • Is any modification to the usual methods of documenting informed consent being requested? Is the request reasonable? (For example, are parents being asked to provide consent for their children, and are the children being asked to assent to participation? Or is a waiver of a signed consent form being requested because the source population has a low literacy rate? Or is a request being made to have no documentation of consent because the existence of a form linking an individual to the study could harm the participant?)
Privacy and confidentiality	• How will privacy and confidentiality be maintained? • What are the plans for the protection of computerized and noncomputerized data?
Safety monitoring	• Does the informed consent statement clearly state how research participants can contact the research team and/or the ethics review board if they have concerns? • What constitutes an adverse event? How will such events be handled?
Conflicts of interest	• How is the project being funded? • Do any financial or personal conflicts of interest need to be disclosed and/or addressed?
Researcher training	• Are the investigators prepared to conduct ethical research?

FIGURE 24-1 (continued)

Category	Considerations
Documentation	• Are copies of all recruitment materials (if any) attached? • Are copies of the questionnaire and/or other assessment tools attached? • Is a copy of the informed consent statement attached? • Are copies of letters of approval from study sites and/or other ethics review committees attached, if applicable? • Is a copy of the grant proposal attached, if applicable? • Are copies of research ethics training certificates for all members of the research team attached?

Proposals for the analysis of existing data may be significantly shorter than proposals for new data collection, but both primary and secondary analysis proposals need to:

- Describe the expected study participants.
- Explain the sample size, the inclusion and exclusion criteria, and the recruitment plans (if applicable).
- Discuss the risks and benefits of the study.
- Describe the plans for seeking and documenting informed consent and monitoring safety (if applicable).
- Explain how confidentiality will be maintained.
- Disclose potential conflicts of interest.
- Provide proof of ethics training.
- Supply all relevant documentation.

For primary studies, the documentation may include a copy of the informed consent statement, the questionnaire, and recruiting materials. For secondary analyses, the application must include evidence that the data are in the public domain or that appropriate individuals or organizations have granted the researcher permission to analyze the data.

24.4 Review Process

Once all application materials have been submitted to a research ethics committee, there are three possible next steps: (1) exemption, (2) expedited review, and (3) full review. The ethics review board decides which action is appropriate.

Exemption from review may be granted—but does not have to be granted—when the research involves the analysis of existing data, documents, or records or stored biological specimens that cannot be linked to individuals. These sources must either be publicly available or anonymized so that study subjects cannot be identified. The U.S. Department of Health and Human Services (HHS) also allows for research protocols to be exempted from review when:

- The study procedures do not involve an intervention.
- Researchers will not interact with participants.
- The participants will not be prisoners, young children, and other individuals in protected populations.
- Individually identifiable information will not be collected.
- Data will be collected using commonly accepted educational practices or tests, established survey or interview procedures, or observation of public behavior, or the study will rely on existing data or biological specimens, data on public benefits or public service programs, or evaluations of taste, food quality, or consumer acceptance.

An exemption can also be granted for data collected as part of routine professional practice that is not intended to contribute to generalizable knowledge. It is important to make a distinction between routine practice activities and intentional research activities. Practice activities include teachers assessing their students' knowledge of class material, clinicians examining their patients, community health organizations initiating monitoring and evaluation projects, and public health officials collecting surveillance data and conducting outbreak investigations. None of these activities requires review by a research ethics committee; all are considered to be within the accepted scope of practice. However, ethics review is required if these practitioners or organizations choose to engage in research activities, such as:

- An educator plans to have students take special pre- and post-tests to assess a new pedagogical approach and hopes to publish the results in a teaching journal.
- A clinician reviews patient records so that they can be presented as a case series at a professional conference.
- The results of a survey of clients of a community organization might later be published in a professional journal.

In such situations, an exemption might be appropriate, but the decision is up to the IRB, not the researcher.

An **expedited review** may be possible when a minor change to a previously approved protocol is requested. Sometimes expedited review is also possible for new studies in which the risk to participants is no greater than what is encountered in ordinary daily life or, in the case of clinical work, during routine examinations or procedures. Exemption from review is not allowed for research with classified vulnerable populations. Expedited review may allow the chair of the ethics committee to approve the protocol without a full meeting of the committee. However, all members must be notified of the decision and given an opportunity to express concerns.

Full review of the research proposal is usually required when an intervention will be tested in individuals or a community, data will be collected through interaction with individuals, identifiable private information will be collected, or other criteria for expedited review are not met.

The ethics review committee has the right to approve each proposal or to deny approval. If a protocol is not satisfactory at initial review, the committee usually informs the investigators of the protocol changes that are necessary to make the proposal acceptable. Some requests may be easy to accommodate, and researchers should simply comply with them. At other times, the requested changes would significantly alter the nature of the project or would be unfeasible given the intended study population. In this situation, the researchers need to present their concerns to the ethics review committee and to try to work with them to find an acceptable resolution. However, the committee does not have to acquiesce to the desires of the researchers. The ethics review board has the right to deny approval of any protocol that does not meet its standards. Furthermore, the board can demand proof that certain standards (for example, standards for data storage or investigator training) are met prior to approving the protocol.

24.5 Review by Multiple Committees

Multiple research ethics committees may be required to review studies that involve researchers from multiple institutions and/or participants from multiple countries or multiple study sites. Additionally, funding agencies may require review by their own ethics boards. For example, a student planning to conduct thesis research in another country must have the research protocol reviewed by, at minimum, two ethics boards: one from his or her own university and one from an ethics committee in the study country (often a local university or a teaching hospital).

At least three issues must be resolved prior to submission of a research proposal to multiple committees: the application documents that will be required, the wording of the informed consent statement, and the order of review.

First, each review board must be consulted about the application materials it wants to receive. Sometimes, submitting the same paperwork to all committees is possible. More likely, each board will require its own unique application materials, perhaps in addition to copies of all documents submitted to other ethics committees. The researchers have the responsibility to ensure that each application packet describes the study objectives and protocol in the same way.

Second, many institutions have their own preferred wording for informed consent statements. The informed consent statement is seen as a legal document, and institutions want to be sure that the wording protects them. However, the preferred wording may differ for each participating institution. A resolution must be reached about how to merge consent statement requirements while making sure that the study participants will understand the language.

Third, the order of review must be established. Sometimes, all the committees independently review the proposal at the same time. At other times, the reviews are conducted "domino" style, with the proposal being independently reviewed and approved by one committee, then passed to the next committee, and so on. Committees commonly stipulate that approval by their institution will be contingent on approval from all other participating institutions, even when they review concurrently. If a modification of the protocol or informed consent document is mandated by one committee, then all other committees must re-review the proposal. A significant amount of extra time for ethics review should be built into the project timeline when multiple research ethics committees will be involved.

24.6 Ongoing Review

Studies that can be completed within 1 year may not require further review by a research ethics committee after initial approval, although most committees require a final report to be submitted that at minimum states the number of participants, affirms that no adverse events occurred, and declares that the project is concluded. However, the research team may be asked to provide mid-year reports about the number of participants recruited in addition to immediately reporting all adverse events to the IRB. Any desired changes to recruiting materials, the informed consent statement, the questionnaire, or other study documents must receive approval prior to being implemented.

All ongoing research protocols must be re-reviewed annually (or more often, at the discretion of the ethics review committee) until the completion of data collection or, in some cases, until the completion of data analysis. The progress report for re-review may need to include (depending on institutional requirements):

- Current versions of the protocol, informed consent statement, questionnaire, and other study documents
- A report on the study population, including the number of participants who have enrolled in the study and who have dropped out, the demographic characteristics of the study population, and basic information about the number of participants who are members of vulnerable populations
- A report of any adverse events, complaints, or unanticipated problems, including details about any issues reported to the ethics committee since the last annual review
- A list of any amendments to the protocol or study materials that are being requested
- A summary of findings (which are especially important for experimental studies that might need to be stopped early if the intervention appears to be harmful or very beneficial)

24.7 Conflicts of Interest

Most ethics review committees and an increasing number of journals require researchers to disclose potential conflicts of interest related to the study. A potential **conflict of interest (COI)** is mostly likely to occur when:

- A new product is being tested, such as a new medication or medical device, and one or more members of the research team earns a salary (or a consulting fee or an honorarium) from or holds equity interests (like stocks or ownership) in the company that produced, developed, or will market the product
- Intellectual property rights (such as the ownership of a patent or copyright) may result in earnings for a researcher or a close family member

When a financial or other relationship could bias the design, conduct, or reporting of the study—or could merely appear to have the possibility of biasing the study—the potential conflict of interest must be disclosed. Several types of relationships might be required to be disclosed to employers, funders, and publishers:

- Personal fees paid as salaries by employers, as honoraria, or as compensation for consulting, lecturing, giving expert testimony, or providing other services
- Financial relationships such as ownership of stocks, shares, or equity
- Income from patents, copyrights, and other intellectual property related to the project, or pending patents that might result in future income
- Nonfinancial support such as donated equipment or supplies, travel support, or writing assistance
- Service on the board of directors of a company doing work related to the research project
- Personal relationships with individuals or organizations that could influence the work, such as having a spouse who works for a company with a direct interest in the research project

The disclosure of a potential conflict of interest is not a confession that bias has occurred or an admission that bias will occur. It is, however, an important assurance of transparency. Most universities, hospitals, and other institutions involved in scientific research have policies about what constitutes a conflict of interest and about when and how potential conflicts need to be disclosed. For example, some universities only require interests exceeding $10,000 to be disclosed to the university, but others have a lower threshold for reporting.

24.8 Is Ethics Review Required?

Ethics review is required for almost every proposal that will involve living human subjects, whether those people will be directly contacted by the research team (in person, by telephone, by mail, by Internet, or via any other method) or their existing personal information will be analyzed. A small subset of projects might be exempted from review, but the decision to exempt a project from review can be made only by the relevant ethics committee(s). Most institutions do not allow researchers simply to declare that their projects do not need to be reviewed. Exemption usually involves a formal process of having an appropriate IRB confirm that a project meets set criteria for exemption from review.

Many incentives are in place to encourage participation in the formal review process. First, institutional approval provides a degree of legal protection to the researcher. An approval letter is evidence that the research plan was deemed reasonably safe by a committee of experts prior to the initiation of data collection and analysis. Another incentive is that some granting agencies will not release funds until a research plan has been approved by a research ethics committee. Finally, an increasing number of journals are requiring that authors provide details about which research ethics committee(s) reviewed the project (even if it was subsequently exempted from review). Some are even requiring copies of the official approval letters. Research protocols cannot be retroactively approved. Therefore, researchers must take the time to undergo a formal review prior to collecting any data or analyzing any data files.

CHAPTER 25

WRITING GRANT PROPOSALS

A proposal is written to request funding or approval for a new research project. The proposal must demonstrate that a new research question is important and that the research plan will yield an answer to that question.

25.1 Identifying Funding Sources

A formal research **proposal** is commonly written for two purposes. One is to seek approval for a project from a supervisor or a review panel, as occurs when a student submits a proposal to a thesis or dissertation committee for review, feedback, and eventual approval. The other is to apply for grant funding. Although not all research projects require financial support, projects sometimes need outside sources of money, or, at a minimum, they would be significantly enhanced by monetary support. The main sources of funding for research include:

- Universities and colleges
- Governmental agencies
- Private foundations and nonprofit organizations
- Businesses

Funds provided by the researcher's school or employer are called **internal grants**. **External grants** and contracts are funded by outside organizations.

A diversity of resources may be useful when searching for funding opportunities:

- Supervisors and mentors may be able to offer advice about sources of internal and external funding that are appropriate for the particular project under development.
- The grant management offices of colleges, universities, health care systems, and other organizations may offer consultations to researchers affiliated with those institutions.
- The websites of funding agencies provide details about the types of research they fund and the eligibility criteria for applicants.

- The newsletters and websites of some professional organizations include lists of new and ongoing funding opportunities relevant to people working within that discipline.
- Some subscription databases compile information about grant opportunities, and these may be accessible through library websites or other institutional offices.

Although receiving a research grant is usually a considerable accomplishment worth celebrating, it is important to remember that getting a grant is not the same as actually implementing the research plan. A grant is merely the opportunity to conduct a particular research project with funding support. Not all research projects require funding. Many projects can be successfully completed without any costs to the researcher beyond the researcher's time. For example, a secondary analysis of existing data or a review of the published literature may require only access to a computer, a statistical software program, and a decent collection of electronic journals. Some primary studies that collect new data incur only relatively minor expenses, such as the cost of photocopying a limited number of questionnaires. Although funding may open up opportunities to conduct more elaborate research studies, researchers without grant funding still have many options for doing meaningful research.

25.2 Selecting Grant Opportunities

There are several factors researchers should consider when selecting which grant opportunities to apply for. These questions include:

- What research areas and types of research questions are supported by this granting organization? Some funders support only projects focused on a particular disease or a very specific population, while others are much more general in scope.
- How much money is available? Some student-focused awards may allow budgets of only a few hundred dollars, while some government agencies offer millions of dollars to established researchers.
- When is the submission deadline? Some funders offer rolling submission deadlines, while others only accept proposals once per year.
- How long after submission of a proposal will an award decision be made? Some granting organizations make decisions about funding as proposals are submitted, while others may require nearly a year to make a decision about whether to fund a project.
- How competitive is the award? Some grants (usually ones open only to students in a particular program) are available to nearly everyone who applies for them, while other agencies may fund less than 1% of submitted proposals.

Funding organizations seeking researchers willing to explore narrow research questions of particular interest to the funder will usually post a **request for**

proposals (RFP), alternatively called a **request for applications (RFA)**, describing the types of projects the selection committee will consider supporting. These funders will often ask researchers to submit a **letter of intent (LOI)**, a **letter of inquiry**, or a **pre-proposal** so that the funder can confirm that there is a reasonable match between the sponsor and the proposed research plan before inviting a full proposal to be written and submitted.

When a funder reaches out to a researcher and asks that person to submit a **solicited proposal**, the organization might offer a contract rather than a grant. A **contract** usually requires that a particular **deliverable**, such as a commissioned report, be submitted to the funding agency by the end of the contract period. The organization might stipulate that the final payment on the contract will not be disbursed until after a satisfactory report is submitted by the researcher.

25.3 Writing a Research Proposal

Research proposals typically include a standard set of components (**Figure 25-1**):

- An abstract or a short summary of the proposal
- A background that explains what is known and what is not known about the proposed study area and justifies the importance of the proposed project
- A statement defining the research goal and specific aims
- A description of the data collection and analysis methods that will be used to answer the research question, and an explanation for why those methods are appropriate
- A plan for the dissemination of the study's findings
- A timeline
- A budget with a justification for each line item
- Information about the researchers

The instructions for the proposal may call various sections by different names. For example, the background may be called a literature review, and the description of the research methods may be called a research plan or a **project narrative**. Additional components may be required, such as an abstract written for a nontechnical audience, a description of the facilities and other resources available to the researcher, a statement about the broader impacts of the research, and letters of support from collaborators.

When writing a research proposal, the researcher should usually assume that readers of the proposal will not know much about the particular research area. It is the writer's responsibility to provide the background information necessary for the proposal to be understood by diverse technical and nontechnical audiences. An effective proposal will clearly answer three questions:

- What is the problem?
- How will the proposed project help solve the problem?
- How will the grant money contribute to achieving a solution?

FIGURE 25-1 Typical Proposal Content

Background
- Brief summary of what is already known about the topic
  - Literature review, with citations of the previous work of other researchers
  - Summary of the researcher's own previous work on the topic and any preliminary results (if applicable)
- Purpose of the new project
- Significance and importance of the new project
- Definition of key terms

Goals and specific measurable or testable aims, objectives, or hypotheses

Methods and procedures
- Study design
- Source population (for new data collection) or data source (for analysis of existing data)
- Sampling methodology and expected sample size
- Recruiting procedures (for new data collection)
- Definition and measurement of key variables
- Data collection procedures
- Laboratory procedures (if applicable)

Analysis plan
- Data management plan
- Data analysis plan

Dissemination plan

References

Timeline

Budget and justification (as allowed by the funding agency.)
- Personnel (such as salaries and benefits)
- Equipment and supplies for the office (such as computers, software programs, and paper) and laboratory (if applicable)
- Communications (such as postage, phones, and Internet access)
- Travel (including mileage on cars, parking, local transportation, and possibly airfare, hotels, and food)
- Other costs (such as publication fees and overhead costs)

Researcher information (such as a biosketch, CV, or résumé)

Optional appendices
- Questionnaire or other survey instrument
- Research ethics review application and supporting documents

The answers to all three of these questions should be clear in the abstract and the narrative, and every component of the submission should answer at least one of these three questions. Each section of the proposal should contribute to substantiating the importance of the health issue that will be studied, justifying the validity of the planned methods, and/or expressing how the proposed work will contribute to advancing knowledge and improving health.

When preparing a funding request, every part of the application must align with the goals of the sponsoring agency and its typical funding level. The goal of a funding request is to demonstrate that the study question is important and that, with funding, the researcher will successfully answer that question. For grant proposals, every component—the title, the narrative, the budget, and all other items—should express why the researcher should be given money for the project. The background needs to say that the health concern that will be studied is an important one that is worth financing. The methods section needs to convince the reader that the proposed approach to answering the study question is a valid and efficient one that is worth bankrolling. The budget needs to show that the researchers will make good use of the money given to them. The biosketches of the researchers need to prove that the research team has the experience necessary to see a project through to successful completion so funds given to them will not be wasted. And the application needs to clearly connect the research idea with the goals of the sponsor.

Guidelines from funding agencies and review committees usually specify how a proposal should be organized, what content should be included in each section of the proposal, and how long each section should be. For example, the instructions may allow only the lead investigator to submit a 2-page résumé or CV, or they may demand that each collaborator create a **biosketch** according to a template from the funding agency. Similarly, the guidelines may restrict the number of references that are allowed to be cited, and they may dictate how those citations should be formatted. It is important for the applicants to carefully follow all the instructions of the organization to which the application materials will be submitted. Neglecting to be compliant with all of the rules about formatting, layout, word length, components, and other details can be grounds for cursory rejection of the proposal. The instructions will also specify whether individuals should submit their own grant proposals or whether submissions must be made by an institution's grant management office.

25.4 Budgets

Granting agencies prioritize funding for research projects that will answer well-defined and significant study questions and that request a budget appropriate for the work that will be done. The budget should cover all the essential costs of the research project without being excessive in total amount or in any category. Each line in the budget may need to be accompanied by an explanation of why the item is necessary and a description of how the budget for that item was determined.

A student or trainee applying for a small grant may be limited to requesting funding for only basic direct expenses, such as travel and printing. Other studies may become quite expensive if they require travel to a distant field site, laboratory testing or other clinical assessments, lengthy durations of data collection, and the hiring of interviewers and data entry personnel. A large grant proposal may request support for a variety of **direct costs**, such as:

- Salaries (or partial salaries) for core members of the research team
- Stipends for consultants and support staff, such as interviewers and laboratory technicians
- Funds for the purchase of equipment and supplies
- Funds for office expenses
- Funds for compensating or reimbursing the expenses of study participants, such as providing a snack and paying for their parking
- Support for dissemination activities like presenting at conferences and paying for publications to be made open access

When developing a budget, money and materials are not the only resources to consider. For many studies, the most important resources are the individuals who are available to contribute their time, expertise, and/or connections to the project. Nonmonetary resources may include:

- Access to potential study participants (perhaps through a community organization or a local healthcare organization)
- Access to data sets (perhaps through a personal contact or a professional organization)
- Use of existing laboratory space, office space, and meeting rooms
- Availability of existing equipment, such as computers and copying machines

These can be highlighted in a grant proposal as part of the description of the research environment available to the researcher.

In addition to providing money to pay for direct costs, some funding agencies will also allow the host institution of the researchers to request a portion of the total grant budget for **facilities and administrative (F&A) costs**, which are alternatively called **indirect costs** or **overhead**. These funds support the institution's costs of maintaining research infrastructure, operating research facilities, purchasing library resources, and administering research functions such as ethics reviews and compliance reporting. Some foundations may not allow any overhead to be charged to the grant; some allow an indirect rate of 10% to 20% or more. Federal grants may allow for a much higher F&A rate to be applied to the grant. When preparing a budget, it is important to carefully read the funding agency's guidelines for what direct costs are allowable and what indirect rate (if any) can be requested.

It is not unusual for the funding cap from a source such as a student research award competition to be lower than the actual amount required for a project. In this situation, the researcher should show in the grant application which expenses will be covered by the new grant, if funded, and which will be supported by other sources. When submitting a proposal, the researcher should also ascertain the absolute minimum amount of support required and should be prepared to turn down offers of partial financial support that are inadequate for that project. For example, if the direct costs of a project will be $800 and funding is secured for only $250, the researcher may decide to use his or her time, energy, and money elsewhere.

25.5 Grant Management

Funders that have decided to support a research project will send an award letter or other notification to the grantee that specifies the amount of money being offered, the opening and closing dates for the grant, and the requirements of the grantee. Grant recipients are usually obligated to submit a series of reports to their institutions (if the grant is an internal one or has been awarded to the institution on behalf of the researcher) and/or to the granting agency. These reports are specific to the grant, and they are in addition to annual reviews of human subjects research protocols and any other paperwork required of all researchers at a particular institution. Grant-related documentation may be required at assigned times throughout the months or years the grant is active, such as:

- Initial paperwork related to accepting the terms and conditions of the grant
- Interim reports, including financial reports and scientific progress updates
- Final paperwork for the **closeout** of the grant, including a final accounting report and a final project outcome report

Keeping careful accounting records and regularly reconciling any differences between the researcher's records and the reports produced by the institution hosting the accounts for the project is of critical importance. Working closely with a budget officer at the host institution can prevent costly mistakes. All primary investigators and others with responsibilities on the grant should follow best practices for money management, including:

- Adhere to all of the policies, regulations, and laws of the funding organization, the host institution, and the government
- Maintain impeccable records of all project-related activities (including time sheets, if salaries or stipends are part of the budget)
- Confirm that every expenditure is an **allowable cost** before making a purchase (such as being aware of policies mandating that equipment be purchased from particular vendors and policies allowing meals but not alcohol to be purchased when traveling for grant-related work)
- Keep receipts for all purchases
- Maintain a log of all equipment and conduct regular inventory checks
- Consult with the granting agency (and any other relevant groups) before reallocating any portion of the approved budget to another area

- Check accounts at least monthly and conduct any **reconciliation** necessary to ensure that the balance in the grant account matches the balance in the financial records
- Conduct regular internal appraisals of accounting paperwork, equipment logs, and other documentation, and be prepared for a possible external **audit**

Financial reports may be required to be submitted to the host institution or funder on a monthly, quarterly, or yearly basis. Technical or performance reports are often also required to be submitted on a quarterly, semiannual, or annual basis. These reports typically provide information about the research activities completed under the grant since the previous report, including summaries of major findings and details about any project-related presentations or publications. (Some funders also request updates on all grant-related dissemination activities that occur in the years after the grant ends.)

If a portion of the budget has not been spent as the end date nears, some (but not all) funding agencies will allow **no-cost extensions** that postpone the closing date without adding new money to the grant's accounts. Others have a "use it or lose it" model and will take back any money that has not been appropriately disbursed within the original dates of the grant. Some funders offer the opportunity for currently funded researchers to apply for **grant renewals** or **grant continuations** that provide additional funding to extend the research project in new directions.

Closeout paperwork must usually be submitted shortly after the closing date for the grant. All grant-related paperwork must be retained for at least several years after closeout, in case the funder, the host institution, or a governmental agency require an audit to be conducted.

STEP

4

ANALYZING DATA

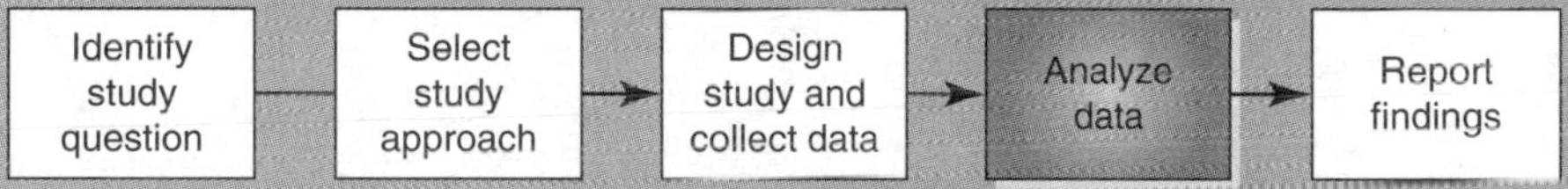

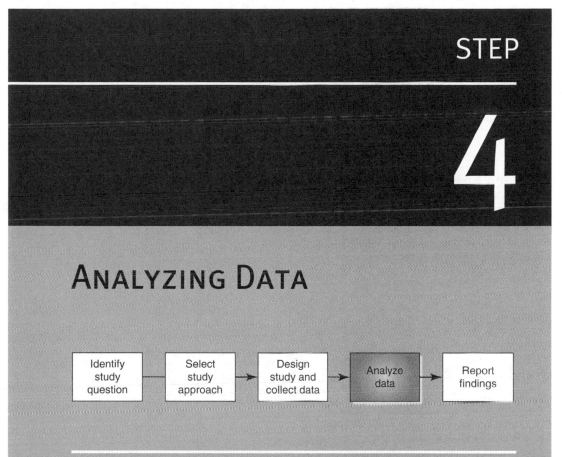

The fourth step in the research process is compiling and analyzing the data that were collected during step 3. Most research projects require only the use of descriptive and perhaps some comparative statistics, but others benefit from the use of advanced analytic methods.

- Data management
- Descriptive statistics
- Comparative statistics
- Regression analysis
- Other analysis tools

CHAPTER 26

DATA MANAGEMENT

Data entry, data cleaning, and recoding are important preparatory steps for data analysis.

26.1 Data Management

Data management refers to the entire process of record keeping, whether tracking articles considered for eligibility in a systematic review, extracting data from patient charts for a case series, logging the responses to a cross-sectional or case-control survey, or recording all the results of clinical assessments conducted during a longitudinal cohort or experimental study. Data managers must take care to protect the confidentiality of protected data and to ensure the integrity of data sets. After data are entered into a database or spreadsheet, the files need to be cleaned and perhaps recoded before beginning statistical analysis.

26.2 Codebooks

Prior to beginning data entry, it is useful to create a **codebook** that describes each variable and specifies how the collected information will be entered into a computer database (**Figure 26-1**). For quantitative surveys, numeric or alphabetical codes can be assigned to the options for the closed-ended response options provided on the questionnaire form. For open-ended questions and qualitative surveys, a codebook is even more essential because it provides clear instructions for how to code and enter free-response comments.

In addition to providing specific instructions about how each piece of information should be entered into the computer file, the codebook should specify:

- The name of each variable (which usually employs only a limited number of capital letters or a combination of capital letters and numbers, and avoids starting with a symbol such as an underscore)
- The variable type
- The wording of the question that was asked

FIGURE 26-1 Example of Codebook Entries

Question Number	Variable Name	Question	Variable Type	Variable Length	Codes
1	INTDATE	{Date of interview}	date	8	• Enter as DD-MM-YYYY
2	AGE	What is your age in years?	numeric	3	• Enter number • *Missing = 999*
3	SEX	What is your sex?	text	1	• Male = M • Female = F • Other/Prefer not to answer = 9 • Missing = {leave blank}
4	WORK	Which of the following categories best describes your work status?	text	10	• Working full time = FULLTIME • Working part time = PARTTIME • Unemployed but want to work = UNEMP • Retired = RETIRED • Student = STUDENT • Homemaker = HOME • Other = OTHER ➔ ***If OTHER go to 4b, otherwise skip to 5***

4b	WORK_OTHER	Other occupational description	text	50	• {Enter text as reported by respondent; only enter for those for whom WORK = OTHER.}
5	STUDENT	Are you currently enrolled in school?	text	1	• Yes = Y • No = N • *Don't know /Missing /Refused = D*
6	ALC	How often do you drink alcohol?	numeric	1	• Never = 0 • Less than 1 time a month = 1 • About 1 time a month = 2 • About 2 times a month = 3 • About 1 time a week = 4 • About 2–3 times a week = 5 • About 4–5 times a week = 6 • Every day or almost every day = 7 • *Don't know* = 8 • *Refused/missing* = 9
7	STD_EVER	Has a doctor ever told you that you had a sexually transmitted disease?	numeric	1	• Yes = 1 • No = 0 • *Don't know* = 7 • *Refused to answer* = 8 • *Missing* = 9

- The options listed on the survey instrument as possible answers to the question
- The way answers should be entered into the computer database
- How to handle missing responses

The codebook is also the place to describe how anticipated data problems will be handled. For example, what should be done if a respondent selects two answers from a multiple choice list when the instructions said to select only one? What if the handwriting on a form is illegible or the person doing the data entry is not absolutely certain about what the words say or which box was checked? If unanticipated quandaries arise, the codebook should be amended to state how the situation was addressed, so that there is a record of the decision and future issues can be resolved in ways that are consistent with that decision.

The codebook will also specify for each variable whether missing answers should be left blank in the database, indicated with a numeric code (such as entering a 9 if the expected entry code is 0 or 1 for a dichotomous variable), or marked with the word "MISSING." The statistical analysis process may need adjustment based on what the codebook says about how missing data were handled. For example, if missing information about age is entered as 999, all of the "999" entries will need to be removed prior to analysis or else the mean age will end up artificially high and the corresponding standard deviation will be very large.

26.3 Data Entry

Data are usually entered into a **database** program (like Microsoft Access). Databases can be designed to be visually appealing, to facilitate consistent entry of the acceptable responses for each question, and to perform automatic skips between questions when such jumps are indicated on the survey instrument. This ensures the uniformity of entries and the completeness of the file.

An alternative option is to enter the data directly into a **spreadsheet** program (like Microsoft Excel). Variable names should be entered in the first row, with one variable per column. Each individual's data should be in a new row, with the first line of data in the second row. The advantage of this data entry approach is that it does not require creating a data entry form, defining fields and variable names, and doing other coding and testing of the data entry system. The disadvantage is that it is easy to accidentally enter new data over an existing row of data or to input inconsistent codes, which makes cleaning the data much more difficult. Both database and spreadsheet files can be uploaded into popular statistical software programs for analysis.

It may be worth doing double-entry of at least some of the completed paper-based survey forms (often a minimum of 10% of them) to confirm the accuracy of data entry. **Double-entry** consists of two individuals entering the same data (or the same person entering the data twice) into two different computer files and then comparing the records in the two files for agreement. Special software programs (such as the Data Compare utility that is part of the U.S. CDC's free Epi Info program) allow the individual records stored in two files to be linked by an ID number or other unique variable and then compared. These programs usually provide statistics about the agreement level. If the agreement is not extremely high, then double-entry of all records is probably required to ensure the accuracy of the final data file. File comparison programs facilitate the creation of a clean final data file after double-entry. They identify disputed entries and allow the researcher to select the best response for the final clean data file after consulting the original survey forms. For example, suppose one of the two database files indicates that a participant was 32 years old, and the other says that the participant was 42 years old. The original form completed by the participant may show that the true age is 42, and 42 can be selected as the correct entry for the cleaned file.

26.4 Data Cleaning

Data cleaning is the process of correcting any typographical or other errors in data files. **Figure 26-2** shows how errors such as extra spaces, typos, and the use of lowercase instead of capital letters can be corrected so that the responses all adhere to the codebook. When paper-based data collection methods are used, fixing incorrect entries sometimes requires looking up the original survey forms. For example, while an "m" or "N" for SEX might reasonably be assumed to be a mistyped "M," it is not clear whether an "R" for STUDENT refers to a "Y" or an "N." Whenever there is doubt about the true value, the respondent's original file should be consulted. Missing

FIGURE 26-2 Example of Data Cleaning

	Before Cleaning		After Cleaning	
Variable	**Response**	**Frequency**	**Response**	**Frequency**
SEX	F	498	F	498
	M	493	M	497
	m	3		
	N	1		
STUDENT	N	899	N	903
	N	2	Y	89
	R	1	[Missing]	2
	Y	87		
	y	1		
	[Missing]	4		

values in a computer database may also require reference back to the original survey forms, because information missing in the computer file may have been written on the survey forms but been overlooked by the data entry person.

The data cleaning steps is also an appropriate time to remove extremely unreasonable responses. For example, suppose a participant's age in years is listed as 192. This number can reasonably be assumed to be a typo, and the original survey form should be consulted for the true age. If the survey form lists the age as 192 or if the survey was computer-assisted and there is no paper trail, then this value should be excluded from analysis because it is clearly an impossible age. However, a study of adults could reasonably include an individual with an age of 105 years. So a value of 105 would not be reasonable to delete or ignore, but it would be worth checking the original survey form for agreement with the entry in the database.

Data cleaning should also ensure that duplicate entries are removed from the database and that the records are complete, with all data from all participants entered into the database.

26.5 Data Recoding

The **recoding** of variables into new categories can be done either prior to or during data analysis. Recoding prior to analysis is often the easiest approach when the intended new categories are known. Database and statistical programs typically offer two mechanisms for creating **derived variables**. One option is to recode based on categories. For example, the variable AGE could be used to create a new variable ADULT that is coded as 0 (no) for any participant younger than 18 years old and 1 (yes) for any participant age 18 or older (**Figure 26-3**). The other option is to calculate new values using mathematical operators. For example, height and weight variables can be used

FIGURE 26-3 Example of Recoding

Original Variable	Derived Variable	Example of coding
AGE	ADULT	
6	0	
29	1	IF AGE < 18, ADULT = 0
43	1	IF AGE > 17, ADULT = 1
14	0	IF AGE = [MISSING], ADULT = [MISSING]
91	1	
50	1	

FIGURE 26-4 Example of Recalculating

Original Variable	Original Variable	Derived Variable	Example of coding
HT_IN	WT_LB	BMI	
66	155	25.0	
73	253	33.4	
59	112	22.6	BMI = (WT_LB / (HT_IN * HT_IN)) * 703
63	159	28.2	
70	180	25.8	
61	98	18.5	

to calculate a derived variable for the body mass index (**Figure 26-4**). Other types of mathematical operators can be used to generate the number of days between two dates and to conduct other types of calculations.

A few basic practices will help protect a cleaned data file. Never do any recoding until an original version of the cleaned data file is safely backed up elsewhere. A saved file allows a researcher to start anew if a file is damaged during recoding. Also, never recode into the same variable; that is, do not replace the original values with the new recoded values. Instead, always recode into a different (new) variable. Having both the original variable and the new variable in the file enables the researcher to compare the original and recoded values and confirm that the recoding was done correctly.

26.6 Data Security

Data security is the process of protecting computer files with passwords and other mechanisms for restricting unauthorized access and use. It is legally and ethically necessary to maintain the confidentiality of any potentially identifiable personal information participants disclose to researchers with the expectation of privacy. It is especially important to be careful with **protected health information (PHI)**, any information about an individual's health history or health status that by law must be kept confidential. One way to maintain confidentiality is to safely store paper records, including signed informed consent statements, in a locked and secure room. Another is to destroy individually identifying information once the records are no longer needed (such as after the data have been entered into a computer file and the files have been thoroughly cleaned) and a research ethics committee has approved the secure disposal of consent statements and other documents.

Data protection also requires the creation of secure computerized data files. In general, no individually identifying information (such as a name or national identity card number) should be included in an electronic file containing other information about participants (such as responses to survey questions or the results of laboratory tests). If there is a need to link records to individuals—something which is rarely necessary unless the study is following participants forward in time across multiple assessment periods—then two separate files linked by a unique study identification number should be maintained. One should contain participant names and contact information. The other should include all other study data. The file containing identifying information should be securely stored separately from the file that contains the other participant data. Access to all files containing sensitive information should be password-protected, and access to them should be limited to essential research personnel. A consultation with an information technology expert prior to data collection can help ensure the security of participant information.

CHAPTER 27

Descriptive Statistics

When used correctly, statistics provide essential information for making sense of health research data. Descriptive statistics describe the basic characteristics of quantitative data.

27.1 Analytic Plan by Study Approach

Statistics can be used to tell a complete and compelling story about the quantitative data collected during a research study. For most research reports, and especially those written by researchers with limited experience in advanced statistics, the goal of analysis should be to use the simplest statistics possible to make the results of the study clear to the researcher and the intended audience for findings. Most research studies do not require the use of complex statistics like regression, and using advanced statistical tests incorrectly is never helpful.

The type of analytic plan that is commonly used with each of the major study approaches is shown in **Figure 27-1**. Each plan starts with a description of the study population. Studies with no comparison group, like case series and cross-sectional surveys, may find that **univariate analysis** describing each key variable without comparing variables is sufficient. Simple statistics like counts (frequencies), proportions, and averages are likely to provide an adequate description of the study population. For studies that compare two or more populations—including case-control, cohort, and experimental studies—the description of the study populations must be completed before moving on to **bivariable analysis**, which uses rate ratios, odds ratios, and other comparative statistical tests to examine the relationship between two variables (one designated as the exposure and one designated as the outcome). **Multivariable analysis** that examines three or more characteristics of participants at one time is usually not required.

FIGURE 27-1 Analytic Plan

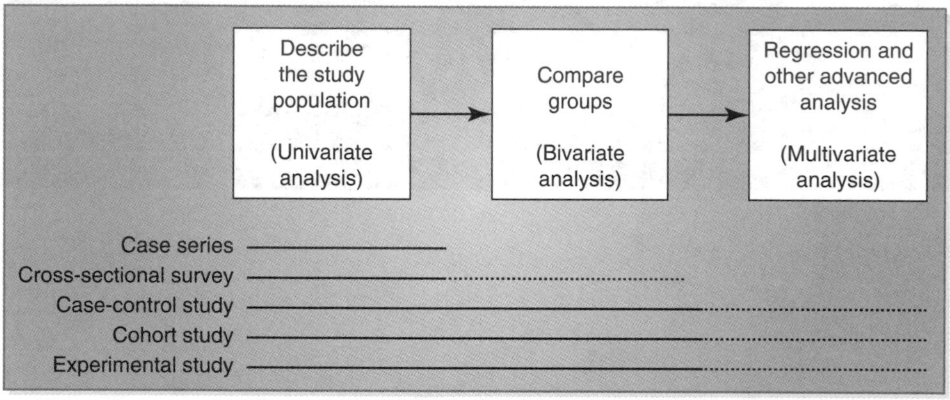

27.2 Types of Variables

A **variable** is a characteristic that can be assigned more than one value. Examples of variables that could be examined during a population health study are age, sex, annual income, languages spoken at home, frequency of alcohol ingestion, cholesterol level, history of chickenpox, and use of contact lenses. The value of a variable for an individual does not have to vary (change) over time, but the response among individuals within a population should be something that might differ.

In most statistical and database programs, responses from individual participants are displayed in rows with each column representing one variable. For example, one column of data may represent sex. One value for sex—such as an F or 0 for females or an M or 1 for males—will be listed in each row. Another column may represent age in years, and one value for age—usually a whole number—will be listed in each row.

There are several ways to classify variables (**Figure 27-2**).

- **Ratio variables** have numeric responses on a scale for which a value of zero indicates "nothing." For example, if height is measured in feet, a measurement of 0 feet tall means that there was no height. As a result, the ratio of heights is meaningful. A person who is 6 feet tall is twice as tall as a person who is 3 feet tall, yielding a ratio of 2 to 1.
- **Interval variables** are also numeric, but they are on a scale for which zero does not stand for "nothing." An outside temperature of 0°C does not mean that there is no heat; if the weather turns colder, the temperature may fall to –10°C or lower. A day with a high temperature of 40°F is not twice as hot as a day with a maximum temperature of 20°F.
- **Ordinal variables**, also called **ranked variables**, order responses from first to last or from best to worst or from most favorable to least favorable. The

FIGURE 27-2 Types of Variables

Variable Type	Definition	Examples
Ratio	Numbers on a scale that has a meaningful zero	Blood pressure, height, weight (If the weight increases from 10 kg to 20 kg, the weight has doubled; so the ratio of 20 kg to 10 kg is meaningful.)
Interval	Numbers on a scale that does not have a meaningful zero	Temperature (°F or °C) (The temperature does not double if it increases from 20° to 40° because 0° does not represent the absence of all heat.)
Ordinal/ranked	An ordered series that assigns a rank to responses (from first to last in the series) but for which the numbers assigned to the values are not meaningful	Highest educational degree earned, scales for never (1) to always (5), scales for strongly disagree (1) to strongly agree (5)
Nominal/categorical	Categories with no inherent rank or order	Employment category, blood type
Binomial	Categorical variables for which only two responses are possible	yes/no, male/female, case/control

rank order can be assigned a number. For example, the responses to a survey that asks participants to indicate their level of agreement with a statement can be coded with agree as "3," neutral as "2," and disagree as "1." Alternatively, responses could be coded with agree as "1" and disagree as "3." Or neutral could be set as "0," agree as "1," and disagree as "–1." No matter what the scale is, the order of the responses is indicated by their numeric values. (Figure 18-4 provides examples of other types of ranked responses.)

- **Nominal variables**, also called **categorical variables**, have responses that represent groups with no inherent rank or order. For example, there is no obvious way to numerically rank the favorite recreational sports activities of participants or their blood types. **Binomial variables** are a subtype of categorical variable with only two possible answers, usually yes and no. These are often called **dichotomous variables**.

Ratio and interval variables can be further classified as either continuous variables or discrete variables.

- **Continuous variables** can take on any value within a range. For example, although height is often rounded to the nearest inch when it is measured, a person's height could actually be 64½ inches or 73¾ inches or 58.1528 inches.
- **Discrete variables** typically result from counting something, so there are gaps between acceptable values. For example, a family can own 2 egg-laying chickens or 17 chickens, but cannot own 2½ chickens or 5¼ chickens.

27.3 Measures of Central Tendency

Descriptive statistics are often used to describe the "average" value of a variable in a population. For numeric variables, the average is often referred to as the **central tendency**. There are several ways to report the average (**Figure 27-3**).

- The sample **mean** is calculated by adding up the values of all responses provided to a question and dividing that sum by the total number of individuals who answered the question.
- The **median** is the middle number when all responses are put in order from least to greatest. Half of the responses in a data set will be greater than the median, and half will be less.
- The **mode** is the most common answer given by respondents.

For ratio and interval variables, the central tendency can be described using means, medians, and modes. For ordinal variables, a median or mode can be reported. A mode can be reported for categorical variables.

FIGURE 27-3 Example of a Mean, Median, and Mode

Values Reported by Participants	Measure of Central Tendency	Value	Calculation
25	Mean	39.5	(25 + 30 + 30 + 40 + 50 + 62) ÷ 6 = 237 ÷ 6 = 39.5
40			
30	Median	35	The two middle values from 25-30-30-40-50-62 are 30 and 40; 35 is halfway between 30 and 40.
50			
30	Mode	30	Two participants provided a response of 30; no other responses were listed more than once.
62			

27.4 Range and Quartiles

Means and medians provide information about the center of a data set, but they do not provide information about how much variability exists in the data set. For example, the participants in a study of adults with a mean age of 50 years may all be 50 years old, or they could range from 18 to 104 years old. That information about the study population is very important when interpreting the meaning of the results. Measures of **spread**, also called **dispersion**, are used to describe the variability and distribution of responses.

For a particular variable, the response with the lowest numeric value is the **minimum** and the response with the highest value is the **maximum**. The **range** for a variable is the difference between the minimum and the maximum. For example, if the youngest participant in a study is 18 years old and the oldest is 104 years old, the range is 104 – 18 = 86 years.

The median marks the value that divides the responses into two halves with equal numbers of observations. **Quartiles** mark the three values that divide a data set into four equal parts. Similarly, **tertiles** divide a data set into three equal parts, quintiles divide a data set into five equal parts, and **deciles** divide a data set into 10 equal parts. The **interquartile range (IQR)** is the range for the 25th to 75th percentiles, which captures the middle 50% of responses.

27.5 Displaying Distributions

A **histogram** is usually the best way to display the responses to a numeric variable like a ratio variable or an interval variable (**Figure 27-4**). On a histogram, the *x*-axis shows the values of responses, and the *y*-axis shows the count of the number of

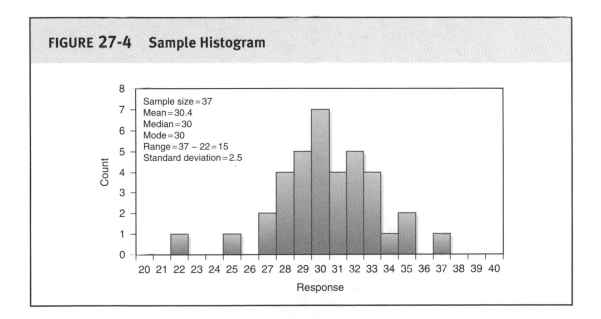

FIGURE 27-4 Sample Histogram

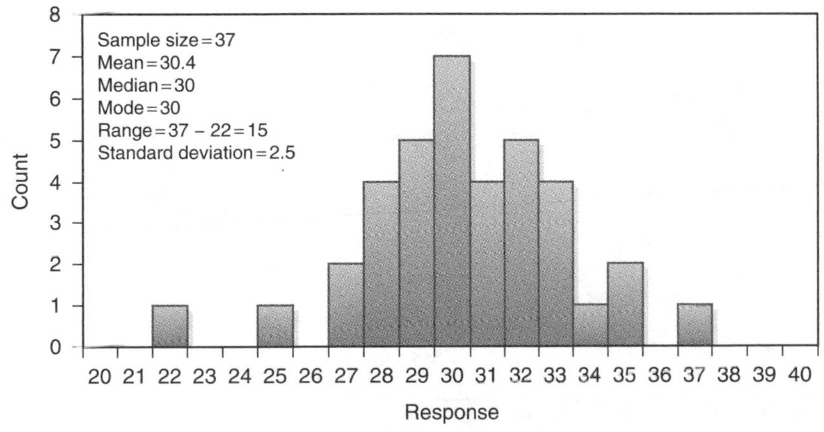

times each response was appears in the data set. For a graph to be considered a histogram, each bar must be the same width. Importantly, there should be no gaps between the bars in the middle of the distribution, where responses are clumped together. (There can be gaps to indicate values of the variable with a count of 0 responses.)

A **boxplot** (also called a box-and-whisker plot) can be used to display information for both ratio/interval and ordinal/ranked variables (**Figure 27-5**). Boxplots can be especially helpful for displaying the distribution of responses when the responses are skewed. Skewing occurs when the "whiskers" on the boxplot extend much farther on one side of the median than on the other side.

For categorical variables, it is not possible to create a histogram or boxplot. The distribution of responses must instead be displayed in a bar chart or, less often, a pie chart. Like a histogram, the *x*-axis of a **bar chart** shows the values of responses, and the *y*-axis shows the count of the times each response appears in the data set. However, for a bar chart the *x*-axis can display either a number or a word. And although histograms require numbered bars to be evenly spaced along a number line, responses on bar charts may appear in any order (**Figure 27-6**). The bars in bar charts can be displayed vertically or horizontally, and there are usually spaces

FIGURE 27-5 Sample Boxplot

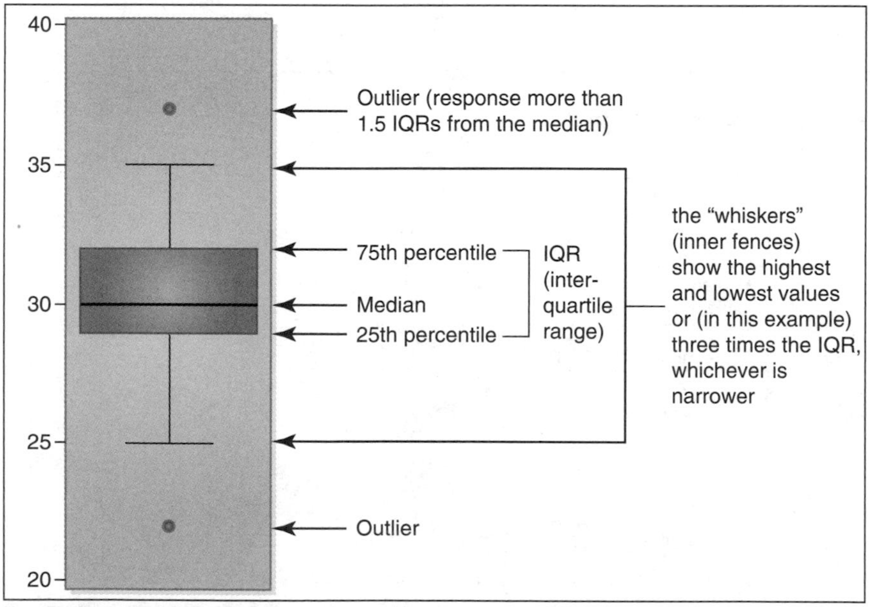

Note: This figure displays the same data as shown in Figure 27-4

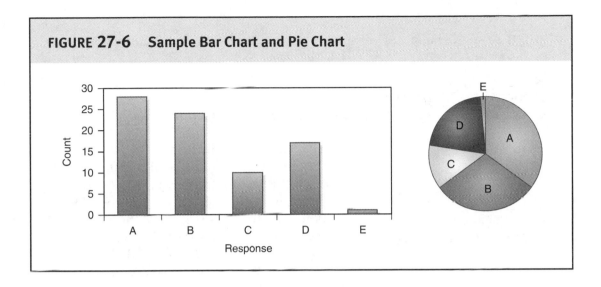

FIGURE 27-6 Sample Bar Chart and Pie Chart

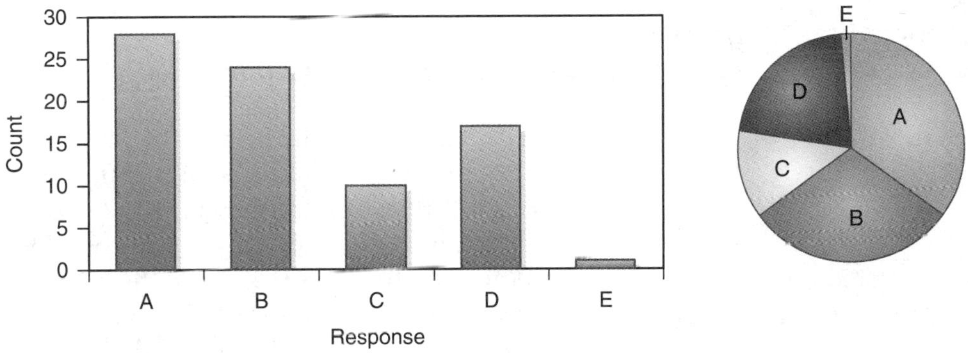

between the bars. A **pie chart** is a circle in which each of the "wedges" or "slices" of the "pie" display the percentage of participants who provided a particular answer to one question. The sum of the percentages for the slices must add up to 100%. Unlike bar graphs, pie charts cannot be used when participants were allowed to select multiple responses to a question.

27.6 Normal Curves, Variance, and Standard Deviation

A histogram showing a **normal distribution** (or **Gaussian distribution**) or an approximately normal distribution of responses will have a bell-shaped curve with one peak in the middle. **Kurtosis** describes how peaked or flat a distribution is: A **leptokurtic** curve is very peaked, a mesokurtic curve is average, and a **platykurtic** curve is flat. However, not all numeric variables have a perfectly normal distribution. The distribution may show **skewness**, with responses that extend farther from the peak on either the left (left-skewed) or the right (right-skewed) side of the histogram. The distribution may have a **bimodal** (two-peaked) distribution instead of being **unimodal** (one peak). Or the histogram may show a **uniform distribution**, with about equal numbers of people providing each response.

For variables with a relatively normal distribution—a reasonably bell-shaped curve—there are three different ways to quantify the narrowness or wideness of the distribution of the responses (**Figure 27-7**). The **variance** is the sum of the squares of the differences between each point and the mean divided by the sample size. The **standard deviation** is the square root of the variance. The **standard error** of the mean is a measure that adjusts for the number of observations in the data set by dividing the variance by the sample size before taking the square root.

FIGURE 27-7 Example of Variance, Standard Deviation, and Standard Error

Values Reported by Participants	Measure of Spread	Value	Equation	Calculation
25 40 30 50 30 62	Variance	201.5	The sum of the squares of the differences between each point and the mean divided by the sample size minus 1 (in a sample drawn from a larger population)	$[(25 - 39.5)^2 + (40 - 39.5)^2 + (30 - 39.5)^2 + (50 - 39.5)^2 + (30 - 39.5)^2 + (62 - 39.5)^2]/(6 - 1) = [14.5^2 + (-0.5)^2 + 9.5^2 + (-10.5)^2 + 9.5^2 + (-22.5)^2]/5 = [210.25 + 0.25 + 90.25 + 110.25 + 90.25 + 506.25]/5 = 1007.5/5 = 201.5$
	Standard deviation	14.2	The square root of the variance	$\sqrt{201.5} = 14.1951$
	Standard error of the mean	5.8	The square root of the variance divided by the sample size	$\sqrt{\frac{201.5}{6}} = 5.7951$

The standard deviation is number most commonly used to describe the spread of normally distributed variables (**Figure 27-8**). When the responses are normal:

- 68% of responses fall within one standard deviation above or below the mean
- 95% of responses are within two standard deviations above or below the mean
- More than 99% of responses are within three standard deviations above or below the mean

A small standard deviation indicates that most responses were fairly close to the mean. A large standard deviation indicates that the distribution of responses was wide. A **z-score** indicates how many standard deviations away from the sample mean the response for an individual from within that population is. For example:

- An individual whose age is exactly the mean age in the population will have a *z*-score of 0.

FIGURE 27-8 Standard Deviations for Normally-Distributed Numeric Variables

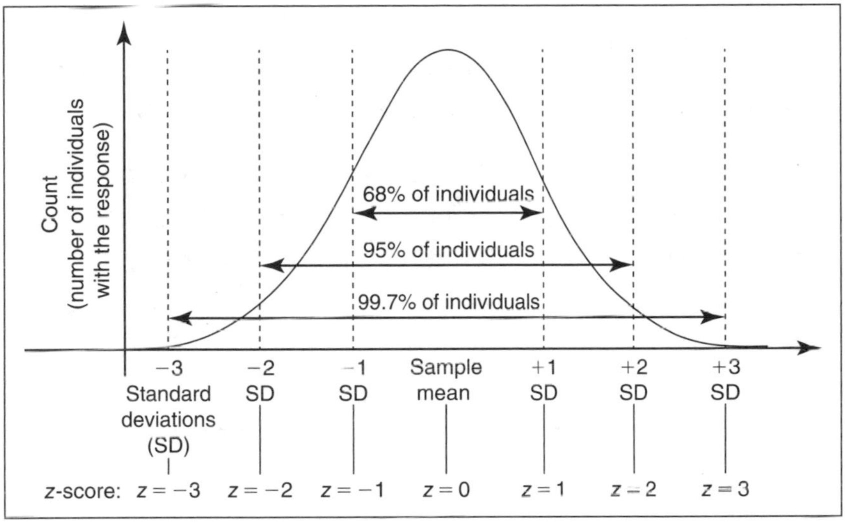

- A person whose age is one standard deviation above the mean in the population will have a *z*-score of 1.
- A person whose age is two standard deviations below the population mean will have a *z*-score of –2.

27.7 Reporting Descriptive Statistics

The goal of **descriptive statistics** is to accurately describe the responses to a variable (**Figure 27-9**).

- For ratio and interval variables, both the mean and the standard deviation are typically reported.
- For ordinal variables (and for ratio and interval variables with a non-normal distribution), the median and interquartile range are often reported.
- For categorical variables, the proportions of participants who provided particular responses are usually used to describe the population.

27.8 Confidence Intervals

Confidence intervals (CIs) provide information about the expected value of a measure in a source population based on the value of that measure in a study population (**Figure 27-10**). For example, if the mean age in a study population

FIGURE 27-9 Common Descriptive Statistics by Variable Type

Variable Type	Common Measure of Central Tendency	Common Measure of Spread	Common Graphical Display
Ratio	Mean	Standard deviation	Histogram
Interval	Mean	Standard deviation	Histogram
Ordinal/ranked	Median	Interquartile range	Boxplot
Nominal/categorical	Mode	—	Bar chart, pie chart
Binomial	Mode	—	—

of 100 people randomly sampled from all workers at a large company is 30 years, the researcher should not assume that the mean age of all employees is exactly 30 years. The 95% confidence interval states how close to 30 years the mean age in the source population (the company) is expected to be. If the 95% confidence interval for the mean age in the study population extends from 26 to 34, a researcher can be 95% confident that the mean age of all employees is between 26 and 34 years.

The width of the interval is related to the sample size of the study. A larger sample size will yield a narrower confidence interval. If every member of the source population is included in the study population, then a confidence interval is not needed because the exact value for the source population will be known.

A 95% confidence interval is usually reported for statistical estimates, and that 95% CI corresponds to a significance level of $\alpha = 0.05$ for a statistical test. This means that 5% of the time a 95% confidence interval is expected to miss capturing the true value of a measure in the source population. Using a 99% confidence interval ($\alpha = 0.01$) would make the confidence interval wider and make it more likely that the value in the source population would be captured within the confidence interval. However, it would also make it more difficult to classify a result as statistically significant because fewer results would be classified as extreme. Alternatively, a 90% confidence interval ($\alpha = 0.10$) could be used. A 90% confidence interval would be narrower and make it easier for a result to be deemed statistically significant because more results would be classified as extreme. However, a 90% confidence interval would be less likely than a 95% confidence interval to capture the true value in the source population.

FIGURE 27-10 Interpreting Confidence Intervals

Statistic	Result with 95% CI	Interpretation
Mean age of all participants (years)	30 (28, 32)	Based on the mean age in the study population (30 years), we are 95% confident that the mean age in the source population is between 28 and 32 years.
Proportion of all participants with a disease (%)	9.0 (7.3, 10.9)	Based on the proportion of individuals in the study population who had the disease (9.0%), we are 95% confident that the prevalence of disease in the source population is between 7.3% and 10.9%.

27.9 Statistical Honesty

Researchers are obligated to describe their data accurately and to correctly report the results of statistical tests. To do otherwise is a form of research misconduct. Three of the most serious forms of research misconduct are:

- **Fabrication**: The creation of fake data, such as creating fictitious rows of data in a spreadsheet for people who never completed a questionnaire or never participated in an experiment
- **Falsification**: The misrepresentation of results, such as modifying extreme data values to improve the results of statistical tests, manipulating photographs or other images collected during laboratory work, or intentionally misreporting a study's methods to make the study look more rigorous than it was
- Plagiarism: The use of other people's ideas, words, or images without proper attribution

Statistical honesty requires more than merely avoiding outright falsification, fabrication, and plagiarism. It also requires adherence to accepted statistical practices. For example, it may be tempting to look for statistical tests that will yield the results the researcher desires, such as ones that are considered statistically significant. However, scientific integrity requires researchers to follow established statistical practices. Consider these examples of unacceptable practices:

- It is not acceptable to run a dozen different types of statistical tests on a data set, hoping that one of them will happen to yield a statistically significant result to feature in a report. Instead, the researcher must select the correct test for the question being asked and the variables being examined.

- It is not appropriate to recode ratio variables into categorical variables by preferentially selecting the cutoff values that yield statistically significant results for tests of the new categorical variable. In general, it is better to use quartiles or other pre-selected divisions when recoding into new categories.
- It is not permissible to ignore **outliers**—unusual responses to a question—where there is not a valid and widely accepted reason for doing so. For example, a recorded birth weight of 80 pounds may be reasonably assumed to be an error in the data file, and it can be removed from analysis. But it is not reasonable to remove an 80-pound adult from the data file because an adult could weigh 80 pounds.

Statistical analysis is about discovering the true story in a data set, not about creatively manipulating data toward a preferred result.

27.10 Consultation and Collaboration

Ideally, the researcher should consult with a statistician during the study design process to ensure that:

- The sampling methods and sample size are appropriate.
- The questionnaire will yield usable data.
- The analysis plan is a reasonable one.

Checking with an expert for the first time later in the research process increases the risk of unfixable flaws in the study data. If answering the study question adequately requires the use of elaborate analytic techniques, invite an expert in that technique to serve as a collaborator and as a coauthor on the resulting research report. An invitation to collaborate should be made as early as possible in the project and in consultation with other coauthors (see Chapter 6).

CHAPTER 28

Comparative Statistics

Comparative statistics compare groups of participants by sex or age, by exposure or disease status, or by other characteristics. Examples of comparative statistical tests include rate ratios, odds ratios, t-tests, and Chi-square tests.

28.1 Comparative Analysis by Study Approach

Comparative statistics categorize study participants into two or more groups and then use tests to compare the characteristics of those groups. For example, the analysis of a case-control study requires using comparative tests to show that the cases (people with the disease) and controls (people without the disease) in the study are similar in terms of age distribution and other demographic characteristics. Then additional comparative tests are applied to determine whether the exposure histories of cases and controls are different. Similar comparative tests can also be used to compare the disease outcomes of exposed and unexposed participants in a cohort study, or to compare the before and after characteristics of participants in an experimental study. **Figure 28-1** summarizes the uses of comparative statistical tests for several common study approaches.

28.2 Hypotheses for Statistical Tests

Comparative statistical tests are designed to test for difference rather than for sameness. Accordingly, the questions driving the selection of hypotheses for statistical tests are usually phrased in terms of differences: Are the means different? Are the proportions different? Are the distributions different? Each question about statistical difference has two possible answers: The values are either different or not different.

The term **null hypothesis (H_0)** describes the expected result of a statistical test if there is no difference between the two or more values being compared. Null means nothing or zero. A **null result** means that there was no statistically significant difference. The **alternative hypothesis (H_a)** describes the expected result if there is

FIGURE 28-1 Analytic Plan for Comparing Groups

Study Approach	First Step	Key Analysis
Case-control study	Show that cases and controls are similar except for disease status	Use odds ratios (ORs) to see whether cases and controls have different exposure histories
Cohort study	Show that the exposed and unexposed are similar except for exposure status	Use rate ratios (RRs) to see whether the exposed and unexposed have different rates of incident disease
Experimental study	Show that the individuals assigned to the intervention and control groups are similar except for exposure status	Use RRs and other measures to see if the intervention and control groups have different outcomes

a difference between the two or more populations being compared (**Figure 28-2**). For example, for a test to compare the mean ages of two groups of study participants, the hypotheses could be as follows:

- H_0: There is *no* significant difference between the two means.
- H_a: There *is* a significant difference between the two means.

A test to compare the distribution of responses to a categorical question in two groups would have as hypotheses:

- H_0: There is *no* significant difference in the distribution of responses in the two populations.
- H_a: There *is* a significant difference in the distribution of responses in the two populations.

28.3 Rejecting the Null Hypothesis

Because statistical tests do not ask questions about sameness, the answers provided by statistical tests do not allow a researcher to say conclusively whether two values are the same. Instead, a researcher must make a decision about whether the results of a statistical test indicate that values are different or not different. The language used to describe this decision is that the researcher will either "reject the null hypothesis" or "fail to reject the null hypothesis."

- Rejecting the null hypothesis means concluding that the values are different by rejecting the claim that the values are not different.

FIGURE 28-2 Examples of Hypotheses for Statistical Tests

Goal	Statistical Question	Null Hypothesis (H_0)	Alternative Hypothesis (H_a)
Test whether the average ages of cases and controls in a case-control study are similar	Are the means *different*?	The means are *not* different.	The means *are* different.
Test whether the mean age of participants drawn from a population with a mean age of 40 years is close enough to 40 years that the study population can be considered representative of the source population	Was the mean age in the study population *different* from 40 years?	The mean is *not* different from 40.	The mean *is* different from 40.
Test whether the proportion of responses to a categorical question about the frequency of flossing was similar for male and female participants in a cohort study	Are the distributions of responses *different*?	The distributions are *not* different.	The distributions *are* different.
Test whether participants, on average, had a change in their scores on a pretest administered prior to an intervention and a post-test administered after the intervention	Are the before scores of participants *different* from the after scores?	The scores are *not* different.	The scores *are* different.

- Failing to reject the null hypothesis means concluding that there is no evidence that the values are different. Functionally, this is like saying that the values are close enough to be considered similar, but failing to reject the null hypothesis should never be taken as evidence that the values are the same.

The decision to reject or fail to reject the null hypothesis is based on the likelihood that the result of a test was due to chance. One way to understand the concept of chance is to consider the variability in sample populations. When a sample population is drawn from a source population, the mean age in the sample population is usually not exactly the mean age of the source population. (See Figure 17-1 for an illustration of the variety of sample means that can occur in different samples drawn from one source population.) The range of expected values for the mean age of sample populations drawn from a source population can be estimated using statistics (**Figure 28-3**). Some sample populations will have mean ages that are very close to the mean in the source population; other sample populations will have mean ages that are quite far from the mean in the source population. No set cutoff defines what will be considered extremely far from the mean age in the source population, but the standard is to say that the 5% of sample means farthest from the true mean are extreme. Thus, by chance, 5% of the samples drawn from a source population will be expected to have an extreme mean.

Similarly, if two sample populations are drawn from the same source population, their mean ages will not be identical even though they are drawn from the same pool of individuals. Comparative statistical tests accommodate this expected difference when testing whether two groups in a study population are different. For example,

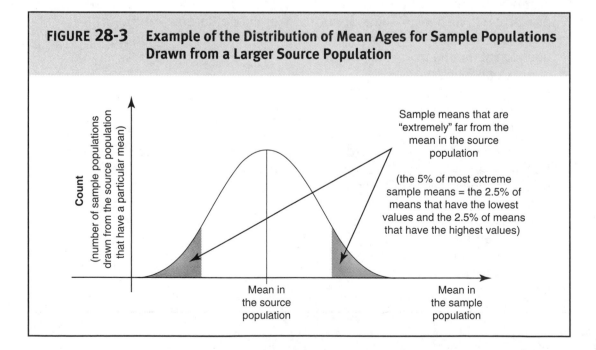

FIGURE 28-3 Example of the Distribution of Mean Ages for Sample Populations Drawn from a Larger Source Population

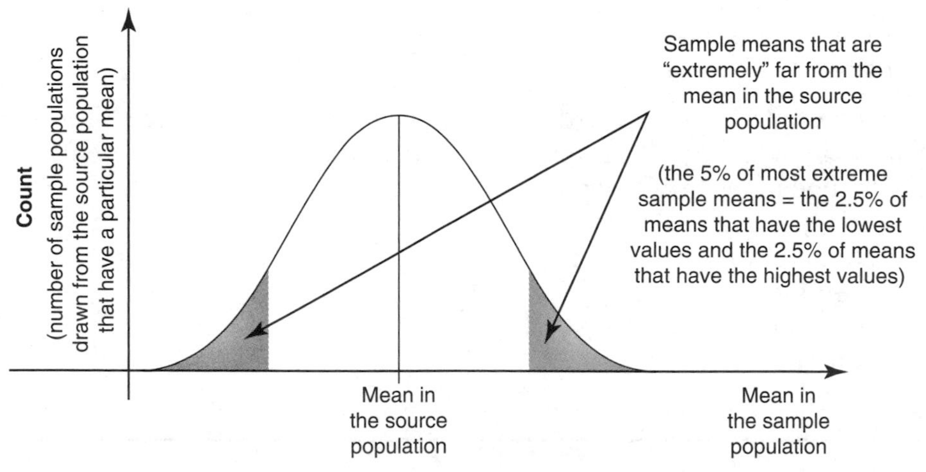

a test that compares the mean ages of cases and controls in a case-control study adjusts for the fact that there will be some difference between the mean ages of cases and controls even when the cases and controls are sampled from source populations with identical mean ages. The test also determines whether the mean ages are so far apart that, if the cases and controls were drawn from source populations with the same mean age, the difference between the mean ages of the cases and the controls would fall among the most extreme differences expected by chance. When the statistical test shows that the mean ages of cases and controls are fairly close, the researcher will fail to reject the null hypothesis and will conclude that the means are not different. When the difference between the mean ages of cases and controls is extreme, the statistical test will show that it is highly unlikely that the group means are not different. The researcher will therefore reject the null hypothesis and conclude that the mean ages of the cases and the controls are different. The difference between the mean ages of cases and controls in the study population will be taken as evidence that the mean age of individuals in the source population for cases and the mean age of individuals in the source population for controls are different. This conclusion assumes that the difference between the source populations is reflected in the sample of cases and controls that happened to be drawn from their respective source populations. Comparative statistics like these are called **inferential statistics** because the researcher does not study an entire population but instead makes inferences—that is, evidence-based assumptions—about the full population based on a sample of members of that population.

28.4 Interpreting *p*-Values

A ***p*-value**, or **probability value**, for a statistical test is used to decide whether the results observed are likely to reflect real differences between groups. The interpretation is similar for all statistical tests: The *p*-value for the study determines whether the null hypothesis (H_0) will be rejected. The standard is to use a **significance level** of $\alpha = 0.05$, or 5%. Any statistical test with a result that is in the 5% of most extreme responses expected by chance when the null hypothesis is true will result in the rejection of the null hypothesis (**Figure 28-4**).

In comparative statistics, a type 1 error occurs when a test indicates a significant difference between two or more populations even though the null hypothesis is true. This type of error will happen 5% of the time if the analyst has selected a 5% significance level. Choosing a significance level of 1% ($\alpha = 0.01$) will reduce the probability of a type 1 error, but will make it more difficult to reject the null hypothesis. Choosing a significance level of 10% ($\alpha = 0.10$) will increase the probability of a type 1 error, causing 1 in 10 tests to indicate "difference" even if there really is no difference in the source population. But a 10% significance level will make it more likely that a test will yield a statistically significant result.

Some *p*-values are reported as being one-sided or two-sided, based on the alternative hypothesis for the statistical test. Although most statistical tests use an alternative

FIGURE 28-4 Interpreting *p*-Values

H_0	Conclusion when $p < 0.05^*$ = reject H_0	Conclusion when $p \geq 0.05^*$ = fail to reject H_0
The means are not different.	The means are different.	The means are not different.
The proportions are not different.	The proportions are different.	The proportions are not different.
The distributions are not different.	The distributions are different.	The distributions are not different.

*Assuming $\alpha = 0.05$.

hypothesis that simply expresses difference (such as "the means are different"), some tests allow for an alternative hypothesis that states the direction of the difference (like, "males have a higher mean age than females") (**Figure 28-5**). If a direction is specified in the alternative hypothesis, then all of the extreme values (all of the shaded area shown in Figure 28-3) will be on one side of the distribution (either all on the left of the distribution or all on the right). When this direction is specified, a **one-sided *p*-value** can be used. In all other situations, a **two-sided *p*-value** should be used to make the decision about rejecting or failing to reject the null hypothesis.

28.5 Measures of Association

Some of the most common types of comparative statistics used in the health sciences are the measures of association explained in the chapters on the various study approaches, such as the correlation used for aggregate studies, the odds ratio (OR) used for case-control studies, and the rate ratio (RR) used for cohort studies.

The OR and RR compare responses to two variables that have each been divided into two levels using what is often called 2×2 analysis. Prior to using a computer to calculate an OR or RR, variables that are not already divided into two categories must be recoded into binomial variables (often coded numerically as yes = 1 and no = 0). In some situations, the cutoff points for the categories are obvious, such as those that divide an ordinal variable into categories for disagreement (strongly disagree or disagree) and agreement (agree or strongly agree). Sometimes the population can be divided into groups of relatively equal sizes using the median, quartiles, or other sample-based cutoff points. Alternatively, biologically or socially meaningful cutoff points can be defined, such as using the 18th birthday to divide a study population into children and adults in countries where legal adulthood begins at age 18. The selected cutoff value will influence whether the exposure and outcome

FIGURE 28-5 Examples of One-Sided and Two-Sided Alternate Hypotheses

Null Hypothesis (H_0)	Two-Sided Alternative Hypothesis (H_a)	Example of a One-Sided Alternative Hypothesis (H_a)
The means are not different.	The means are different.	The mean of cases is higher than the mean of controls.
The proportions are not different.	The proportions are different.	The proportion of the intervention group is lower than the proportion of the control group.
The scores are not different.	The scores are different.	The after scores were, on average, higher than the before scores.

have a statistically significant association. Accordingly, the decision about how to define categories should be justifiable.

The results of 2×2 analyses are often presented using tables like the one shown in **Figure 28-6**. The reference group for an odds ratio or rate ratio should be specified. In the example, males are compared to females (the reference group), those with a waist circumference greater than 35 inches to those with smaller girths, former smokers to never smokers, and current smokers to never smokers. Two separate odds ratios were calculated for tobacco use because the variable for tobacco use had three possible responses instead of just two.

The 95% confidence interval provides information about the statistical significance of the tests. For example, the 95% confidence interval for the odds ratio comparing the sex distribution of cases and controls contains OR = 1. This means that it is not clear from the test whether cases are more likely or less likely than controls to be male. The conclusion is, therefore, that there is no statistically significant difference in the proportion of cases and controls by sex.

28.6 Interpreting Confidence Intervals

Confidence intervals (CIs) provide more information about a statistic than can be conveyed by a *p*-value. For example, the confidence intervals for odds ratios and rate ratios indicate whether the populations being compared are different or not different, and they also provide information about how well the test statistic captures the true value of that measure in the source population (**Figure 28-7**). A 95% confidence interval (95% CI) corresponds to a significance level of $\alpha = 0.05$. For odds ratios and rate ratios, a 95% confidence interval that does not overlap 1—one for which the full range is below 1 or the full range is above 1—is equivalent to having a *p*-value of $p < 0.05$. If the confidence interval overlaps 1, that is the equivalent of $p > 0.05$.

FIGURE 28-6 Example of Odds Ratios for a Case-control Study

Exposure		**Percentage of Cases (Acute Myocardial Infarction) (*n* = 150)**	**Percentage of Controls (no AMI) (*n* = 250)**	**OR (95% CI)**	**Interpretation**
Sex	Female	39.3%	42.4%	Reference group	Cases and controls in the study did *not* have significantly different proportions of males.
	Male	60.7%	57.6%	1.14 (0.75, 1.72)	
Waist circumference >35 inches	No	37.3%	51.2%	Reference group	Cases had greater odds than controls of having a waist circumference greater than 35 inches.
	Yes	62.7%	48.8%	1.76 (1.16, 2.67)*	
Tobacco use	Never smoked	68.0%	73.6%	Reference group	Cases and controls in the study population did *not* have significantly different smoking histories.
	Former smoker	11.3%	10.8%	1.14 (0.58, 2.18)	
	Current smoker	20.7%	15.6%	1.43 (0.84, 2.44)	

*Statistically significant at $\alpha = 0.05$ level.

Suppose that the point estimates for the incidence rate ratios calculated from two cohort studies are both RR = 3.0. One study has 200 participants and a 95% confidence interval ranging from 1.6 to 5.8. This is usually written as RR = 3.0 (1.6, 5.8). The other study has 1000 participants and a rate ratio of RR = 3.0 (2.2, 4.0). In the first study, the researcher can be 95% confident that the true value of the RR in the

FIGURE 28-7 Interpreting Confidence Intervals

Statistic	Result with 95% CI	Interpretation
Odds ratio (OR)	1.7 (0.6, 5.3)	Based on the OR in the study population (OR = 1.7), we are 95% confident that the OR in the source population is somewhere between 0.6 and 5.3. Because this overlaps with OR = 1, we conclude that there is no association between the exposure and disease status.
Relative risk (RR)	1.6 (1.1, 2.4)	Based on the RR in the study population (RR = 1.6), we are 95% confident that the RR in the source population is between 1.1 and 2.4. Because this range does not overlap with RR = 1, we conclude that the exposure is associated with an increased risk of disease.

source population is a number between RR = 1.6 and RR = 5.8. There is a 5% likelihood that the actual RR is less than RR = 1.6 or greater than RR = 5.8. In the second study, the one with the larger number of participants, the 95% CI is narrower, and there is more certainty about the true value. Because the 95% confidence intervals for both of these studies do not overlap 1, the *p*-values for both are $p < 0.05$. For both studies, the conclusion is that the incidence rates in the two populations being compared are different. However, there is more certainty about the level of difference in the larger study.

Other types of confidence intervals can also be calculated. A 90% confidence interval corresponds to a significance level of $\alpha = 0.10$. A 99% confidence interval corresponds to $\alpha = 0.01$. A 90% confidence interval for an odds ratio (OR) is less likely to overlap OR = 1 than a 99% confidence interval. The 90% CI is also less likely than the 99% CI to capture the true odds ratio in the source population. The 90% CI is more likely than the 99% CI to be deemed "statistically significant" and to lead to the conclusion that there is an association between the exposure and the outcome being examined (**Figure 28-8**).

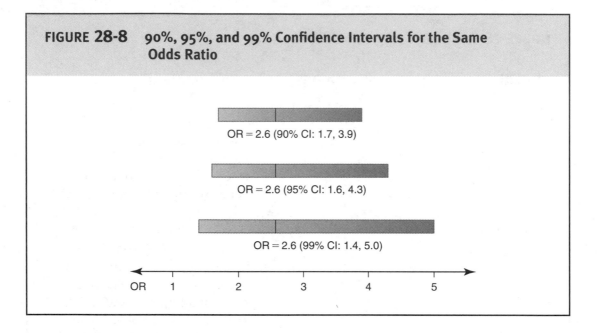

FIGURE 28-8 90%, 95%, and 99% Confidence Intervals for the Same Odds Ratio

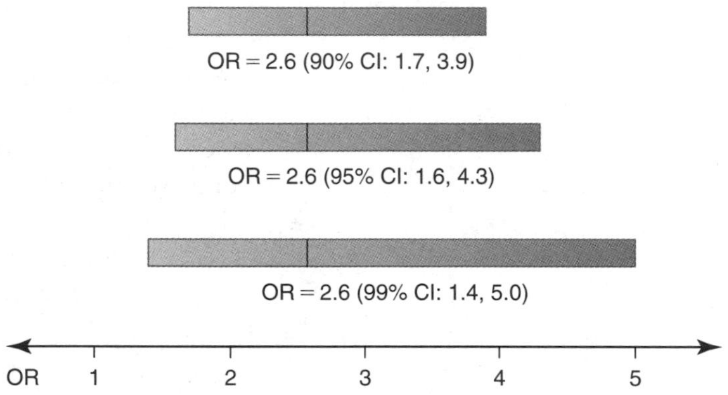

28.7 Selecting an Appropriate Test

For statistical comparisons more complex than 2×2 analysis, analysts must select a test that is appropriate for the goal of the analysis and the types of variables being analyzed. The steps for identifying and using a statistical test are summarized in **Figure 28-9**.

First, the variables to be compared should be selected and the goal of the test clearly stated. The goal could be:

- To compare the mean ages of males and females. The key variables for this test are age (a ratio variable) and sex (binomial).
- To see whether the proportion of cases and controls with various blood types is similar. The key variables for this test are blood type (a nominal variable) and disease status (binomial).
- To compare the responses of older and younger adults to a question about how often the participant eats dark chocolate as per a 5-point frequency scale ranging from "never" to "every day." The key variables are age group (binomial) and the frequency of chocolate consumption (an ordinal variable).
- To determine whether participants with higher HDL cholesterol levels tend to have lower heart rates. Both of these variables are continuous variables (ratio variables).

Then select a test that is appropriate for the types of variables being examined. Some tests require the variables being examined to have particular distributions or other characteristics. The researcher must confirm that the variables meet these **assumptions** of the test prior to running the test and interpreting the output.

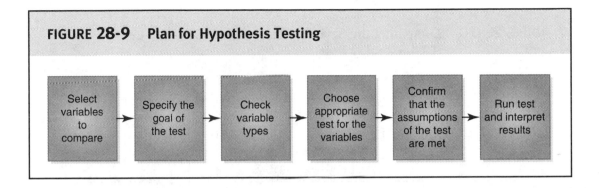

FIGURE 28-9 Plan for Hypothesis Testing

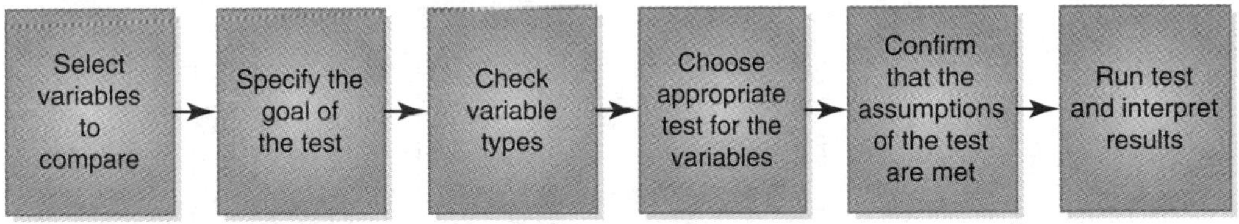

Statistical tests are often classified as being either parametric or nonparametric. The basic difference between these two types of tests is that parametric tests make more assumptions about the variables being examined than nonparametric tests.

- **Parametric tests** assume that the variables being examined have particular distributions, often requiring the variables to have normal or approximately normal distributions. These tests may also require that the variance for the variables of interest—the spread of observations around the mean—be equal or at least similar in the population groups being compared.
- **Nonparametric tests** do not make assumptions about the distributions of responses.

Parametric tests are typically used for ratio and interval variables with relatively normal (bell-shaped) distributions of responses. Parametric tests tend to be more statistically powerful than nonparametric tests, so the preference is to use a parametric test whenever the variable being examined fits reasonably well with the assumptions the test makes about sample size, distribution, and the equality of variances.

Nonparametric tests are often used for ranked variables, such as the responses to surveys that ask participants to indicate preferences using scales from 1 (strongly disagree) to 5 (strongly agree), and for categorical variables, including variables with just two groups (such as cases and controls, males and females, or children and adults). They are also used when the distribution of a ratio or interval variable is non-normal.

28.8 Comparing a Population to a Set Value

The goal of some statistical tests is to compare the value of a statistic in a study population to some set value. For example, suppose that participants in an experimental study are students at a university at which the mean age of undergraduate students is 21 years. The researcher wants to confirm that the mean age of the study participants is reasonably close to 21 years. If the distribution of ages in the study population looks like the distribution in Box A of **Figure 28-10**, then 21 years is captured within two standard deviations of the study's mean age. The conclusion would be that the sample mean is not so far from 21 that the means

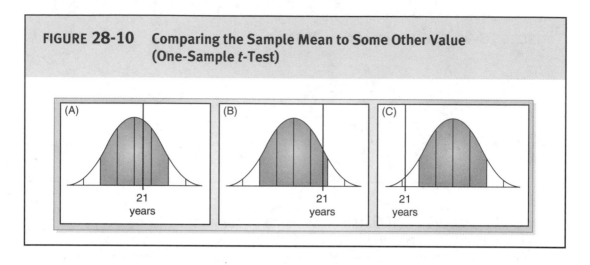

FIGURE 28-10 Comparing the Sample Mean to Some Other Value (One-Sample *t*-Test)

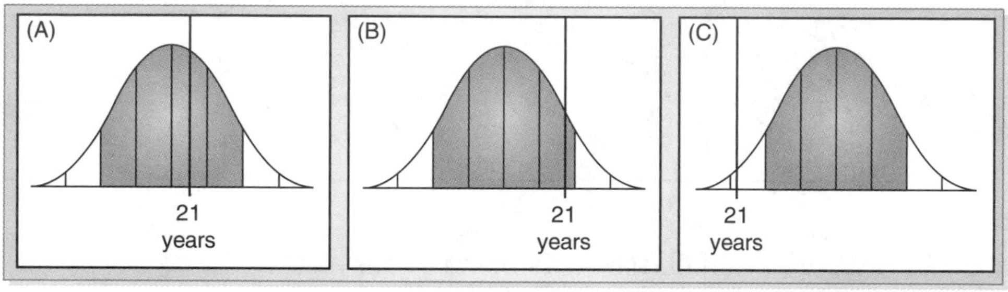

would be considered different. In other words, the sample shown in Box A fails to reject the null hypothesis that the means are not different. The *p*-value for this **one-sample *t*-test** is $p > 0.05$. The conclusion is that the means in the study population and the university student population as a whole are not significantly different. Box B also captures 21 years within the 95% confidence interval, even though the mean age of study participants is farther from 21 than it was in Box A. The *p*-value for this test is also $p > 0.05$. In Box C, however, the study participants were several years older than the average student at the university, and 21 years does not fall within the 95% confidence interval. The *p*-value for this test is $p < 0.05$. In this situation, the null hypothesis is rejected, and the conclusion is that the study population mean is different from 21 years. This test result indicates that the study population may not be adequately representative of the university's undergraduate student population.

28.9 Comparing Independent Populations

Sometimes study participants are grouped into **independent populations**, which are populations in which each individual can be a member of only one of the population groups being compared. For example, if the populations being compared are divided by age, the population of adults ages 18 to 49 will not overlap with the population of adults ages 50 to 79. Each individual participant in the study population can be assigned to no more than one of these groups, so the populations are independent.

A variety of statistical tests can be used to compare independent populations. The appropriate test to use depends on the type of variable being examined (**Figure 28-11**). For example, an **independent-samples *t*-test** (also called a **2-sample *t*-test**) could be used to compare the mean ages of cases and controls participating in a case-control study. A **Fisher's exact test** could be used to examine whether the proportions of males in the exposed and unexposed groups

FIGURE 28-11 Common Tests for Comparing Two or More Groups

	Type of Variable Being Examined			
	Ratio/ interval (parametric tests)	**Ordinal/rank (nonparametric tests)**	**Binomial**	**Nominal categories**
Statistic being evaluated	mean	median	proportion	proportions
Test for whether the statistic in one population is different from a hypothetical value	one-sample *t*-test	one-sample median test	binomial test	Chi-square (χ^2) goodness-of-fit test
Test for whether the statistic differs in two populations	independent-samples (2-sample) *t*-test	Mann–Whitney *U* test (Wilcoxon rank sum test)	Fisher's exact test	Chi-square (χ^2) test of independence
Test for whether the statistic differs in three or more populations	one-way ANOVA (*F* test)	Kruskal–Wallis *H* test	Chi-square (χ^2) test	Chi-square (χ^2) test of independence

of a cohort study are similar. A **Chi-square test** could be used to determine whether the distributions of participants by race or ethnicity are similar for the intervention and control groups of an experimental study.

A variety of measures of correlation can be used to examine the relationships between two variables. The correct test for the types of variables being compared must be used. Pearson's product-moment correlation (r) examines the association between two ratio or interval variables. Spearman's rho (ρ_s) and **Kendall's tau (τ)** are measures of the correlation between two ordinal or rank variables. The **phi (ϕ) coefficient** calculates the correlation between two binomial variables. **Cramér's *V*** quantifies the correlation between two nominal variables or between one binominal variable and one nominal variable. Some tests of correlation allow for comparison of different types of variables. Eta (η) and eta squared (η^2) are measures of the correlation between one ratio or interval variable and one nominal variable. The point-biserial r_{pb} correlation (or η or η^2) calculates the correlation between one ratio or interval variable and one binomial variable. The Glass rank biserial r_{rb} measures the correlation between one ordinal or rank variable and one binominal variable. Epsilon squared (ε^2) quantifies the correlation between one ordinal or rank variable and one nominal variable.

When running statistical tests, it is often beneficial to create a table of basic information about the variables of interest for each of the comparison groups as well as the result of the statistical tests used to compare those populations. **Figure 28-12** shows sample output for tests of whether responses differed for the male and female participants of a cohort study. Additional columns might be added for details such as the value of the **test statistic** (such as the *F*-stat or *t*-stat) and the **degrees of freedom (df)** for each test, which is a number related to the sample sizes of various groups being compared. In this example, the males have a significantly greater average age than the females because the *p*-value for the independent-samples *t*-test is $p < 0.05$. However, the proportion of males and females who smoke is not significantly different because the *p*-value for Fisher's exact test was $p > 0.05$.

The table shown in Figure 28-12 includes more information than is usually included in published manuscripts. However, it allows the researcher to double-check that the correct tests were used and that the correct interpretations were made. It also facilitates the writing of the statistical methods portion of the research report. A more succinct comparison table is usually prepared for the final report. A sample results table is shown in **Figure 28-13**.

28.10 Comparing Paired Data

A different set of tests is used when the goal is to compare before-and-after results in the same individuals (**Figure 28-14**). If the goal is to see whether, on average, a participant in a cohort study gained weight between the baseline exam and the 1-year follow-up exam, a **matched-pairs *t*-test** can be used. If the goal is to see whether a safe driving course improves the pass rates for a driving licensure exam, **McNemar's test** can be used to examine how many participants switched from failing a pretest to passing a post-test, how many switched from passing a pretest to failing a post-test, and how many had no change in status. McNemar's test can also determine whether the differences indicate that the course had a significant impact on exam pass rates.

Figure 28-15 shows sample output for paired tests. In this example, participants in a 3-month exercise program lost weight during the study period because the *p*-value for the matched-pairs *t*-test was $p < 0.05$, but the participants did not increase their ability to run 1 mile in less than 10 minutes because the *p*-value for McNemar's test was $p > 0.05$, which indicates that there was no difference in this variable during the study period.

FIGURE 28-12 Examples of Tests for Comparing Males and Females in a Study Population

Variable	Report	Males (n = 200)	Females (n = 200)	Variable Type	Test of Comparison	p-Value for Test	Interpretation
Age	Mean (SD)	43.7 (7.8)	40.1 (8.1)	Ratio (normal)	Independent-samples t-test	<0.01	The means are different.
Current smokers	%	12%	10%	Binomial (yes / no)	Fisher's exact test	0.52	The proportions are *not* different.
Home district:	n (%)			Nominal	Chi-square (χ^2) test	0.86	The proportions are *not* different.
North		90 (45%)	87 (44%)				
Central		50 (25%)	48 (24%)				
South		60 (30%)	65 (33%)				

FIGURE 28-13 Simplified Version of Figure 27-12

Characteristic		Males (n = 200)	Females (n = 200)	p-Value
Age	Mean (SD)	43.7 (7.8)	40.1 (8.1)	<0.01*
Current smokers	%	12%	10%	0.52
Home district:	n (%)			
North		90 (45%)	87 (44%)	0.86
Central		50 (25%)	48 (24%)	
South		60 (30%)	65 (33%)	

*Statistically significant at $\alpha = 0.05$ level.

FIGURE 28-14 Common Tests for Comparing Matched Populations

	Type of Variable Being Examined			
	Ratio/Interval (Parametric Tests)	Ordinal/Rank (Nonparametric Tests)	Binomial	Nominal Categories
Test for whether value of the variable is different in one population measured twice (such as "before" and "after" in the same population) or in two paired groups	matched-pairs (paired, dependent) t-test	Wilcoxon (matched-pairs) signed-rank test or sign test for matched pairs	McNemar's test	McNemar's test
Test for whether the value of the variable is different in three or more matched groups	repeated-measures ANOVA	Friedman test	Cochran's Q test	Cochran's Q test

FIGURE 28-15 Examples of Tests for Comparing Pre-Test and Post-Test Results for Participants in a 3-Month Exercise Program

Variable	Report	Pretest	Post-Test	Difference	Variable Type	Test of Comparison	*p*-Value for Test	Interpretation
Sample size	*n*	40	40	0	Count	—	—	—
Weight (pounds)	Mean (SD)	178 (19)	172 (18)	–6 (6)	Ratio (normal)	Matched-pairs *t*-test	<0.01	Individuals, on average, had pre- and post-test weights that were significantly different.
Able to run 1 mile in less than 10 minutes	*n* (%)	12 (30%)	16 (40%)	6 no-to-yes, 2 yes-to-no, 32 no change	Binomial	McNemar's test	0.29	The pre- and post-test ability for an individual participant to run 1 mile in less than 10 minutes was, on average, *not* different.

CHAPTER 29

REGRESSION ANALYSIS

This chapter provides a brief overview of the most commonly used advanced statistical techniques, including linear and logistic regression models.

29.1 Regression Modeling

Regression models seek to understand the relationship between an **independent variable** (or **predictor variable**) and one **dependent variable** (or **outcome variable**). When multiple independent variables are included in the model, the effect of one predictor variable on the outcome can be examined while controlling for other predictor variables by keeping those other values constant. The two most common types of regression are linear regression and logistic regression, which are discussed in the following sections. The steps for model fitting are similar for both types of models and are summarized in **Figure 29-1**.

In general, statistical software programs require the analyst to:

- Select a variety of specifications for the model, such as the particular estimation technique (often, an ordinary least squares, generalized least squares, or maximum likelihood estimation model).
- Choose the method the computer will use to select variables for inclusion in the model. For example, a **simultaneous multiple regression** model includes all predictor variables in the model. A **stepwise multiple regression** model systematically adds or removes predictor variables to the model to find the best fit. A forward stepwise method instructs the computer to add the best predictor variables to the model one at a time until adding an additional variable does not significantly improve the fit of the model. A backward stepwise method deletes variables from the model until deleting a variable significantly reduces the fit of the model.
- Check the fit of the model by examining its residual terms and the results of statistical tests of the **goodness-of-fit** for the model that indicate how well real data match the values predicted by the model.

FIGURE 29-1 Steps in Fitting a Regression Model

Step	
1	Select one outcome (dependent) variable.
2	Identify the appropriate type of regression (such as a linear or logistic model) for the outcome variable.
3	Select one or more predictor (independent) variables.
4	Check to make sure that any assumptions required for the model (such as the variable types or distributions of outcome and predictor variables) are met.
5	Choose a selection method for helping the computer to decide which set of predictor variables will produce the "best-fit" model (the model that the computer determines is the best at explaining the relationship between the predictor variables and the outcome variable).
6	Examine the model for potential problems. For example, examine residuals for possible autocorrelation, check for possible interaction between predictor variables (such as the multicollinearity that might occur when two predictor variables are highly correlated), and look for other potential problems that might need to be addressed.
7	Interpret the results of the regression model, and consider whether they fit with the theoretical framework for the analysis (for example, confirming that all necessary covariates are included and all illogical ones are excluded).

A statistics reference guide or a statistician should be consulted for detailed information about these and other advanced analytic techniques.

29.2 Simple Linear Regression

A linear regression model is used when the outcome variable is a ratio or interval variable. **Simple linear regression** models examine whether there is a linear relationship between one predictor variable and the outcome variable. The relationship between the predictor and outcome variables in a simple linear regression can be visually displayed using a scatterplot. Each point from a data set is plotted on the graph, and a best-fit line is drawn through those points.

An **ordinary least squares (OLS)** approach is typically used to find the best-fit line in linear regression. OLS fits a line to the data points from a study with the goal of minimizing the average vertical distance from each point to the line. Suppose that a regression model is being fit for the relationship between body mass index (BMI) on the *x*-axis and cholesterol levels on the *y*-axis, and the fitted line describing that relationship indicates that a person with a BMI of 24 is predicted to have a total cholesterol level of 180. If one of the study participants being analyzed had a BMI of 24 but a cholesterol level of 195, that individual's data point will be 15 units of cholesterol distant from the line. That distance of 15 units—the vertical distance from the point to the line—is the **residual** for the data point. OLS calculates the residual for each data point in the full data set, squares each distance, and then adds up all of the squared residuals. The best-fit regression line is the one that minimizes the sum of the squared residuals (often shortened to SSR).

Figure 29-2 provides an example of how to interpret the results of a simple linear regression. The coefficient for the predictor variable (often designated as β or beta in the output of statistical software programs) is the slope of the line. The constant in the regression model is the *y*-intercept for the line. These values can be used to write an equation for the best-fit line, and that equation can be used to predict the expected value of the outcome variable for different values of the predictor variable. The r^2 for the model, which is the square of the correlation coefficient, provides information about how well the regression model predicts the variation in

FIGURE 29-2 Example of a Simple Linear Regression Model

The output for the regression model is:

	β (coeff.)	SE (standard error)	*p*-value
Predictor_1	3.1	0.4	0.01
Constant	0.9	6.4	0.89

The r^2 for the regression line is $r^2 = 0.79$, which means that the predictor variable explains 79% of the variation in the values of the outcome variable. This is a strong model.

The equation for the regression line is:

OUTCOME = 3.1*PREDICTOR_1 + 0.9

Predictor_1 value	Expected outcome value
10	30.9
15	47.4
28	87.7

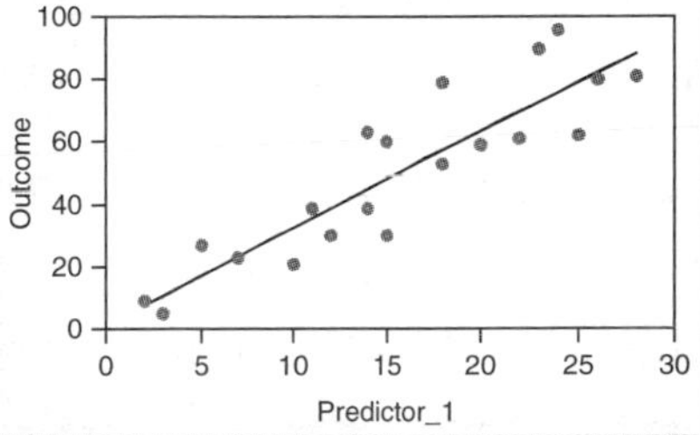

the values of the outcome variable. The value of r^2 ranges from 0 to 1, with values closer to 1 indicating a better model fit.

29.3 Simple Logistic Regression

Logistic regression models (sometimes called **logit regression models**) are used when the outcome variable is a dichotomous variable. Logistic regression models predict the probabilities of the outcome occurring. Logistic regression is commonly used in case-control studies, for which the outcome variable is usually case status, with case = 1 and control = 0. For outcome variables that are other types of yes/no variables, it is typical to let yes = 1 and no = 0. Predictor variables for a logistic regression model can be categorical (when the categories are coded with numbers) or continuous. A **maximum likelihood estimation (MLE)** approach is used to find the coefficient values that best explain the outcome.

The β (beta) coefficient for a predictor variable in a logistic regression model is the natural log of the odds ratio, ln(OR). The odds ratio for the association between that predictor variable and the outcome variable can be found by calculating the exponential of the coefficient, exp(β). The odds ratio for each predictor variable represents the change in the odds of the outcome—typically, the odds of being a case or being classified as a "yes"—for a 1-unit change in the predictor variable. The confidence interval for the odds ratio can be calculated using the value of the coefficient and its standard error.

Figure 29-3 provides an example of the output for a simple logistic regression. The value of the coefficient for sex, which was coded as female = 0 and male = 1, is β = 0.644. The point estimate for the odds ratio is the exponential of beta,

FIGURE 29-3 Example of a Simple Logistic Regression Model

The output for the regression model predicting being a case (not a control) is:

	β	SE	OR (95% CI)	p-value
Sex	0.644	0.204	1.90 (1.28, 2.84)	0.002
constant	–0.584	0.109		0.000

OR for Sex = $\exp(\beta) = \exp(0.644) = 1.904$

Lower bound of 95%CI: $\exp(\beta - 1.96 * \text{SE}) = \exp(0.644 - 1.96 * 0.204) = 1.276$

Upper bound of 95%CI: $\exp(\beta + 1.96 * \text{SE}) = \exp(0.644 + 1.96 * 0.204) = 2.842$

Multipliers: 1.645 for a 90% CI, 1.96 for a 95% CI, and 2.576 for a 99% CI

exp(0.644) = 1.90. The 95% confidence interval can be calculated using beta, the standard error, and a multiplier of 1.96 (because 95% of the area under a normal curve falls within 1.96 standard deviations of the mean). Because the confidence interval of (1.28, 2.84) does not overlap with OR = 1, with the entire range greater than 1, sex is considered to have a statistically significant association with being a case. In this example, being male rather than female (that is, a 1-unit increase in the value of the sex variable) is associated with 1.90 times greater odds of being a case. Likelihood ratio tests, the Wald statistic, the Hosmer–Lemeshow test, and other goodness-of-fit tests can confirm the soundness of a logistic regression model.

29.4 Confounding and Effect Modification

One of the main reasons researchers use multivariable statistical models—that is, analyses of three or more variables at one time—is to examine the interactions that may occur among variables. This can be especially helpful when a **third variable** (also called an **extraneous variable** or **lurking variable**) may be concealing or distorting the true relationship between two other variables. Several different types of third-variable effects might occur, including confounding and effect modification.

A **confounder** may make the association between an exposure variable and an outcome variable appear more or less significant than it truly is. For example, suppose that the crude (unadjusted) odds ratio for the relationship between sedentariness and a first heart attack shows that the odds of physical inactivity in the past year are four times higher (OR = 4) among adults who have had a recent heart attack than among adults who have no history of heart disease. Yet age may confound this association. Older adults are more likely than younger adults to be inactive, and older adults are also more likely to have a heart attack. Age-specific analysis may show that the odds ratio for this association is OR = 2 among young adults and it is also OR = 2 among older adults. The discrepancy between the crude association (OR = 4) and the age-specific associations (both OR = 2) is a sign that age is confounding the association between sedentary behavior and myocardial infarctions. The confounder is hiding the true association between physical inactivity and heart attacks. When a third variable like age is shown to be a confounder, an adjusted measure of association, such as an age-adjusted odds ratio, should be reported for the association between the exposure and the outcome. In the example, instead of reporting a crude odds ratio of $OR_{cr} = 4$, it would be more accurate to report an age-adjusted odds ratio of $OR_{adj} = 2$.

An **effect modifier** (sometimes called an **interaction term**) is a third variable that often defines groups of individuals who might experience different biological responses to various exposures. For example, menopausal status may be an effect modifier for some studies about women's health. Suppose that heavier weight is associated with a decreased rate of breast cancer in premenopausal women but it has the opposite effect, an increased rate of breast cancer, in postmenopausal women. Grouping all women together without accounting for menopausal status might make it look like weight is not a risk factor for breast cancer, even though it is a significant risk factor in both pre- and post-menopausal women. Reporting that there was no association between weight and breast cancer would hide a potentially important biological difference in breast cancer risk that may be related to hormonal status. If a third variable is shown to be an effect modifier—one in which the stratified measures of association are different in populations with different biological characteristics—it is usually best to report separate stratum-specific measures of association for each level of the effect modifier, such as separate results for premenopausal and postmenopausal women. Pooling the results for the biologically different groups would hide meaningful differences, so an adjusted or crude measure of association should not be reported when effect modification is occurring.

Figure 29-4 summarizes the steps required to identify confounders and effect modifiers. To be a confounder or effect modifier, the third variable must be independently associated with both an exposure (or predictor) variable and an outcome variable. These two relationships should be confirmed. Then, a crude odds ratio (or other measure of association) for the relationship between the exposure and the outcome should be calculated, along with a separate measure of association for each level of the third variable, such as separate odds ratios for males and females.

FIGURE 29-4 Confounding and Effect Modification

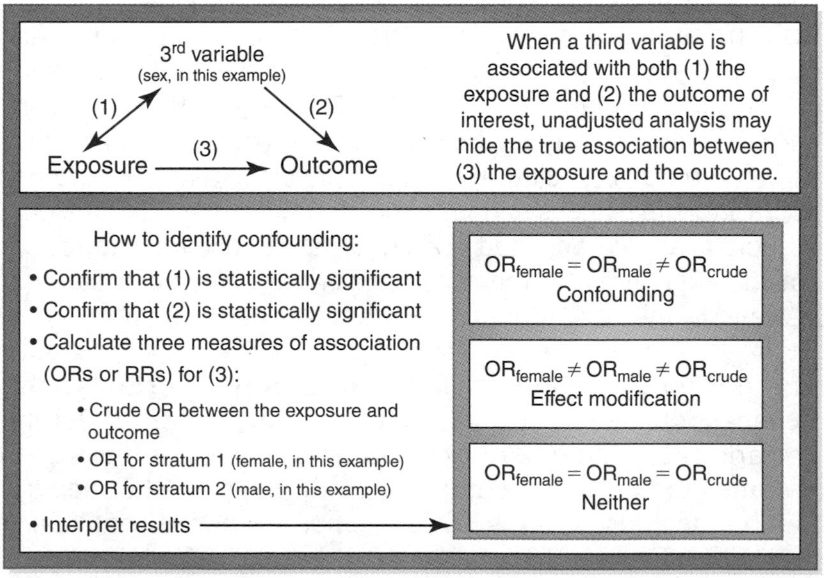

The crude and stratum-specific measures are compared using a **Breslow-Day test** for the homogeneity of the stratum-specific measures of association, a –2 log likelihood test, or another appropriate statistical test. After running a suitable test, the interpretation is as follows:

- If the stratum-specific measures of association are not different but they are different from the crude measure of association, the third variable is a confounder. Report an adjusted measure. Report an adjusted measure, such as a **Mantel-Haenszel** adjusted odds ratio.
- If the stratum-specific measures of association are different from one another and they are also different from the crude measure of association, the third variable is likely an effect modifier. Report stratum-specific measures.
- If the crude and stratum-specific odds ratios are all similar, then neither confounding nor effect modification is occurring. Report a crude (unadjusted) measure.

29.5 Multivariable Comparisons of Means

Several tests are used to compare means in independent populations (**Figure 29-5**). One-way **ANOVA (analysis of variance)** is used to compare the mean values of a continuous variable among independent groups of people, such as comparing the mean age of patients at three different family practices who do not share any patients. **Two-way ANOVA** compares the mean values of a continuous variable across two factors. For example, two-way ANOVA could compare mean ages by sex and smoking status (never smoker, past smoker, current smoker). This analysis would involve six comparison groups: female never smokers, male never smokers, female past smokers, male past smokers, female current smokers, and male current smokers.

Both of these types of ANOVA require several assumptions to be met before the tests are used. The populations being compared must be independent, with each study participant assigned to only one of the groups being compared. The dependent variable—the variable for which the mean values are being compared—must be approximately normally distributed. There can be no significant outliers in the variables included in the ANOVA analysis, and **Levene's test** must demonstrate the homogeneity of the variances of the different groups. Suppose that mean ages of patients at a family practice and a pediatric practice are being compared. The family practice is likely to have a wide spread of ages, while the pediatric practice will have a narrow distribution of ages among its patients. In this example, Levene's test would show that the variances were different ($p < 0.05$), so ANOVA would not be an appropriate test of comparison to use.

Several extensions of ANOVA allow for more complex analyses of the differences of means in independent populations. **Analysis of covariance (ANCOVA)** can be used to control for confounding variables when comparing the means of two or more groups. **Multivariate analysis of variance (MANOVA)** can be used to test for differences in group means when there are multiple dependent

FIGURE 29-5 Examples of Tests for Comparing Means in Two or More Groups

Name	Independent Variable(s)	Dependent Variable(s)
One-way ANOVA (analysis of variance)	1 nominal variable	1 ratio/interval variable
Two-way ANOVA (analysis of variance)	2 nominal variables	1 ratio/interval variable
ANCOVA (analysis of covariance)	1+ nominal variable and 1+ ratio/interval and/or nominal covariate	1 ratio/interval variable
One-way MANOVA (multiple analysis of variance)	1 nominal variable	2+ ratio/interval variables
Two-way MANOVA (multiple analysis of variance)	2 nominal variables	2+ ratio/interval variables
MANCOVA (multiple analysis of covariance)	1+ nominal variable and 1+ ratio/interval and/or nominal covariate	2+ ratio/interval variables

variables. **Multivariate analysis of covariance (MANCOVA)** controls for potential confounders when comparing multiple dependent variables.

29.6 Dummy Variables

The predictor variables in regression models can take a variety of forms, but they must have numeric responses. Nominal categorical variables have responses that cannot be ordered, so they cannot be assigned a rank. However, a set of **dummy variables** can be created to convert categorical responses to a series of dichotomous (0/1) variables that can all be included in the same regression model. Dummy variables can also be used to convert ratio and interval variables into a set of derived categories, so that a series of odds ratios for the levels of the derived categorical variable can be estimated with a logistic regression model.

Figure 29-6 provides an example of how this type of recoding is done. If the original categorical variable has "n" possible responses, then "n – 1" dummy variables are required to capture all the responses to the original question. In the

FIGURE 29-6 Dummy Variables

If the response to the original question was...	Then the values of the dummy variables are... B_Dummy (Was B the response to the original question?)	C_Dummy (Was C the response to the original question?)	D_Dummy (Was D the response to the original question?)	Conclusion based on the dummy variables
A	0 (no)	0	0	The response was not B, C, or D, so it was A.
B	1 (yes)	0	0	The response was B.
C	0	1	0	The response was C.
D	0	0	1	The response was D.

example in the figure, there were four possible responses, so three dummy variables are required. If there were nine categorical responses instead, then eight dummy variables would be required. In some modeling approaches, all of the "n – 1" variables are routinely included in a regression model, even if some would otherwise be eliminated during a stepwise selection process. A statistician can provide guidance on appropriate use.

29.7 Multiple Regression

A variety of analytic approaches can be used to test relationships among three or more variables while adjusting for possible confounders (**Figure 29-7**), including both linear and logistic regression models.

Multiple linear regression models examine the effects of several predictor variables on the value of the outcome variable. Multiple linear regression models can have both continuous and categorical predictor variables, as long as the responses to categorical variables are expressed by numbers and all of the key assumptions of this type of model are met. The relationship between the independent and dependent variables must be linear. The independent variables in the model must have reasonably independent errors, with the tolerance index,

FIGURE 29-7 Examples of Multivariable Analysis Approaches for Testing Relationships Among Three or More Variables

Name	Independent Variable(s)	Dependent Variable(s)
Multiple linear regression	2+ ratio/interval and/or nominal variables	1 ratio/interval variable
Multiple logistic regression	2+ ratio/interval and/or nominal variables	1 nominal variable
Discriminant analysis	2+ ratio/interval and/or nominal variables	1 nominal variable
Canonical analysis	2+ ratio/interval and/or nominal variables	2+ ratio/interval and/or nominal variables

the **variance inflation factor (VIF)**, and other tests showing that the predictor variables are not too intercorrelated. The presence of **multicollinearity** or **autocorrelation** might mean that the model outcomes are inaccurate. The residuals for all variables must be normally distributed, as per a Kolmogorov–Smirnof test or another goodness-of-fit test. (Log transformations can sometimes be used to change nonlinear variables into ones that will result in a normal distribution.) And a plot of residuals must show that the error terms demonstrate **homoscedasticity** (rather than **heteroscedasticity**) by having variances that are evenly distributed. Although it is easy to use a statistical software program to generate multiple regression models, researchers must carefully check all of the related output before concluding that the model is a valid one.

Figure 29-8 provides an example of how to interpret the output for a multiple linear regression model with two continuous predictor variables. The constant and the coefficients (the betas) for the predictor variables can be used to write an equation for a best-fit line. That equation can be used to examine the individual effect of each predictor variable on the outcome variable. To make this assessment, the value of one of the two predictor variables is kept constant so that the effect of a 1-unit change in the value of the other predictive variable on the expected outcome value can be ascertained.

Figure 29-9 shows how to interpret models with multiple types of predictor variables that do not interact. In the example, a 1-unit increase in the value of the "Predictor_2" variable is associated with a 2-unit increase in the value of the outcome (because the coefficient for "Predictor_2" is $\beta = 2.0$). This relationship between Predictor_2 and the outcome is the same for both males and females, even though males have an 18.7-unit higher value for the outcome than females (because the coefficient for sex is $\beta = 18.7$).

FIGURE 29-8 Example of a Multiple Linear Regression Model with Two Continuous Variables

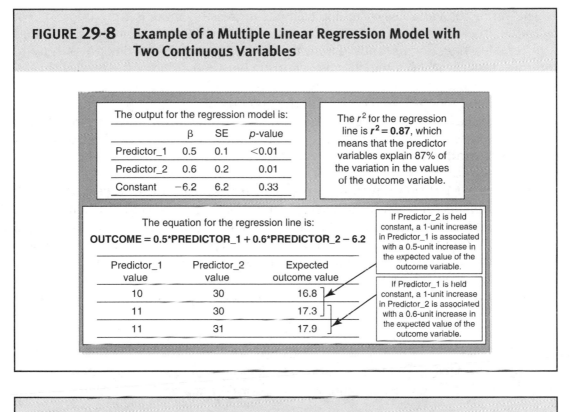

The output for the regression model is:

	β	SE	*p*-value
Predictor_1	0.5	0.1	<0.01
Predictor_2	0.6	0.2	0.01
Constant	−6.2	6.2	0.33

The r^2 for the regression line is $r^2 = \mathbf{0.87}$, which means that the predictor variables explain 87% of the variation in the values of the outcome variable.

The equation for the regression line is:

OUTCOME = 0.5*PREDICTOR_1 + 0.6*PREDICTOR_2 − 6.2

Predictor_1 value	Predictor_2 value	Expected outcome value
10	30	16.8
11	30	17.3
11	31	17.9

If Predictor_2 is held constant, a 1-unit increase in Predictor_1 is associated with a 0.5-unit increase in the expected value of the outcome variable.

If Predictor_1 is held constant, a 1-unit increase in Predictor_2 is associated with a 0.6-unit increase in the expected value of the outcome variable.

FIGURE 29-9 Example of a Multiple Linear Regression Model with One Continuous and One Categorical Variable with No Interaction

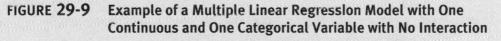

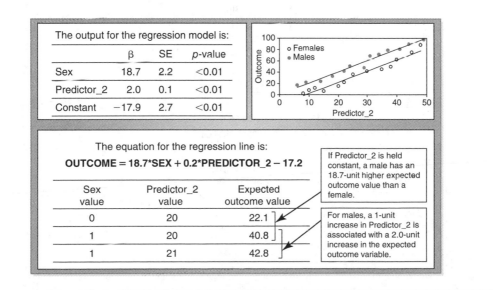

The output for the regression model is:

	β	SE	*p*-value
Sex	18.7	2.2	<0.01
Predictor_2	2.0	0.1	<0.01
Constant	−17.9	2.7	<0.01

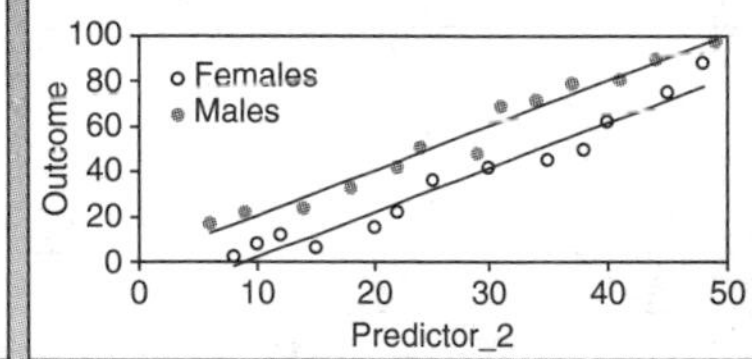

The equation for the regression line is:

OUTCOME = 18.7*SEX + 0.2*PREDICTOR_2 − 17.2

Sex value	Predictor_2 value	Expected outcome value
0	20	22.1
1	20	40.8
1	21	42.8

If Predictor_2 is held constant, a male has an 18.7-unit higher expected outcome value than a female.

For males, a 1-unit increase in Predictor_2 is associated with a 2.0-unit increase in the expected outcome variable.

The predictor variables in multiple linear regression models may interact. For example, interaction may be occurring when the best-fit regression lines for males and females have significantly different slopes. **Figure 29-10** illustrates how to interpret models when interaction is occurring between some of the predictor variables. In the example, a 1-unit increase in the value of Predictor_2 is associated with a 2.4-unit increase in the value of the outcome for females but only a 1.2-unit increase for males. The equation for the regression model expresses this interaction through the use of a special interaction term. A **hierarchical model** (also called a **multilevel model**) adjusts for different levels of exposure, such as for both census tract and county.

Figure 29-11 shows how to interpret a **multiple logistic regression** model. Multiple logistic regression models can have both continuous and categorical predictor variables, and the predictor variables do not have to have a normal distribution, be linearly related, or have equal variances. A model with two predictor variables generates adjusted odds ratios for both variables. In the example, the food-adjusted OR for sex has $p = 0.23$, which means that males and females did not have different likelihoods of being a case of gastroenteritis rather than

FIGURE 29-10 Example of a Multiple Linear Regression Model with One Continuous and One Categorical Variable with Interaction

The output for the regression model is:

	β	SE	*p*-value
Sex	28.0	4.1	0.01
Predictor_2	2.4	0.1	0.01
Sex*Predictor_2	−1.2	0.1	0.01
Constant	−20.3	2.8	0.01

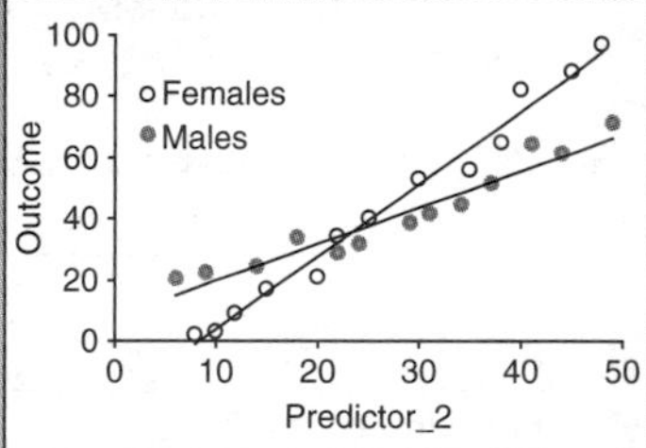

The equation for the regression line is:

OUTCOME = 28.0*SEX + 2.4*PREDICTOR_2 − 1.2*SEX*PREDICTOR_2 − 20.3

Sex value	Predictor_2 value	*Expected* outcome value
0 (female)	20	27.7
0 (female)	21	30.1
1 (male)	20	31.7
1 (male)	21	32.9

For females, a 1-unit increase in Predictor_2 is associated with a 2.4-unit increase in the expected value of the outcome variable.

For males, a 1-unit increase in Predictor_2 is associated with a 1.2-unit increase in the expected value of the outcome variable.

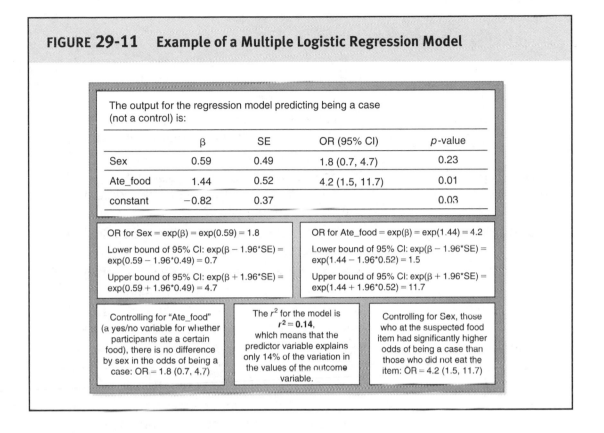

FIGURE 29-11 Example of a Multiple Logistic Regression Model

The output for the regression model predicting being a case (not a control) is:

	β	SE	OR (95% CI)	*p*-value
Sex	0.59	0.49	1.8 (0.7, 4.7)	0.23
Ate_food	1.44	0.52	4.2 (1.5, 11.7)	0.01
constant	−0.82	0.37		0.03

OR for Sex = exp(β) = exp(0.59) = 1.8

Lower bound of 95% CI: exp(β − 1.96*SE) = exp(0.59 − 1.96*0.49) = 0.7

Upper bound of 95% CI: exp(β + 1.96*SE) = exp(0.59 + 1.96*0.49) = 4.7

OR for Ate_food = exp(β) = exp(1.44) = 4.2

Lower bound of 95% CI: exp(β − 1.96*SE) = exp(1.44 − 1.96*0.52) = 1.5

Upper bound of 95% CI: exp(β + 1.96*SE) = exp(1.44 + 1.96*0.52) = 11.7

Controlling for "Ate_food" (a yes/no variable for whether participants ate a certain food), there is no difference by sex in the odds of being a case: OR = 1.8 (0.7, 4.7)

The r^2 for the model is **$r^2 = 0.14$**, which means that the predictor variable explains only 14% of the variation in the values of the outcome variable.

Controlling for Sex, those who at the suspected food item had significantly higher odds of being a case than those who did not eat the item: OR = 4.2 (1.5, 11.7)

a healthy control. The sex-adjusted OR for eating the suspected culprit food has $p = 0.01$ and an odds ratio of OR = 4.2 (1.5, 11.7), which indicates that people with gastroenteritis had four times greater odds of eating the suspect food item than those who were not sick.

29.8 Causal Analysis

Although multiple regression models cannot prove that an exposure caused an outcome, they can provide insights about the **etiology** (or cause) of a disease or other health disorder. **Path analysis** uses regression models to examine causal patterns among variables, assuming a **recursive model** in which all causality is unidirectional. **Structural equation modeling (SEM)** uses maximum likelihood estimation to examine causal patterns with a **nonrecursive model** approach that allows for more complexities in the directionalities of the path diagram.

A statistical **association** between two or more variables is not proof that a causal relationship is present. Researchers are often cautioned with the reminder that correlation does not equal causation. However, results of regression models can be used as part of qualitative considerations of **causality** derived from the **Bradford Hill criteria** and other more recent adaptations (**Figure 29-12**). There

FIGURE 29-12 Criteria for Causation

Temporality	Did the exposure happen before the onset of disease?
Strength of Association	Is the measure of association (such a rate ratio or odds ratio) between the exposure and outcome strong?
Dose–Response Relationship/Biological Gradient	Do people with a higher level of exposure have a higher risk of the outcome than people with a lower level of exposure?
Cessation	Does stopping the exposure reduce the risk of the outcome?
Specificity	Are the exposure and outcome both narrowly defined rather than general concepts?
Theoretical Plausibility	Is there a reasonable biological explanation for why the exposure might cause the outcome?
Consistency	Has a potentially causal relationship between the exposure and outcome been observed in other studies and other populations?
Coherence	Is a causal relationship between the exposure and outcome congruent with other knowledge about the variables?
Consideration of Alternate Explanations	Are there reasons why what appears to be a causal relationship might not actually be causal?
Experimentation	If it is ethical to conduct an experimental study of the exposure and outcome, has experimental testing confirmed a causal relationship?

is no requirement that all causal criteria must be met for an exposure to be considered the cause of an outcome, but the likelihood that a relationship is causal increases when more criteria are met. Most researchers are very cautious about using language that claims or implies causality, and any use of these terms must be carefully justified.

29.9 Survival Analysis

Survival analysis examines the distribution of the durations of time that individuals in a study population experience from an initial time point (such as the date of enrollment in a study or the date of diagnosis of a particular condition) until some well-defined event, which can be death, discharge from a hospital, or some other outcome. Some survival measures are based on **cumulative probability**, the probability of an event occurring by the end of a particular observation period. Others are based on **conditional probability**, the probability of an event occurring given that some prior event has already occurred. A cumulative survival study might ask what percentage of people born in the early 1900s lived to age 95, while a conditional survival study might determine the percentage of people who have already lived to age 90 who survive 5 more years to age 95. Common measures of survival include:

- Median survival time
- Cumulative survival at set times after enrollment or diagnosis
- **Life tables** that record conditional and cumulative probabilities of survival
- **Kaplan-Meier plots** that display cumulative survival rates in a study population (**Figure 29-13**)
- **Log-rank tests** that determine whether survival rates are longer in one population than another
- **Cox proportional hazards regression**, which estimates a **hazard ratio** that compares durations of time to an event (such as death) in two populations

29.10 Cautions

Only a very limited number of studies require regression analysis or any of the other advanced statistics that are described in this chapter. User-friendly statistical

FIGURE 29-13 Example of a Kaplan-Meier Plot

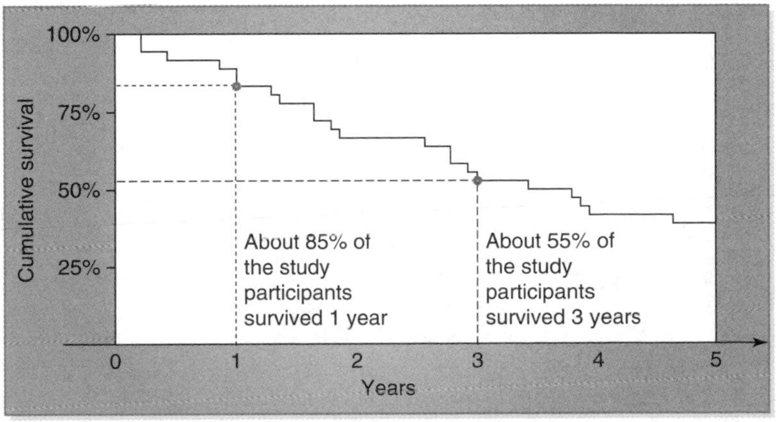

software programs have made it possible for nearly everyone to run advanced statistical analyses, but these programs still require the user to select appropriate tests and decipher what the output means. Researchers should not use these tests without first knowing when to use them, what conditions have to be met to make their use appropriate, how to run them, and how to interpret them. Advanced statistical tests should be used only when they are necessary for the research question. Specialty statistical references and experienced statisticians need to be consulted before attempting to implement any of these methods. Expert consultations are especially helpful for making decisions about how to handle missing data and about which sensitivity tests to confirm the robustness of study results will be helpful.

CHAPTER 30

Additional Analysis Tools

This chapter provides a quick reference to some of the advanced quantitative analysis techniques being used to enhance health science research.

30.1 GIS and Spatial Analysis

If global positioning system (GPS) coordinates or other geographic data have been collected as part of primary research or are available in secondary data sets, then special software programs may be useful for conducting spatial analyses. Once the geographic data have been incorporated into a **GIS (geographic information system)**, it is possible to map the locations of events, to examine the spatial distribution of events, to search for patterns like disease clusters (using a statistic like Moran's *I* coefficient, which tests for spatial autocorrelation, which is a measurement of how similar one location is to nearby places), and to test for possible associations between various social and physical environmental characteristics and health status. A medical geography or health geography reference should be consulted for assistance with spatial analysis.

30.2 Mathematical Modeling

Mathematical modeling explores the relationships between selected theoretical or real-life populations. For example, **SIR models** in epidemiology are models of infection transmission that describe patterns for how the susceptible (S) individuals in a population may become infected (I) and then eventually recover (R) with immunity. An SIR model is a **compartmental model** in which each member of a population exists in one of the three states—susceptible, infectious, or removed—at one time, but over time these individuals can move between compartments. Complexity can be added to the model by creating additional compartments, such as separate S, I, and R compartments for each age group or for different exposure groups. **Ordinary differential equations (ODE)** or other types of equations are used to describe the flows between compartments over time. For example, one equation might describe the infection rate, which is the rate at which individuals move from the S compartment to the I compartment. Another equation might describe the rate at which individuals age from one age group compartment to the compartment for the next oldest age group. To add more realism to a model, the distribution of population members among the compartments and the rates of flow between compartments usually are based on data from field studies. Some models are **deterministic models**, which means that the outcomes of the model will be the same every time the model is run with the same inputs. Some are **stochastic models** that have parameters that vary according to a probability distribution, so the outcomes differ every time the model is run. A distribution of the outcomes can be generated by re-running the model hundreds of times. **Sensitivity analysis** examines the robustness of statistical methods and the results of models. A variety of **sensitivity tests** of mathematical models can help ensure that a model has reasonable validity and provides insights into how the real world works.

30.3 Agent-Based Modeling

Agent-based modeling, sometimes called **agent-based simulation** or **individual-based modeling**, uses computers to simulate the actions and interactions of various individuals (agents) in a population. After identifying a set of assumptions about how the agents in the model behave and how they relate to one another, those assumptions are written into the model's code. Specialized software is then used to run the simulation. Agent-based models can assist with developing and testing new theories as well as with understanding complex data.

30.4 Machine Learning

Machine learning is a method of data analysis derived from artificial intelligence (AI). As a computer runs and re-runs many rounds of analysis, the computer "learns" more about the patterns in the data. Machine learning is used to create and evaluate neural networks, decision trees, and a host of other emerging applications. For example, machine learning can assist with **natural language processing**, which is used in analysis of qualitative and social media data to examine how people speak and write in real-life situations.

The machine learning algorithms generated by this iterative process are often used for predictive analyses. Explanatory and causal models seek to explain observed associations by examining the strength of association between variables. Predictive models have a different goal: They aim to determine which variables best predict group membership. In modeling, **discrimination** is the ability of a model to distinguish between independent groups. For example, **discriminant analysis** (or **discriminant function analysis**) and **canonical analysis** make predictions about membership in groups by identifying the set of variables that most accurately predicts group membership. **Propensity score matching** is a common method for predicting the probability of group membership while adjusting for covariates.

30.5 Cost-Effectiveness Analysis, QALYs, and DALYs

A diversity of health economics methods are useful tools for health research. For example, **cost-effectiveness analysis (CEA)** compares the health gains from an intervention (in the **numerator** of the CEA ratio, which is the top number in the ratio) to the financial costs of that intervention (in the **denominator** of the CEA ratio, which is the bottom number in the ratio). Health gains are often quantified using **quality-adjusted life years (QALYs)**. One QALY is equivalent to one year in perfect health. Diseases and disabilities reduce health status to less than perfect. Premature death (death at ages younger than the target life expectancy in the population) reduces the QALY for that individual to 0. Health interventions—prevention campaigns, screening tests, clinical procedures, rehabilitative therapies, and others—can restore the QALYs that in the absence of intervention would have been lost to illness and can prevent the QALYs that would otherwise have been lost to death. The average cost per QALY can be used to evaluate the cost-effectiveness of an intervention.

The **disability-adjusted life year (DALY)** is a metric similar to the QALY that is frequently used for **burden of disease** studies and health impact assessments. DALYs define disability as any reduction in health status, whether that is an acute infection, a chronic noncommunicable disease, a mental health condition, physical impairment stemming from an injury, or some other cause of diminished health. DALYs are the sum of **years of life lost (YLL)** to premature death and **years lived with disability (YLD)**, with YLDs determined based on assigned disability weights. Other measures of quality of life (QOL) and health-related quality of life (HRQOL) can also be used for economic analyses. Specialty references from health economics, health services research, and related disciplines should be consulted about how to estimate these measures.

STEP

5

Reporting Findings

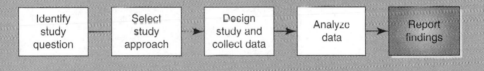

The fifth and final step in the research process is writing a research report and disseminating the results through presentation and publication. This section provides tips for writing, revising, presenting, and publishing findings.

- Posters and presentations
- Article structure
- Citing
- Critical editing
- Writing success strategies
- The manuscript submission, review, and publication process

CHAPTER 31

POSTERS AND PRESENTATIONS

Research results are often publicly shared for the first time during an oral presentation or a poster session at an academic or professional conference.

31.1 Purpose of Conferences

The primary benefit of most professional and academic conferences is the networking that occurs during the gathering: meeting new people working in the same field of interest, catching up with former classmates and colleagues, and making and nurturing professional connections that may be helpful in the future. Conferences are a place to exchange ideas: to be inspired by the discoveries others in the field are making, to learn new methods and techniques in a discipline, and to share current work with others and receive advice from experts. Presenting new research in the form of a poster or an oral presentation can be a particularly useful way to get feedback on a project before submitting the work for review by a journal. Sharing findings is a way to gauge the strengths and weaknesses in the initial presentation that can be enhanced or corrected in the subsequent manuscript.

31.2 Structure of Conferences

Some conferences are annual events sponsored by professional organizations that draw thousands of attendees. Others are small gatherings of a few dozen scholars working in a narrow field of study. Most conferences include a mix of:

- Plenary sessions for all attendees, which often feature keynote addresses
- Concurrent sessions in which multiple panels of oral presentations are held at the same time in different rooms
- Poster sessions in which attendees can mingle while reviewing research posters
- Exhibitions where attendees can visit informational displays set up by partner organizations, vendors, and other sponsors
- Business meetings run by the officers of the host organization

Presenters are usually assigned to deliver either an oral presentation or a poster presentation. Oral presentations are generally considered to be more prestigious than posters, in part because there are usually more slots for poster presenters than for oral presenters. **Oral presentations** usually require delivering a prepared presentation and then participating in a question-and-answer (Q&A) period with the audience and other panelists. This interaction can be so helpful in improving the work prior to publication that some presenters are disappointed when no one in the audience points out a weakness in their work. However, oral presentations can be very stressful for those who are not experienced public speakers.

Poster sessions usually do not require the presenters to make a formal speech. Instead, they are designed to facilitate one-on-one and small group conversations. Posters may be taped along the walls of a room or displayed on long rows of easels, and attendees can browse through the posters at their own pace and interact with presenters if they want more information about a project. These relatively private conversations may allow for a more fruitful exchange of ideas than is possible during the Q&A time at the end of an concurrent session. Another benefit of posters is that they can be displayed in the hallway of an academic department or workplace for several months after the conference. However, posters often require more preparation time than oral presentations, and they may be expensive to print and a hassle to transport.

31.3 Submitting an Abstract

Researchers who want to present at a conference usually are required to submit an abstract for consideration by the organizing committee. The planning committee and other reviewers will:

- Rate the submitted abstracts
- Decide which researchers will be invited to present
- Select who will give an oral presentation as part of a panel and who will be assigned to a poster session

Abstracts selected for a conference are usually printed in a bulletin that attendees use to decide which sessions to attend and which posters to seek out. A good health research abstract includes key methods and results while also conveying one clear health message that is appropriate to the audience expected at the conference. If the conference focuses on clinical practice, the abstract's applied message should be readily translatable into improved patient care. If the conference focuses on research theories and methods, the abstract should emphasize the novelty of the approaches used and their applicability to other research topics. If the conference focuses on health policy, the abstract should have a clear policy implication.

At the time of abstract submission, applicants may be asked about their preferred presentation formats. Those who indicate a willingness to make either an oral presentation or a poster may increase the likelihood that their abstracts will be accepted for the conference.

Abstracts often are due many months before a conference, yet it is not uncommon for conference guidelines to prohibit the submission of abstracts for studies that will be published in a journal prior to the conference. Thus, the ideal timing is to have preliminary results ready to include in the abstract, to prepare the final results for presentation at the conference, and then to use the feedback from the conference to finish the full-length manuscript that will be submitted for publication.

In a few scientific subdisciplines, it is common for article-length research reports to be published as **conference papers** in a book-length volume of conference proceedings. In those fields, conference papers are considered equivalent to peer-reviewed journal articles. However, in most population health disciplines the only written outputs from a conference are abstracts that are not complete enough to be considered part of the formal scientific literature. When only an abstract from a conference is published, researchers are encouraged to consider the conference presentation as an intermediate step toward publication and not as an end product.

Submitting an abstract implies a commitment to attend the conference if selected to be a presenter. The sponsoring organization may (or may not) keep track of dropouts and absentees and not allow them to present at future conferences. The fine-print instructions for the conference often specify the other expectations of applicants. Most conferences require presenters to pay a registration fee (often several hundred dollars) as well as cover all of their own travel expenses. Some schools and employers may reimburse some or all of these expenses for researchers who will present their work at a conference, but if funds are not available the researcher will bear these costs.

31.4 Preparing a Poster

Conference attendees are drawn to visually appealing, symmetric posters. Researchers preparing a poster must give attention to both the content and the design of the poster (**Figure 31-1**). Posters should be well organized and have focused content, a pleasing balance among text, images, and "white space" (background of any color that is not covered with words or images), and an inviting color palette.

Posters can be created by using either specialized graphic design software or a presentation software program (like Microsoft PowerPoint). The size of a slide or page can be adjusted so that the dimensions match those required by the conference. A sample layout is shown in **Figure 31-2**, and the Internet has many examples of other poster designs. Asking several people to check both the content and the design of the poster before it is printed will improve the product. Prior to having the poster printed, the researcher should inquire about:

- Printing costs (which will vary significantly depending on the size of the poster, the amount of color, the type of paper or fabric, and any special options like laminating or mounting)
- The amount of time required for printing
- Whether a special carrying case is needed

FIGURE 31-1 Checklist for Poster Content and Design

Content	• Keep the content focused on one core message. • Choose a descriptive title. • Include the names of all coauthors, brief author affiliations, and contact information for at least one author. • Do not list information about the conference (such as name, dates, or location) on the poster. • Consider skipping the abstract to save space. • Clearly state the main goal, the specific objectives or hypotheses, and the importance of the study. • Use a structured format, with introduction/background, methods, results, and conclusion/discussion sections (and a reference list, in small font, if previous studies are cited). • Be concise. Use short sentences and bulleted lists when possible. • Images like graphs, tables, flowcharts, photographs, and maps are more effective than words at conveying information.
Design	• Find out the size and shape (horizontal or vertical) of the display area that the conference organizers will provide and create a poster to fill the space. • Decide whether to print one large poster (preferred) or smaller panels that can be joined together at the conference venue. • Organize content into three or four columns or another structure with a logical flow. • Use boxes, color, and/or lines to group the information. • Select a visually-pleasing color palette. • Ensure adequate contrast between the background (usually light) and content (usually dark). • Use large and consistent fonts that can easily be read several steps back from the poster. • Simplify graphs and make sure that they can be read from a distance (which may require adding a title and directly labeling lines or bars rather than using a key). • Use high-resolution images (and remember that enlarged photographs become fuzzy).

FIGURE 31-2 Sample Poster Layout

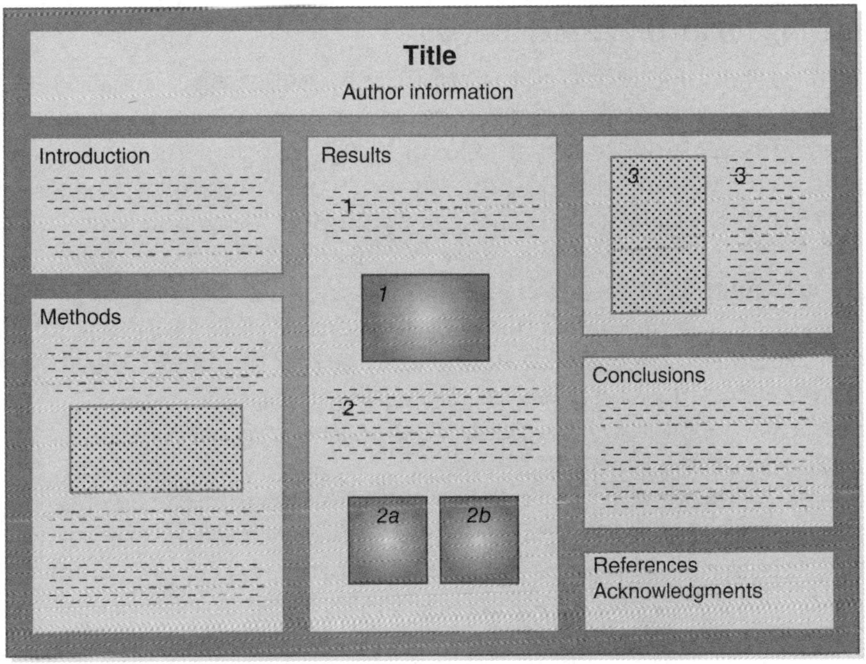

31.5 Presenting a Poster

At most conferences, the poster presenter is responsible for setting up the poster at an assigned time. Although some conference organizers provide all the necessary supplies, this is not always the case. Because a variety of display setups may be used, poster presenters should come prepared with binder clips (for clipping a poster to a stiff board set on an easel), pushpins (for pinning a poster to a corkboard), and tape (for taping a poster to a wall). The presenter is also responsible for taking down the poster at an appointed time. It is considered bad form to take down a poster early or to leave it up after the assigned time, when someone else may be waiting to set up a poster for the next session.

Some conferences designate poster session times when presenters are expected to stand by their posters and interact with attendees for an hour or two. These sessions provide valuable time for one-on-one conversations with interested individuals. It is appropriate to greet each person who stops to view the poster, and it is acceptable not to interact with those who are merely passing by. Becoming so engaged with one person that all others with questions or comments are ignored—or, conversely, allowing only superficial banter—is a missed opportunity to network.

Some presenters prepare a handout that is either a page-sized printout of the full poster or a sheet with highlights. Most presenters have business cards with contact information available for distribution.

31.6 Preparing for an Oral Presentation

A typical oral presentation time slot is about 15 minutes long. Because a minute or two is required for setup at the beginning and for questions at the end, about 10 to 12 minutes of this time slot are available for the actual presentation. Most presenters at health science conferences prepare a set of computerized slides (typically using PowerPoint) that will guide their talks and provide visual information to the audience. Because most presenters can describe 1 or 2 slides per minute, about 12 to 20 slides are appropriate for a 10- to 12-minute talk (**Figure 31-3**). The slides should not attempt to reproduce a paper on the screen; they should highlight the key message of the presentation using images in place of words as often as is appropriate. Figures and tables of statistical results usually need to be very simple to be readable during a presentation. A credit must be provided for all images not created by the coauthors; only images that are in the public domain, licensed for reuse, or otherwise approved for public use by the presenter should be projected. References for any previous publications mentioned in the slide show can be listed in small font at the bottom of the relevant slides. **Figure 31-4** provides a checklist for the content and design of slides for a presentation slide show.

FIGURE 31-3 Sample Distribution of Slides for a 10- to 12-Minute Talk

Content Area	Number of Slides
Title slide with author names and contact information for the presenter	1
Research goal	1–2
Background	2–4
Methods	2–4
Results	4–8
Strengths and limitations	1
Future directions	0–1
Conclusions	1
Acknowledgments and/or invitation for questions	0–1
Total	12–20

FIGURE 31-4 Checklist for Presentation Slide Show

Content	• Graphs, tables, photographs, and other images are used in place of words as often as is appropriate. • Key words and phrases are used instead of full sentences. • The number of slides is appropriate for the scheduled presentation duration (about 1–2 slides per minute, excluding time set aside for questions). • There are no more than about six lines of text per slide. • All bulleted phrases on one slide use a consistent voice (for example, all start with the word "to" or all start with an "-ing" word). • All words are spelled correctly, and all phrases are grammatically correct. • The content of each slide is accurate. • Every slide is relevant. • The slides are in a logical order. • Citations, references, and image credits are provided (if applicable).
Design	• The background is simple and not distracting. • All tables and figures are easy to interpret. • A consistent, readable, and adequately large font size is used for text, tables, and figures (which may require simplifying images and enlarging the font of various components). • There is an adequate contrast between the background and the text (either dark letters on a light background or light letters on a dark background). The contrast is adequate under different lighting conditions (for example, when overhead lights are on or off). • A consistent and pleasant color scheme is used throughout. • The slides are not cluttered. • Unnecessary effects like sounds, animated components, and fancy slide transitions are avoided.

Preparing the slide show is only the first step in preparing for an oral presentation. **Figure 31-5** provides a list of content-, voice-, and performance-related items to practice extensively in the weeks before a presentation. Consider video-recording a practice performance, reviewing it, and identifying areas for improvement.

FIGURE 31-5 Items to Practice Before the Presentation

Content	Opening lines	Practice the exact opening sentences; these need to capture the attention of the audience.
	Message	Master the content of each slide enough to describe each one without referring to notes.
	Phrasing	Use relatively short, precise sentences with active verbs.
	Flow	Practice transitions from one slide to the next.
	Closing lines	Practice exact closing sentences about key conclusions.
Voice	Pace	Speak at a moderate to slow rate.
	Volume	Speak relatively loudly.
	Pitch	Vary your voice inflection.
	Enunciation	Speak clearly.
	Pronunciation	Check on the pronunciation of technical words and names.
	Fillers	Try to avoid fillers (such as "um, ... ah, ... like ... you know").
Performance	Engagement	Smile and make eye contact with members of the audience.
	Posture	Stand tall or sit straight.
	Delivery	Do not just read the slides or read from a script.
	Movement	Try not to fidget, sway, pace, or make other distracting gestures or movements.
	Technology	Become comfortable with advancing slides (using a mouse, keyboard, and/or clicker) and with using a pointer, if applicable; face the audience when using these tools, if possible.

Ask for honest feedback from colleagues and mentors. No one can plan for everything that might be encountered at the conference, including nerves, but practice makes a positive experience more likely.

A few weeks before the conference, check on the equipment that will be provided in the presentation room (such as a computer and an LCD projector).

- Some conferences expect presenters to bring their own laptop computers.
- Some conferences require presenters to upload their presentation files to a website in advance of the conference.
- Some ask presenters to email their files to the session moderator.
- Some expect presenters to have the file on a flash drive.

No matter what format is preferred, always bring a backup copy of the presentation file in an accessible format.

31.7 Giving an Oral Presentation

Figure 31-6 summarizes the key tasks for the day of the presentation. Conference organizers often advise presenters to:

- Arrive at the presentation room at least 15 minutes before the panel begins (not 15 minutes before an individual presentation time)
- Check in with the moderator
- Set up the computer and projector or confirm that slides are ready to be projected

Presenters must remember to be considerate of other presenters in their session by strictly adhering to their assigned time limits.

At most conferences, time is allotted for questions from the audience, either after each presentation or after all the panelists in the session have spoken. If a microphone is not available for those asking questions, the respondent should repeat the question before answering it. The appropriate etiquette is usually to:

- Keep responses short
- Thank those who offer suggestions for improving the work
- Acknowledge the limitations of the project while highlighting its strengths
- Be respectful to everyone

At the end of the session, one-on-one or small group conversation about the research may continue. Presenters should have business cards available to share with those who have overlapping interests. When contact information is exchanged, it is appropriate for the presenter to send a follow-up email after the conference that expresses an interest in continued communication and possible collaborations.

FIGURE 31-6 Checklist of Tasks on the Day of the Presentation

Time	Tasks	
Fifteen minutes before the assigned presentation panel is scheduled to begin	Moderator	Check in with the session moderator or chair, if there is one.
	Q&A	Ask the moderator whether the question-and-answer time will take place after each presenter or after all of the presenters are finished.
	Time	Confirm the amount of time for the presentation, and ask the moderator whether there is a timekeeper and what sort of warning signs will be given when the allotted time is nearly finished. If there is no timekeeper, ask a friendly person in the front row to serve as one.
	Computer	If using a computer and/or projector, check to be sure that the devices are set up and that the presentation is loaded on the computer and ready to use.
	Pointer	If using a pointer and/or clicker, check to be sure that they are working.
	Microphone	If using a microphone, conduct a sound check.
	Water	Bring a bottle of water and have it easily accessible to you during your presentation.
	Co-presenters	Greet other presenters in the session.
During other presenters' talks in the session	Listen	Pay attention to the other talks; do not focus on personal notes or preparation during this time.
	Connect	Listen for points of connection between the research talks being presented, especially if the question-and-answer period comes at the end of the session.

FIGURE 31-6 (continued)

Time	Tasks	
During the talk	Relax	Trust that practice will result in a proficient presentation.
	Be calm	Be alert to nervous behaviors, such as adding fillers to speech or swaying the body.
	Keep time	Do not exceed the allotted time period.
After the talk	Thanks	Thank the moderator, timekeeper, technology support person, and fellow presenters.
	Belongings	Check to be sure that personal items are not forgotten.
	Conversations	Wait in the room for at least a few minutes in case anyone has follow-up questions; move the discussion into the hallway as soon as the presenters for the next session begin setting up their talks.

CHAPTER 32

Article Structure

Research articles almost always have the same structure: abstract, introduction, methods, results, and discussion.

32.1 Writing Checklists

The most common information included in each section of a scientific article is shown in **Figure 32-1**. Several checklists have been developed for the specific content to include in reports about various types of studies. Some of the most widely used checklist like the **STROBE**, **CONSORT**, **COREQ**, and **PRISMA** statements are listed in **Figure 32-2**. A sample outline for an article 18 paragraphs in length about a primary observational or experimental study is shown in **Figure 32-3**. Outlining a paper down to the paragraph level before writing allows authors to track progress toward a complete manuscript and to ensure that no critical information is inadvertently omitted.

32.2 Abstract

The abstract is a paragraph-length summary of the article. Its most important function is to serve as an advertisement for the manuscript, catching the eye of potential readers. Even when researchers have access to the full text of an article, they will not be likely to read past the abstract if the summary does not draw their attention. An abstract must convey the key message of the paper in a compelling way while also including critical information about the person, place, and time characteristics of the study as well as the exposure, disease, and/or population that were studied. Writing an accurate and reasonably complete synopsis can be a challenge when most journals limit abstracts to a maximum of 150 to 250 words.

A **structured abstract** uses subheadings, like Objective, Methods, Results, and Conclusion, to highlight content. An **unstructured abstract** usually follows the same outline but does not list the section titles. Most journals' author instructions

FIGURE 32-1 Key Content for Articles Reporting on Analysis of Individual-Level Data

Section	Content
Abstract/ summary	• Summarize the article using key words.
Introduction/ background	• Provide essential background information. • State the objectives of the study (or, for experimental studies, the hypotheses tested). • Identify the study design (including, for experimental studies, the randomization method). • Describe the source population (including selection methods and eligibility criteria and, if applicable, recruiting methods), the setting, and the dates of the study.
Methods	• Define key exposures, key outcomes, and other variables. • Explain how data were collected. • Describe how the required study size was estimated. • Discuss ethical considerations (such as which research ethics committees approved the project, whether an inducement was offered, and how informed consent was documented). • Describe the statistical methods used for analysis.
Results	• Describe the study population, including the sample size (using a flow diagram to show the number of individual participants at each stage of the study if that will be helpful). • Report relevant results (using tables and figures when possible). • Summarize key findings and how they relate to the study objectives (or hypotheses). • Discuss the limitations of the study.
Discussion	• Summarize (briefly) the key findings and state how they achieved the goals of the study. • Describe the key implications of the study for changes in practice, policy, and/or future research.
Endmatter	• Provide the information requested by the target journal, such as a description of each author's contributions, acknowledgments of the contributions of those who did not meet the authorship criteria, funding sources, and possible conflicts of interest. • References.

FIGURE 32-2 Common Reporting Guidelines

Study Approach	Checklist	
Case series	CARE	*Ca*se *Re*port
	STARD	*Sta*ndards of *R*eporting of *D*iagnostic Accuracy
	TRIPOD	*T*ransparent *R*eporting of a multivariable prediction model for *I*ndividual *P*rognosis *O*r *D*iagnosis
Cross-sectional survey Case-control study Cohort study	STROBE	*S*trengthening *t*he *R*eporting of *Ob*servational Studies in *E*pidemiology
Experimental study	CONSORT	*Con*solidated *S*tandards *o*f *R*eporting *T*rials (for randomized controlled trials)
	SPIRIT	*S*tandard *P*rotocol *I*tems: *R*ecommendations for *I*ntervention *T*rials
	SQUIRE	*S*tandards for *Qu*ality *I*mprovement *R*eporting *E*xcellence
	CHEERS	*C*onsolidated *H*ealth *E*conomic *E*valuation *R*eporting *S*tandards
	TREND	*T*ransparent *R*eporting of *E*valuations with *N*onrandomized *D*esigns
Qualitative studies	COREQ	*Co*nsolidated Criteria for *Re*porting *Q*ualitative Research
Systematic review Meta-analysis	PRISMA	*P*referred *R*eporting *I*tems for *S*ystematic Reviews and *M*eta-*A*nalyses (for evaluations of interventions)
	MOOSE	*M*eta-analysis *o*f *O*bservational *S*tudies in *E*pidemiology

(and most calls for abstracts for conferences) will specify whether a structured or unstructured abstract is preferred. Many authors find it easiest to write the abstract after the rest of the paper has already been written and the focus, key results, and conclusions are clear. Other authors find it helpful to write the abstract first, so that it can guide the way they present their key message in the full manuscript.

FIGURE 32-3 Sample Outline for an 18-Paragraph Paper

	Section	Paragraph
1	Abstract	Summary
2	Introduction	Set the stage
3		Justify the importance of the study
4		Main study question and 3 specific aims
5	Methods	Sampling and recruiting
6		Survey instrument
7		Ethics
8		Statistical methods
9	Results	Description of participants (Table 1)
10		Key finding #1 (Table/Figure 2)
11		Key finding #2 (Table/Figure 3)
12		Key finding #3 (Table/Figure 4)
13	Discussion	Answer to the main study question
14		Commentary on key finding #1
15		Commentary on key finding #2
16		Commentary on key finding #3
17		Study strengths and limitations
18		Implications and conclusions
	Endmatter	References
		Table/Figures

Most research databases and Internet search engines have access only to abstracts. A carefully constructed abstract will include a diversity of likely search terms in order to maximize hits from computerized searches. For example, although the MeSH (medical subject header) dictionary considers the terms "hypertension" and "high blood pressure" to be synonyms, abstract databases might not. If an abstract about hypertension includes only the word "hypertension," then someone searching for "high blood pressure" might not find the article. A stronger abstract will include both "hypertension" and "high blood pressure" among its words. Similarly, if a study about a particular country has relevance to a wider region, it is advantageous to include both the country name and regional terms. For example, an abstract on Lebanon might benefit from inserting terms like "the Middle

East" and "the Eastern Mediterranean" (the name of the World Health Organization region that encompasses North Africa and the Middle East) into its objectives or conclusion statements.

32.3 Introduction

The **introduction section** (or **background section**) provides critical information a reader must know to understand the methods and results of the article. This section often includes important definitions, the foundational theories that informed the design of the study, and contextual information about the study's key exposures, diseases, and populations, including details about the study location. The section may also include a paragraph justifying the importance, significance, and novelty of the new study. The introduction section usually ends with a paragraph spelling out the overall goal and the specific aims, objectives, or hypotheses that the paper will address.

The length of the introduction section compared to the discussion section varies according to the target publication venue. For some journals, a typical introduction might consist of only one or two paragraphs, but a lengthy discussion section is expected. For other journals, the introduction might be several pages long, but the discussion section is relatively short. For example, a long introduction section might include a comparison to previous studies and a discussion of what is novel about the new study, but that content often appears in the discussion section instead.

32.4 Methods

The **methods section** should begin by clearly identifying the study design used. If person, place, and time characteristics and definitions for the key exposures, outcomes, and other variables were not provided in the introduction, they should be listed in this section. For example, for a case-control study, the case definition should be spelled out; for an experimental study, the intervention and control should both be described in detail. For some studies, supplying the exact phrasing and order of questionnaire items, along with the steps taken to validate the survey instrument, are important.

For primary studies, the methods used to identify, sample, and recruit participants should be described, and the inclusion and exclusion criteria should be listed. The methods for collecting data should also be described, including interview techniques and (if relevant) laboratory methods, physical examination checklists, and measurement methods. For secondary analyses, the report should state who collected the data originally, how the data were collected, and how the data files were acquired for secondary analysis.

The methods section must describe how data were coded for analysis, cleaned, and analyzed, and how missing data were handled. The various statistical tests used in the analysis are often listed in this section, and information about the interpretation of uncommon tests may be included. Studies that include laboratory analyses and other assessments should describe those procedures in adequate detail, providing references to critical methodological papers as appropriate.

The methods section should provide information about ethical considerations, such as whether inducements were offered, how informed consent was documented, whether community groups were consulted, and which research ethics committees reviewed the project. Ethical issues may also be included in the endmatter, depending on the preference of the journal.

The methods section of a paper can often be written even before data collection begins, because most of the methods are finalized before data collection starts.

32.5 Results

The **results section** should start with a description of the study population that clearly identifies the sample size and the demographics of the participants. Additional results of quantitative and/or qualitative analyses should then be provided, using tables and figures when possible. Most studies do not require multivariate statistics or other types of advanced analyses. The results of a statistical test should not be reported unless the authors fully understand when that test can be used and how it should be interpreted.

One common organizational strategy for this section is to match results paragraphs to the specific aims of the study. For example, if there are three specific aims, then the results section might have four paragraphs: one that describes the characteristics of the study population, one that presents the results most relevant to the first objective, one with results for the second objective, and one for the third objective (**Figure 32-4**). Another organizational approach is to write one paragraph about each table and figure. The first table typically describes the study population and is the first paragraph of the results section. The remaining tables and figures are presented in an order that best aligns with the specific aims or hypotheses.

FIGURE 32-4 A "Follow the 3s" Approach to Storytelling in a Scientific Paper

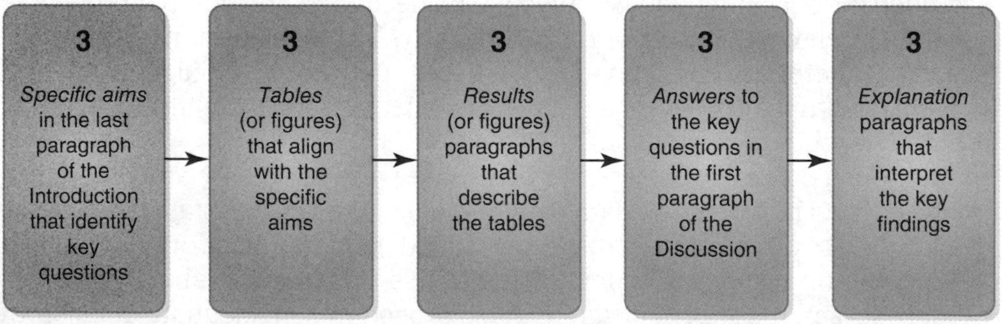
3
Specific aims in the last paragraph of the Introduction that identify key questions
3
Tables (or figures) that align with the specific aims
3
Results (or figures) paragraphs that describe the tables
3
Answers to the key questions in the first paragraph of the Discussion
3
Explanation paragraphs that interpret the key findings

32.6 Discussion

The **discussion section** usually begins with a brief summary of the key findings of the new study. The key findings should align with the aims, objectives, or hypotheses spelled out in the last paragraph of the introduction section. Ideally, the answer to the main research question posed at the end of the introduction section should be answered in the first sentences of the discussion section. The ensuing paragraphs should compare the new study to previous studies and include a thorough discussion of the relevant existing literature along with an adequate number of citations.

Every paper needs to include at least one paragraph about the strengths and limitations of the study. The limitations paragraph should identify potential types of bias and other problems that could make the study results inaccurate, invalid, or not generalizable beyond the study population. The discussion section sometimes also explains the steps taken during the study's design, implementation, and analysis to minimize the likelihood of encountering serious problems. Fixable problems should have been corrected long before the discussion section is written. This is the place to describe the issues that could not be avoided and to offer an honest appraisal of how those remaining concerns might have biased the results.

The final paragraph of the discussion should state the conclusions and implications of the study. All conclusions must stem directly from the results of the study. For example, a paper reporting on the results of an experimental test of a new prostate cancer therapy should have a conclusion about cancer treatment that stems directly from that study's results. It should not have a conclusion about screening or diagnosis or some other therapy. A study about risk factors for sports-related injuries should have a conclusion about sports injury prevention that is closely related to that study's results.

The appropriate conclusions vary by discipline and journal, but they might include recommendations for new preventive, diagnostic, or therapeutic practices and policies; a summary of the new theories that emerge from the analysis; or calls for future research. In general, a suggestion about the need for further research on the topic is the weakest conclusion that can be made. It is better to end with a specific key message directed at improving clinical or public health policy and practice, especially if the recommended action is a cost-effective one that could reasonably be implemented in the target population.

32.7 Endmatter

Some journals list information between the conclusion and the reference list. This **endmatter** may include:

- The affiliations of the authors and their contact information (if this is not listed on the title page)
- The specific contributions of each author to the paper
- Acknowledgments of people who assisted with the study but who did not meet authorship criteria

- Information about some ethical aspects of research, such as a declaration that each participant gave informed consent along with the names and locations of the committees that reviewed and approved the project
- A list of all funding sources
- Disclosures of the presence or absence of possible conflicts of interest, including personal financial conflicts of interest as well as potential conflicts related to being employed by an organization having a financial interest in the study

Some journals provide this information in the final published version of the paper but request that it be removed from the submitted manuscript because they use a blind review process and this information could reveal the identities or affiliations of the authors. The author guidelines of each journal will indicate what information should be provided in the endmatter of submissions.

32.8 Tables and Figures

Many health journals limit the number of tables and figures allowed for each article, often to a maximum total of four (tables and figures combined). This limit means that the content for tables and figures must be carefully selected to highlight the most important aspects of the study. **Tables** should be used to organize and present statistical results that cannot easily be listed in the text in a sentence or two. Graphs, maps, photographs, and other **figures** should be used when a visual presentation of the material is more effective than words or numbers at conveying a result. Any images used should be meaningful, not merely decorative. There is no need to repeat information in the text that is provided in a table or figure, but a **callout** for each table and figure—that is, a phrase like "Figure 1 shows…" or a notation in parentheses like "(Table 2)"—should be placed in the text to indicate when the reader should refer to the table or figure.

A table should provide enough information so that it can be independently interpreted and understood even in the absence of the text (**Figure 32-5**).

- The title of the table should provide a brief but complete description of the content.
- The rows and columns should each have a descriptive label and, when applicable, provide units and/or sample sizes (which are often designated by *n* for the number of participants).
- For each statistic, provide a confidence interval, *p*-value, and/or other measure of uncertainty, such as a standard deviation or standard error for a mean or an interquartile range for a median.
- A note just below the table (or just after the title) should explain the meaning of asterisks (*) and other symbols (such as †, ‡, and §) commonly used to denote statistical significance and other items of interest.
- Consistent fonts, spacing, and number of decimal points should be used for all tables in the manuscript. Do not provide more numbers (digits) after the decimal (that is, **significant figures**) than are appropriate for the sample size.

FIGURE 32-5 Sample Table Describing the Participants in a Case-control Study and Showing that the Case and Control Populations Are Similar

Characteristic		Cases $n = 102$	Controls $n = 237$	X^2 *p*-value
Sex	Female	54 (53%)	138 (58%)	0.37
	Male	48 (47%)	99 (42%)	
Home district	North	33 (32%)	62 (26%)	0.47
	Central	33 (32%)	89 (38%)	
	South	36 (35%)	86 (36%)	
Current smoker	Yes	18 (18%)	31 (13%)	0.28
	No	84 (82%)	206 (87%)	

A **graph** should provide enough information in the title, figure, and/or legend or key for a reader to be able to interpret the graph even without reading the related portion of the text. **Figure 32-6** highlights some of the features that may make a graph easier or more difficult to interpret correctly, including the selection of an

FIGURE 32-6 Examples of Correct and Problematic Graphs

Correct:

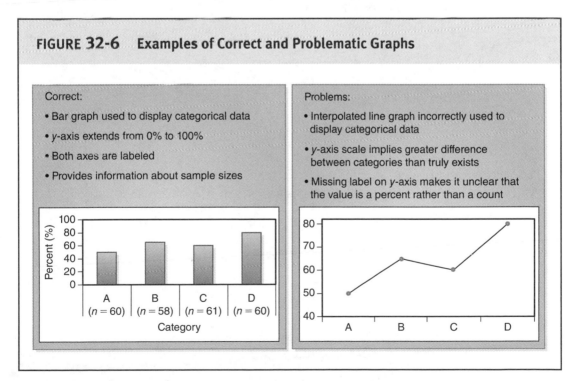

- Bar graph used to display categorical data
- *y*-axis extends from 0% to 100%
- Both axes are labeled
- Provides information about sample sizes

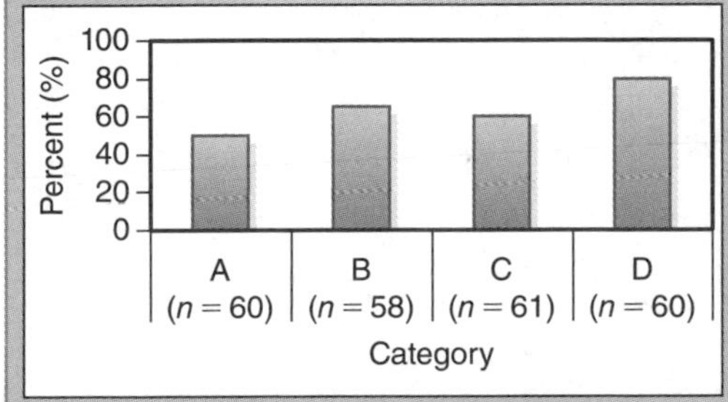

Problems:

- Interpolated line graph incorrectly used to display categorical data
- *y*-axis scale implies greater difference between categories than truly exists
- Missing label on *y*-axis makes it unclear that the value is a percent rather than a count

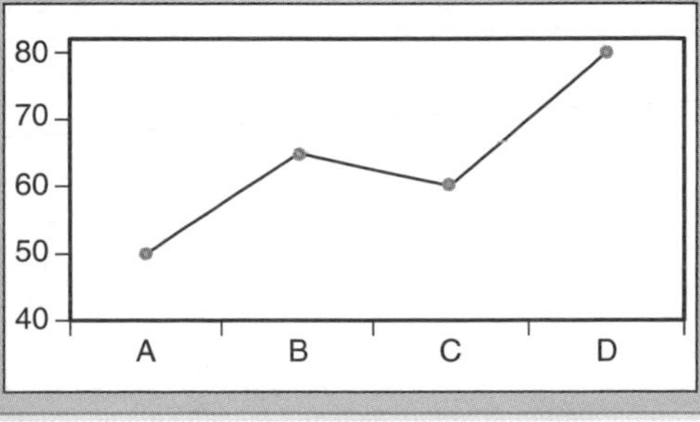

appropriate type of graph, the use of appropriate scale and labels for axes, and the inclusion of other relevant information about the data being presented.

High-resolution photographs, maps, flowcharts, and other images provided by the authors can also be used as figures. Photographs of study participants are usually not allowed to be published without the written permission of the subject or subjects. This is true even when a black bar covers the eyes or other features. Clinicians who are considering writing a case report or case study and are documenting the progression of a patient's disease with photographs should usually secure written permission to use those images prior to taking the first photo.

CHAPTER 33

CITING

Research reports must contain accurate reference information about the sources that informed or supported the methods, findings, and conclusions of a new study.

33.1 Referring to the Scientific Literature

The authors of every scientific paper need to explain how their new investigation fits with previous studies. The introduction section of a manuscript usually provides the background necessary to understand the importance of the new work. The discussion section typically provides an extensive comparison of the results of the new study and the results of previously published works. A typical article in the health sciences refers to about 25 or 30 other articles published in peer-reviewed journals, although some cite only a handful and some (especially review articles) may cite hundreds.

Pertinent articles can be found by searching electronic databases and by looking at the reference lists of articles already identified and determined to be helpful. (See Chapter 3 for more information about how to find relevant articles.) Most of the articles that will be cited in the text of the paper and then included in the reference list at the end of the document should provide evidence that supports the importance, validity, and conclusions of the new study. References can also be used to acknowledge alternative methodological approaches that could have been used, to identify areas where the new findings appear to contradict previous studies, and to provide varying perspectives on the policy and practice implications of the study.

The best articles to cite are ones that present results and key findings that are directly relevant to the new study. Authors should be cautious about citing commentary from the introductions and discussions of other papers, especially when the pertinent commentary is citing other sources. Suppose that "Paper 1" makes an interesting comment in its discussion section about the findings of "Paper 2" and

"Paper 3." In that situation, the best option is to look up both "Paper 2" and "Paper 3" so that their methods and results can be examined and then cited if relevant. "Paper 1" does not need to be cited, because the supporting evidence for the new paper does not derive from the results of "Paper 1" itself. Or suppose that "Paper 4" cites 8 articles at the end of a sentence as evidence that many previous studies have identified a particular exposure to be a risk factor for a particular disease. The best option in that situation may be to look for a review article about that association. The results section of most systematic review articles presents a summary and synthesis of the full body of literature on the selected topic. That analysis will clarify whether there is consensus about the effects of the exposure, or whether 8 studies have found a significantly risky association but 80 others have found no association. A review article is a more helpful and concise citation to provide than either "Paper 4" or a lengthy list of references.

Citing an article is an endorsement of its authors—except in the rare instances when specific flaws in prior work need to be pointed out—so it is important to read the full text of every cited article and make sure that the methods and conclusions are sound. (Reading the full article carefully is even more important when criticizing the work.) Do not trust abstracts to be reliable. Abstracts may incorrectly or incompletely summarize the methods and results of a study. For example, abstracts may omit critical information, like a very small sample size, a very low participation rate, or the use of a data set that is many decades old. Or they may report only the statistics that are most congruent with previous studies or the most shockingly different from them. Additionally, abstracts often state conclusions that the study's data do not support. Before citing any article, read and understand the full article. (If an **erratum** has been issued to correct an error in the article, be sure to read the updated version of the manuscript.)

Journal articles are the preferred source of evidentiary support for scientific articles, although books, book chapters, and scientific reports (such as those published by governmental agencies and international organizations) are also acceptable **formal sources**. **Figure 33-1** summarizes the characteristics of formal reports. Fact sheets, websites, and other **informal sources**, that have not been peer-reviewed and then published by a trusted organization should be cited only when a more reliable and permanent source of information is not available (**Figure 33-2**).

33.2 Writing in One's Own Words

Almost no scientific articles quote directly from another source word for word. There are many reasons to avoid quoting from another publication. One of the most important reasons is that borrowing phrases and sentences from other writers often makes the writing in a document choppy. Some people who use quotations do so because they feel that the original works were so perfectly written that the new authors could not express the same thought equally well using different words. This is not true. Communicating the same idea in one's own writing style usually is better for the new work because it allows the entire article to have a consistent voice.

FIGURE 33-1 Characteristics of Formal Scientific Reports

Formal Scientific Reports ...

- Are published in a peer-reviewed journal (or sometimes a peer-reviewed report or book), not on a website, in a newspaper, or in a popular magazine
- Describe the study design and explain why it was appropriate for the objectives of the study
- Explain how the study population was selected and demonstrate that the sample size was sufficiently large
- Explain how exposures and outcomes were defined and assessed
- Describe the analytic approaches used and present results using easily interpreted tables and graphs
- Draw conclusions that are reasonable and based on the study's data
- Discuss the limitations of the study
- Compare the new study to previous studies
- Follow a standard outline and other conventions for scientific writing

Another benefit of paraphrasing is that it helps ensure that the article being cited has been understood. Paraphrasing accurately requires a level of comprehension that direct quoting does not. Using a quotation that is not fully understood is never a good idea.

Paraphrasing does not remove the requirement to cite the original source; it just means that quotation marks do not have to be used. When a direct quotation is lifted from a paper and reused, the entire quotation must be in quotation marks (or indented from the left margin, depending on the length of the quote and journal formatting preferences). Additionally, an in-text citation must be provided. When the ideas or findings of other scholars are paraphrased, quotation marks are not used because the words are not being copied, but an in-text citation for the source of the original information must still be provided. **Figure 33-3** illustrates the difference between a quotation and a paraphrase.

33.3 Common Knowledge and Specific Knowledge

Any **specific knowledge**, such as a statistic or the result of a particular field or laboratory study, must be cited when it is referred to in a scientific paper. However, some types of information do not require a citation. **Common knowledge** (also called **general knowledge**) refers to what a typical person in the discipline knows. In scientific writing, common knowledge does not refer to what a randomly selected person from the general

FIGURE 33-2 Citable Sources

Source	Formal or Informal?	Citable?	Remarks
Website or fact sheet	Informal	Rarely	Websites and fact sheets may be helpful starting places for informal research but should only be cited in a formal manuscript if they are from a trusted organization and no formal article or report provides the same information.
Newspaper or popular magazine	Informal	Rarely	Popular media items should be referred to only when no formal scientific article or report provides the same information.
Statistical database	Formal	Yes	Cite statistical databases and reports only when information is provided about how, when, and where the data were collected.
Official report	Formal	Yes	Reports are usually cited only when they are formal publications (with assigned publication years and/or other bibliographic information) from trusted organizations.
Book or book chapter	Formal	Yes	Although most scientific communication occurs through journals rather than books, scientific books are acceptable sources for formal manuscripts; general textbooks are rarely appropriate sources, but some highly technical textbooks are appropriate to cite.
Abstract	Formal	No	Cite only full-text articles (and be sure to read the full text before citing them).
Article	Formal	Yes	Articles from peer-reviewed journals are the preferred references for formal manuscripts.

FIGURE 33-3 Examples of Quoting and Paraphrasing

Quotation (almost never used in journal articles)	Paraphrase (often used)	Reference (always required for either a quotation or a paraphrase)
A case-control study examining risk factors for ovarian cancer in Canadian women found that "age at first full-term pregnancy was not associated with risk of ovarian cancer."[1]	A case-control study of Canadian women found no association between ovarian cancer and the ages of participants at the time of their first full-term pregnancies.[1]	1. Risch HA, Marrett LD, Jain M, Howe GR. Differences in risk factors for epithelial ovarian cancer by histologic type: results of a case-control study. *Am J Epidemiol* 1996; 144:363–72.
The authors acknowledged that "since we did not adjust for depth of inhalation and age at smoking onset, the RR for women, compared with that for men, due to smoking was likely to have been underestimated by our results."[2]	The authors of the study pointed out that it was possible that they might have underestimated the magnitude of the increased risk of lung cancer in female smokers compared to male smokers because they had not statistically adjusted for smoking behaviors, such as the depth of inhalation.[2]	2. Zang EA, Wynder EL. Differences in lung cancer risk between men and women: examination of the evidence. *J Natl Cancer Inst* 1996; 88:183–92.
The investigators noted that "cholera is usually considered to be a water-borne disease, but, in this outbreak, the available evidence indicates that a food item served as part of a meal was the most likely vehicle of infection."[3]	The investigators concluded that the most likely cause of the cholera outbreak was food served to passengers on the airplane.[3]	3. Sutton RG. An outbreak of cholera in Australia due to food served in flight on an international aircraft. *J Hyg (London)* 1974; 72:441–51.

population knows. For example, health professionals generally know that influenza is caused by a virus and that Germany is located in Europe. This is common knowledge in the discipline. Both of these facts are well established, and a quick search for papers on influenza or about studies conducted in Germany would show that this information is not usually accompanied by a citation. In contrast, a statistic about the proportion of Germans who seek clinical care for influenza in a typical year and the results of a particular epidemiological study of influenza in Germany are both specific knowledge, and the sources of those details would need to be cited. When in doubt about whether a bit of information is common knowledge, err on the side of using a citation. Also, any disputed fact should be well supported by one or more reliable sources.

33.4 Avoiding Plagiarism

Plagiarism occurs when someone's wording, thinking, image, or creative output is repeated in a new document without attribution. Copying the exact words of another person without using quotation marks and providing a full citation, engaging in "thesaurus plagiarism" that swaps in synonyms for words in an original source in order to avoid the need for quotation marks, paraphrasing a unique theory or observation without providing a citation, and using an image without permission and an acknowledgment are all forms of plagiarism. Failing to fully acknowledge the source of the original work deprives the author or creator of the material the recognition that person deserves, and it may result in the plagiarist getting credit for work that he or she did not do.

Plagiarism is a major violation of scholarly integrity, and it can have a damaging long-term impact on a professional career. For example, a published article with extensive plagiarism must be retracted, and a **retraction** notice will be issued by the journal to remove the article from the accepted scientific literature and to serve as a permanent open record of wrongdoing. For students, plagiarism can result in expulsion from school. For employees, plagiarism can result in the loss of a job. The other consequences of plagiarism and other forms of research misconduct, such as redundant publication or the fabrication or falsification of data, are discussed in detail on the website of the Committee on Publication Ethics.

Several habits can be adopted to ensure that plagiarism does not occur. One helpful practice is never to cut and paste information from a website, article, or any other source into a document file that contains any draft material for an article. It is far too easy for those words, phrases, or even whole sentences or paragraphs to be unintentionally incorporated into the text of a manuscript—and "unintentional plagiarism" is still plagiarism, and it carries the same penalties. When browsing websites and other electronic for background material, take the time to paraphrase the information instead of cutting and pasting the content for later review.

Another good habit is to always include a full reference alongside all research notes derived from particular sources. For example, if an article presents a theory that explains the findings of the new project, do not just make a note about the theory. Jot down the theory and put a bracket with the author and year next to it, as is typically done in journal manuscripts, and then add in the full bibliographic information for the article so that the source of the theory can be easily identified later on when writing is under way and a citation is required.

33.5 Citation Styles

Most of the citation styles used in the health sciences require two types of notations about each source of information:

- In-text citations where the sources of information are briefly identified in the text
- A reference list at the end of the document that provides full bibliographic information for each source

Every article listed as a citation requires a full reference. Every entry in the reference list must be cited at least one time in the main text.

No one citation style is used across the health sciences. The two most common ones are **APA style** and **AMA style**. Many social science and nursing journals use APA (American Psychological Association) style. Many medical and public health journals use a version of a style alternatively called AMA (American Medical Association) style, Vancouver style, ICMJE (International Committee of Medical Journal Editors) style, or NLM (National Library of Medicine) style. The journals that require an AMA-type citation usually provide a guide to their own customized preferences for which variation (or **house style**) to use. Sometimes other styles are required, such as MLA (Modern Languages Association) style, Turabian style, or Chicago style. Reference manuals and style guides are available for all of the widely used styles, and most journals provide an author's guide on their websites that spells out the journal's own style preferences. Articles recently published in the target journal provide additional examples of the journal's preferred style. When preparing a manuscript for publication or writing a less formal report, the goal should be to use a consistent citation and reference style throughout the document.

In-text citations are abbreviated bits of information about the cited work that allow the full reference to be located in the reference list at the end of the article. Examples of formats for in-text citations are shown in **Figure 33-4**. (Some journals will convert bracketed citation numbers to superscript numbers during the editing and layout process, so the author guidelines must be carefully examined to see which submission style is preferred.)

The reference list at the end of the article presents cited works either alphabetically in order of the first authors' last names or in the order of first appearance of the cited work in the text of the article. Sources appear only one time in each reference list. In AMA style, the first article cited is referred to as reference [1] any time it is cited in the manuscript. In APA style, the authors' names are listed in the in-text citation every time the article is cited. The only change that occurs when an article is cited more than one time is that an article with three, four, or five authors will list all of the authors in the first in-text citation but for subsequent in-text citations will list only the first author's last name with "et al." (the abbreviation for the Latin phrase *et alia*, which means "and others") after it.

FIGURE 33-4 In-Text Citation Styles

Number of Citations for the Sentence	1 Source	2 Sources	3 Sources
First author's last name and publication year	... [Ruiz, 2014].	... [Ruiz, 2014; Yamamoto, 2001].	... [Ivanov, 2008; Ruiz, 2014; Yamamoto, 2001].
Author(s) and publication year	... (Ruiz, 2014).	... (Ruiz & Sanchez, 2014; Yamamoto et al., 2001).	... (Ivanov, 2008; Ruiz & Sanchez, 2014; Yamamoto et al., 2001).
Number in brackets (square brackets)	... [1]. ... .[1]	... [1, 2]. ... .[1, 2]	... [1–3]. ... .[1–3]
Number in parentheses (round brackets)	... (1). ... .(1)	... (1,2). ... .(1,2)	... (1–3). ... .(1–3)
Superscript number	... .^{1}	... .^{1,2}	... .$^{1-3}$

When preparing a manuscript for submission to a journal, check the document carefully for compliance with the journal's style specifications. Journals using AMA style or a variant typically list authors by last name and first initials (with no periods after them), then the title (with capital letters only for proper nouns), an abbreviated journal name (which uses a formal journal title abbreviation as specified in *Index Medicus*), the publication year, volume, and page numbers. The components may be separated by periods (full stops) or by semicolons or commas. However, the journals may make minor adjustments to these components. Some journals expect all authors to be listed no matter how many there are; some journals use an abbreviated version for six or more authors, such as listing only the first three authors followed by "et al." Some use abbreviations for journals; others use the full journal name. Some list journal issue numbers; most do not. Some list the full page numbers (such as 202–209), and others use a slightly shorter elided version (such as 202–9). Some use italics or bold type for some parts of the bibliographic entry.

Authors need to be careful to use a consistent style across all entries in the reference list. A sloppy reference list may cause reviewers of a submitted manuscript to worry that the authors were similarly careless in their data collection and analysis. It is worth taking the time to compile, check, and re-check an impeccable reference list.

CHAPTER 34

Critically Revising

Once a complete manuscript has been drafted, it needs to be revised and polished.

34.1 Organization

Research writing is not just about getting facts on paper. Every scientific report should convey one key message, and that "storyline" should be supported by every section, every paragraph, and even every sentence. The paper should have a well-structured "plot" that establishes a research question, presents a sequence of compelling information about it, and then answers that question.

The storyline should be able to be summarized in a single sentence. Indeed, some journals require a **précis** that is 35 words or less. The abstract for the report should tell the entire story in one compelling paragraph. And the whole manuscript must convey a cohesive message with a strong plotline (**Figure 34-1**). The first step in editing is to make sure that the big picture message is being clearly communicated.

The introduction section of a paper in the health sciences should spell out the core question—the "mystery"—that the paper will explore and answer. In some disciplines, it is common to start a manuscript by writing "In this paper, I/we will show that..." and then revealing the key argument. Most papers in the health sciences take a different approach, posing a question in the introduction that will not be answered until later in the paper.

The methods and results sections provide the evidence that will allow the "mystery" to be solved. These sections say what the researchers did and what they observed. They provide all the necessary "clues" for answering the main research question, and they demonstrate that those observations are valid, sufficiently comprehensive, and reasonably unbiased.

The discussion section should tie all the parts of the "story" together, neatly presenting the solution to the "mystery." Many fictional mystery stories end with a detective revealing the culprit and succinctly explaining how this determination was made. A similar approach is often used in nonfiction science writing.

FIGURE 34-1 Does the Paper Tell a Compelling "Story"?

- Does the paper have a clear "storyline"? Can the "plot" be summarized in one sentence?
- Does the title of the paper reflect the key message of the study?
- Does the abstract summarize the key parts of the story?
- Do the opening paragraphs draw the reader into the story?
- Does the introduction overtly ask the main research question?
- Does the methods section explain how the study design allows the main research question to be answered?
- Does the results section provide all the evidence necessary to answer the study question?
- Does the discussion section overtly answer the main research question?
- Are there any missing parts of the story that need to be added so that it is complete and compelling? Do any gaps in logic need to be addressed?
- Are any parts of the manuscript redundant or peripheral to the main story? Can these be removed to tighten the storyline?
- Are the conclusions fully supported by the results?

Some paper drafts do not read well because the authors present many related observations but they have not clearly identified one key message. These papers improve when the authors select one storyline, delete all of the sentences and paragraphs that are not central to the core theme, and then rewrite the remaining components of the paper to align with the narrative. Other paper drafts read poorly because there are two or more plotlines, and none of those stories is presented completely. One paper must tell one story, not several stories. Sometimes it is better to write two well-organized and persuasive papers on related but distinct topics than to try to fit all of the results into one unfocused paper.

34.2 Structure and Content

Once the paper's storyline is clear, the next step is to check the structure and content of the manuscript (**Figure 34-2**). The paper should be well organized. Each paragraph must have one clear theme, and that theme must be an essential part of telling the paper's story. The paper must accurately describe what the researchers did and what they observed, and it must be complete yet concise.

The final paper must not exceed the word limits of the target journal. Full-length reports in the health sciences are often capped at 3000 or 3500 words (excluding

FIGURE 34-2 Checklist for Structure and Content of the Paper

- Is the paper well organized? Is the content focused?
- Does every paragraph have one theme? Does every sentence within a paragraph fit with that paragraph's theme?
- Does the order of paragraphs within each section support the plotline?
- Does the introduction provide all essential background information? (For example, are the person, place, and time details listed somewhere in both the abstract and the text?)
- Does the introduction make the research project appear necessary and important? Does the introduction say why the study is novel?
- Are the methods described in adequate detail?
- Is enough statistical analysis presented? Is each statistic included in the paper necessary?
- Are the tables and figures well designed?
- Are all statistics presented either in the figures/tables or in the text, but not in both?
- Does the discussion provide a concise summary of key findings and then place the new findings in the context of previous research?
- Does the discussion section avoid redundancy with the results section? (No statistical results should be repeated in the discussion section.)
- Does the discussion adequately address the potential limitations of the study?
- Is every claim in the discussion section supported by citations? Should additional references be added to further support the key message of the paper?
- Is every reference listed important and necessary? Can any entries in the reference list be cut?
- Has the paper been double-checked to ensure that no part of it is plagiarized or paraphrased without proper attribution?
- Is every part of the paper truthful? (For example, does the paper report the methods that were actually used rather than an idealized version of them? Does it report the results of the most appropriate statistical tests rather than results from less appropriate tests that happened to produce statistically significant results?)
- Is the paper's word count within the specifications of the target journal?

the abstract, references, tables, and figures). Short reports may be limited to 1500 or 2000 words, or as little as 800 or 1000 words, with only one table or figure allowed. Being aware of these restrictions prior to beginning a draft allows an appropriately focused narrative to be crafted.

34.3 Style and Clarity

In a final check, look at each word, sentence, paragraph, and section, examining style and clarity (**Figure 34-3**):

- Words must be used carefully.
- Sentences must be concise and clear.
- The voice must be consistent, and it must match the style of the target journal.
- Grammar and spelling must be correct.

FIGURE 34-3 Checklist for Style and Clarity

- Are words used precisely? (For example, are terms like "associated," "correlated," and "caused" used appropriately? Are "incidence" and "prevalence" used correctly?)
- Is unnecessary jargon avoided? Are definitions provided for all key terms?
- Are all abbreviations introduced at first use?
- Is the tone of the writing appropriate? Is the writing style fact based rather than emotion based?
- Does the article consistently use a third-person voice or, in rare situations, consistently use a first-person ("I" or "we") voice? Is the voice correct for the target journal?
- Do all subjects (nouns or pronouns) agree with their associated verbs? (For example, since "data" is a plural word, is "data are..." used rather than "data is..."?) Are all other grammatical conventions followed?
- Are active verbs rather than passive verbs used whenever possible?
- Is the verb tense consistent? (For most papers, the past tense is used rather than the present tense because the data were collected in the past.)
- Is each sentence clear? Are phrases as concise as possible?
- Are all words spelled correctly? (Each report should consistently follow the spelling conventions of one country.)
- Is all punctuation correct? (For example, are there extra or missing commas?)
- Does the paper adhere to the specifications of the target journal?

CHAPTER 35

Writing Success Strategies

This chapter provides tips for moving through the writing process successfully.

35.1 The Writing Process

By the time a researcher is ready to write a final report about a project, the vast majority of the work on the project has been completed. A study question has been identified and refined, a study approach has been selected and a protocol developed, and data have been collected and analyzed. The end of the project is in sight, but the prospect of creating a report that is intended to be disseminated beyond those immediately involved in the project can be intimidating. Putting off the writing process is easy. The writing can drag on, and in some cases it is never completed.

Few writers have the ability to sit down and crank out a complete manuscript in one burst of productivity. Most writers experience cycles of high motivation and productivity followed by periods of limited or no interest in their work. **Figure 35-1** illustrates a typical writer's productivity levels during the writing process. The durations of each stage vary among writers and for different papers, but most writers need strategies for motivation at three key times:

- First, writers must overcome the barriers to getting started.
- Second, writers must find ways to prolong the period of high productivity that often occurs at the start of a writing project.
- Finally, most writers become fatigued during the writing process and at some point lose all desire even to think about their projects. At such points, they must find the motivation to persevere and to complete the manuscript.

35.2 Getting Started

By the time a researcher has defined a study question, designed a study, and collected and analyzed data, there should be sufficient information to answer the key study question and explain the findings. At that point, the only way to get started

FIGURE 35-1 Typical Variations in Productivity During the Writing Process

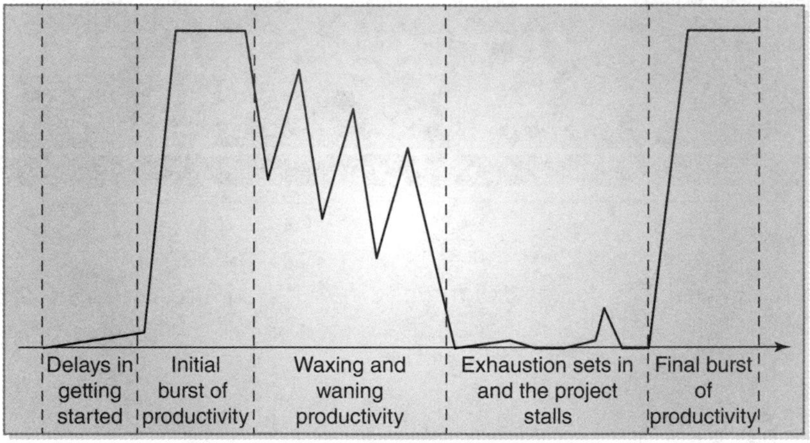

on a writing project is to start writing. Because scientific papers follow a standard outline, an easy way to start filling pages is to:

- Put a working title for the paper at the beginning of the file, along with the names of all the coauthors
- Add in the headers for the Abstract, Introduction, Methods, Results, Discussion, Acknowledgments, and References
- Fill in the names of the people to thank in the acknowledgments section
- Paste in a table or figure that was created during the analysis process and will be included in the final report
- Paste in some relevant lines about methods from the protocol

Then start filling in the gaps. Perhaps find a model article from the target journal and use it as a template to create a detailed outline that specifies exactly what each paragraph in the paper will cover. For example, the headers for paragraphs on statistical methods and ethical considerations can be inserted at the end of the methods section. A brief list of what to cover in each of those paragraphs can then be added based on what was reported in the model article. (Be careful not to plagiarize any ideas or phrases from the model article.) Then write a sentence or two for each of those key points: a sentence about informed consent, a sentence about ethics committee review, a sentence about the significance level used for statistical tests, and so on.

The content of the manuscript does not need to be added in any particular order. Many authors of scientific papers find it easiest to start with the methods, then to write the results, then the introduction and discussion, and finally the abstract, but

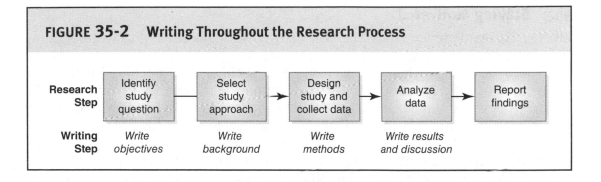

FIGURE 35-2 Writing Throughout the Research Process

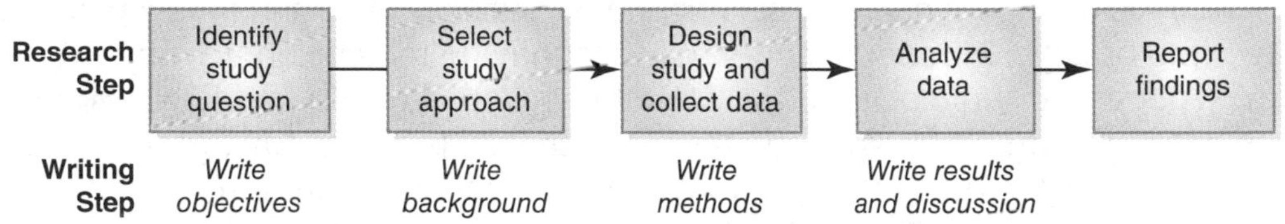

that order is not required. Many authors skip around in the paper, adding a few sentences at a time here and there. Some authors find it helpful to write throughout the research process (**Figure 35-2**). They may draft the introduction as soon as the study question and approach have been selected, the methods once the study is designed, and the results as soon as data have been analyzed. Then they draft the discussion section and edit the earlier sections of the manuscript to ensure that the paper tells a focused story. In short, when getting started on a paper, a good plan is to first write whatever part of the paper is ready to be put into words. Then just keep on writing.

If the barrier to getting started is not having a clear sense of how best to tell the "story" of the paper, it may help to try an oral, visual, or kinesthetic method for moving toward writing productivity.

Researchers who process their thoughts best by talking about them should seek out opportunities to have conversations about their research with coauthors, colleagues, and friends. Answering the questions these audiences ask will provide valuable practice describing and explaining the project. Try developing an "elevator pitch" that tells the main lesson learned from the project in 30 seconds. Try narrating the story of the paper aloud to oneself and recording it; then, transcribe those words as a first step toward drafting a paper. It may be easier to edit spoken language into more formal written language than it is to start from scratch on a formal report.

Researchers who are visual processors may find it helpful to create a poster about the research project or to create a slideshow for a presentation about it. Organizing a poster or presentation helps clarify the flow of the storyline and the relationships among the study's objectives, methods, results, and conclusions. Presenting at a research seminar or conference is an excellent way to receive feedback that will improve the subsequent manuscript. An added benefit is that the visuals created may become figures for the paper.

Researchers who are kinesthetic learners may find it helpful to take a long walk away from a computer and to use that time to think through the story that needs to be written. Walk, then write. Consider using a standing desk or walking desk (a desk with a treadmill) if that activity improves the writing experience.

35.3 Staying Motivated

Most writers experience times when they have a strong desire not to write. A number of steps can help a writer to regain motivation.

Sometimes changing habits or scenery helps, such as writing in a new place or at a new time of day. However, a better practice may be to develop a writing routine, and to write at the same place at the same time every day. Writing daily, even when one is not in the mood to write, means making daily progress toward project completion. Remove distractions from the writing area, including banning music, videos, computer games, and email if those are barriers to productivity. Ensure that the writing space has a supportive chair and other provisions to make writing comfortable.

A manuscript can be completed relatively quickly when the author writes a small fraction of the draft daily. Writing 100 words each weekday will yield a complete draft of a 3000-word manuscript in 6 weeks. If the daily writing time during the following 2 weeks is used for editing, the manuscript can be completed and ready to submit in about 2 months. Writing just one paragraph each day (or making one table or figure during the daily writing time) will yield a complete manuscript in about 1 month. Because most journal articles in the health sciences follow the same outline, it is possible to know exactly which paragraphs are needed for a draft even before the first word is written. These paragraphs can be written in any order. When stuck on a particular paragraph, move on to another one and write that one instead. To maximize productivity, end each day with a plan for what paragraph to write the next day.

Setting a timeline for completing portions of a paper is often helpful. A timeline can include a schedule of events to celebrate intermediate successes on the way to a completed paper. Writers can select rewards that they will give themselves if they achieve their writing targets. It may be helpful to ask others to aid in enforcing those self-imposed deadlines. A supervisor can mandate a particular level of output, but coauthors and other motivators can also serve in this role. Some writing groups are excellent about propelling their members to productivity. (Be cautious about support groups that validate excuses for not writing rather than equipping members to become productive.) Mentors can also help with accountability, if that is the way the relationship has been defined.

35.4 Conquering Writer's Block

Writer's block occurs when an author encounters sustained struggles with writing. This creates a negative thought cycle that can be difficult to break. The underlying issues leading to writer's block are often fear of being judged and fear of failure. Acknowledging these worries is an important step toward getting back to writing. But writers also need to initiate new behaviors to facilitate success, and they need to stop engaging in writing avoidance behaviors. **Figure 35-3** lists various types of writer's block and the realities that challenge them. Writer's block can be overcome when an aspiring writer makes writing a priority. The completed manuscript will not

FIGURE 35-3 Forms of Writer's Block and Writing Avoidance

Reason to Avoid Writing	Reality Check
"I don't know how to write a scholarly paper."	The best way to learn how to write is by writing. A writing support group, coauthors, and/or mentors can help with this process.
"I don't have time to write."	Almost everyone can find 15 or 30 minutes a day to write if that is a priority. Do not use "busyness" as an excuse to avoid writing.
"I only write well when I'm under pressure from a deadline."	Most people do not do their best work when they are stressed.
"I don't know how to get started." "I don't know what to do next."	Coauthors and mentors will be happy to offer advice about how to move forward.
"This project was not interesting so it is not publishable."	If the topic was interesting enough to merit designing a study and collecting data, then it is probably interesting enough to present and publish. Check with a mentor about options for appropriately disseminating the findings.
"This research project had some flaws."	Every study has flaws, but few are fatally flawed. Ask a mentor about how to address the limitations of the study. Write a paragraph about the strengths and weaknesses of the project for the discussion section, and then move on to writing the rest of the paper.
"This study isn't going to change the world."	Most studies make only minor contributions to moving a field forward, but the only way to make any contribution is to publish.
"I'm stuck on this one section, and I can't work on anything else until I finish this part."	Writing and rewriting the same section over again is a waste of time. Work on another section of the paper or ask a coauthor or mentor for assistance.
"I need to read some more articles and run some more tests before I start writing."	These are both stall tactics. There is always one more article that could be read and one more test that could be conducted, but these are not good reasons not to write.

FIGURE 35-3 Forms of Writer's Block and Writing Avoidance (continued)

Reason to Avoid Writing	Reality Check
"I don't want to disappoint or be criticized by my professor or supervisor."	Supervisors want a paper to be as good as it can be, and they are obligated to make suggestions about critical revisions if they are coauthors. Ask a writing support group member or a trusted friend to critically review manuscript drafts before they are shared with a supervisor. Procrastination will only increase anxiety about being evaluated.
"If I submit this paper and it is rejected, I will be embarrassed."	Comments about a paper are not criticisms of the person who wrote it. The only people who will know about the status of a manuscript are those whom the authors choose to tell about it. Research supervisors know that many papers are submitted to several journals before they are accepted for publication. Procrastination will only delay the start of the review process and the possibility of acceptance and publication.
"If this paper is published, someone might discover a flaw in it, and that would be embarrassing."	Coauthors, reviewers, and editors will not let an obviously flawed or badly written article proceed to publication. No paper is perfect, and at some point the authors need to stop revising and finish the manuscript.
"I'm not a good writer." "I'm not good at writing in English."	Coauthors, colleagues, and friends can help polish the manuscript, but only after it has been drafted.

be perfect. No paper is perfect. By the time a report is written, there are likely to be several imperfections in the study design and implementation that cannot be fixed. These flaws are normal and expected. Authors cannot remedy or hide those issues, but they can ensure that they:

- Fully explain the actual methods used
- Conduct all the appropriate analyses
- Honestly identify the limitations of the study and explain what was done to address them

- Include a helpful set of references that support the results
- Polish the prose
- Ask coauthors, mentors, and others to provide feedback on drafts

Most people will always be able to find something they would rather do than write. It is easy to allow distractions to crowd out writing time. But researchers who want to disseminate their work must force themselves to stop planning, stop working on other tasks, and just write. Being a consistently productive writer often is easiest when authors:

- Have a regular writing routine
- Set deadlines for making progress toward a complete manuscript
- Identify and address the excuses they use to avoid writing
- Have mentors, coauthors, and others who support their writing goals
- Focus on the story they want to tell and the population that will be served by that story being shared

Figure 35-4 summarizes a diversity of strategies for getting started on a writing project, staying motivated, and seeing a paper through to completion.

FIGURE 35-4 Thirty Examples of Strategies for Writing Success in the Health Sciences

Focus on the Story	1. Identify the "mystery" and the "plot" of the paper.
	2. Identify the most important practice or policy implication supported by the results of the project. Write a paper that justifies this call to action.
	3. Develop an "elevator pitch." Be able to tell the story of the project in 30 seconds. Use that as the starting point for writing.
	4. Tell the story of the project in images. Start by making tables and figures.
	5. Write a précis (one sentence) and an abstract (one paragraph) that summarize the storyline before starting on the full paper.
	6. Make a poster that tells the story of the project.
	7. Make a slideshow that tells the story of the project, focusing on the order in which different parts of the story are presented.
	8. Tell the full story of the project to others, focusing on the mystery, the evidence, and the solution. Talk, then write.
	9. Record yourself telling your "story," transcribe the recording, and then edit the transcript into formal written language.

FIGURE 35-4 Thirty Examples of Strategies for Writing Success in the Health Sciences (continued)

Be Organized	10. Use a recent article from the target journal to create an outline for the new paper.
	11. Use a writing checklist (like CONSORT or STROBE) to create an outline.
	12. Create an outline that "follows the 3s" (see Figure 32-4) from the objectives through the methods and results to the conclusions.
	13. Start by outlining the paragraphs within each section, and then outline the sentences within each paragraph.
Make Steady Progress	14. Write throughout the research process.
	15. Write a set number of minutes every day.
	16. Write a set number of words (or one paragraph) every day.
	17. Set deadlines for when each part of the paper is "due." Reward yourself for meeting those deadlines.
	18. Write whatever is easy to write on a particular day rather than writing the paper in order from the first paragraph to the last paragraph. To maintain writing momentum, end each writing session by deciding which paragraph to write during the next writing session.
Learn from Others	19. Read other people's papers. Pay attention to how they frame their arguments, present their evidence, and support their conclusions.
	20. Seek mentorship.
	21. Join a writing support group.
	22. Welcome feedback from coauthors, colleagues, supervisors, conference attendees, reviewers, editors, and others.
Be Persistent	23. Have a writing routine. Write at the same time and place regularly.
	24. Try something new when stuck. Try a new writing place or a different writing strategy, and make that part of your revised writing routine.
	25. Walk, then write. Step away from the computer to compose your thoughts, and then return to type up the ideas developed while being physically active.
	26. Remove distractions when writing. Turn off videos, music, phones, and the Internet.

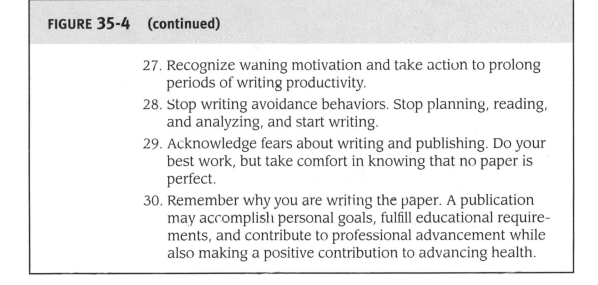

FIGURE 35-4 (continued)

27. Recognize waning motivation and take action to prolong periods of writing productivity.
28. Stop writing avoidance behaviors. Stop planning, reading, and analyzing, and start writing.
29. Acknowledge fears about writing and publishing. Do your best work, but take comfort in knowing that no paper is perfect.
30. Remember why you are writing the paper. A publication may accomplish personal goals, fulfill educational requirements, and contribute to professional advancement while also making a positive contribution to advancing health.

CHAPTER 36

Reasons to Publish

Many professional and personal benefits accrue from publishing research findings in peer-reviewed journals.

36.1 Scientific Dialogue

Publishing in peer-reviewed journals is the way scientists publicly communicate with one another. Submitting a manuscript to a journal for review is a first step in a series of conversations about a research report. The initial discourse occurs among authors, editors, and reviewers. After the article is published, the conversation continues as other researchers read, discuss, cite, and apply the work. It is typical for experienced authors writing new papers to cite the papers that cited their previous publications. Maps of these citation networks often illuminate vigorous written exchanges between research groups. Having one's work cited by others is a permanent record of participation in the dialogue about a particular health issue.

Presenting research findings at conferences is a helpful part of the scientific conversation, but presentations are not entered into the permanent record of scholarly discourse. The abstracts published from conferences are generally not cited in future publications because they are so incomplete. (An exception to this occurs in fields that publish full-length conference papers in book-like conference proceedings.) Conference abstracts are generally considered to be previews of works in progress, and not final products like published journal articles.

If the results of a research study are not published, for all practical purposes it is as if the research was never done. The findings do not become part of the conversation among scientists because there is no formal record of the project. Although the researcher may have learned from the project even if it is never formally written up, an unfinished report does not further scientific knowledge or improve clinical or public health practices and policies.

36.2 Critical Feedback

The peer-review process is an opportunity to receive expert and constructive feedback about a draft report. Reviewers are usually quite adept at identifying weaknesses in a manuscript and asking authors to carefully think through the problem areas and to fix to them. Responding to suggestions from reviewers and editors requires authors to:

- Understand and appreciate different perspectives
- Balance conflicting sets of advice about what would strengthen a paper
- Rewrite the parts of the paper that were confusing to reviewers
- Recover from negative comments and demonstrate resiliency by moving forward

All of these are skills that make authors better researchers and better health professionals, not just better writers. Gaining alternative perspectives about a research area may improve the design and implementation of subsequent studies while also providing new insights about how to serve diverse patients, clients, and communities. Weighing competing points of view and charting an acceptable path forward are valuable skills for primary investigators and also for team leaders working in any sector. Learning how to explain a procedure or decision better improves communication in any workplace. And building resilience and compassion in response to unkind words and rejections can be beneficial for professional and personal growth.

But the most valuable part of critical feedback is that it improves science. Reviewers who identify weaknesses in a paper and propose solutions for them, refer authors to helpful resources, and challenge authors to tell their story better are equipping researchers to do their best dissemination work. The kind of detailed and specific feedback provided by journals is not usually available after a conference presentation. Subjecting a manuscript to criticism and possible rejection can be intimidating and unpleasant, but the peer-review process produces better scientists and stronger manuscripts.

36.3 Respect for Participants and Collaborators

When participants donate their time to a project, the researcher has an ethical obligation to make sure that their time is not wasted. One way to fulfill this responsibility and to show respect for the contributions of these volunteers is to share the results of the study widely. If a project finds a statistically significant outcome, that finding should become part of the scientific literature. If a well-designed study fails to reject the null hypothesis, those results should also be published, even if it is often more challenging to publish a null results study than it is to publish a study that finds a strong association. A complete record of research results improves scientific knowledge and allows other scientists not to waste time and resources on a redundant project. Statistically insignificant papers can still be quite meaningful.

Seeing a research project through to completion also shows respect for collaborators and mentors. Naming minor contributors in the acknowledgments section of a paper is a nice public gesture of appreciation. For major contributors, being a coauthor on a published article is often the only "compensation" received for the time invested in the project. A lead author who fails to see a research project through to publication is denying all of the coauthors public recognition of their involvement in the project and an additional line on their CVs or résumés. Conversely, a publication in a respected journal is an achievement shared by the entire research team, and mutual respect and appreciation results from a successfully concluded project.

36.4 Personal Benefits

Publishing enhances the authors' CVs and résumés. A published article proves that a researcher is part of the scholarly community, can see a project through to completion, and has the ability to handle constructive criticism. A published article becomes a part of each coauthor's permanent record, because the paper will be indexed in abstract databases for decades and certainly for the length of each author's career. And although authors of scholarly journal articles are not paid for their writing—and, in fact, are often happy when they do not have to pay fees for publication—the payoff often comes in terms of improved job opportunities and promotions. Scientific publishing is unlikely to bring a person fame and fortune, but it does provide a tangible product after all the many hours that the author spent reading, planning, collecting data, running statistical and laboratory analyses, and writing. A published paper is evidence of the author's professional expertise and commitment to improving health for individuals and communities.

For those seeking to build and grow focused research portfolios, publications provide opportunities to gain expertise and recognition in a particular area. The research process does not necessarily end when a first report is published. The research process is a cycle in which data analysis and reporting naturally feed back into the formation of new study questions (**Figure 36-1**). Publishing marks an important step

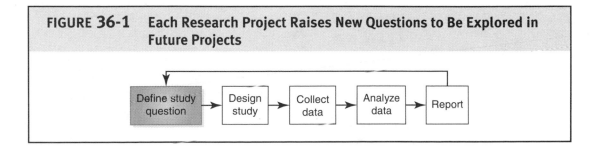

FIGURE 36-1 Each Research Project Raises New Questions to Be Explored in Future Projects

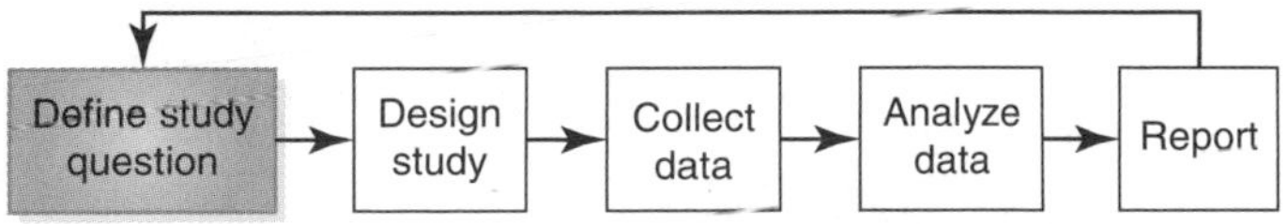

in this cycle. The next goal is not to publish the same results again—especially since redundant publication is a violation of professional standards and may result in the retraction of both of the duplicate articles—but to expand the research in a new but related direction. For example, some aspects of the data set that were not covered in the first publication might be worth exploring or some newly identified gaps in the literature could be investigated. A published paper provides the momentum to launch into examining new study questions raised by the published report.

CHAPTER 37

SELECTING TARGET JOURNALS

The culmination of a well designed and carefully conducted health research project is often the dissemination of results through an appropriate publication.

37.1 Choosing a Target Journal

Researchers who want to publish their findings must identify one or more journals that could reasonably be expected to disseminate their reports. Selecting a **target journal** early in the writing process makes it easier to hone the paper's message for the journal's audience. An examination of recent articles published in the target journal provides guidance about:

- The best outline to follow
- How to divide commentary between the introduction and discussion sections
- What subsections to include in the methods section
- The appropriate voice and writing style
- The amount of technical detail to include
- The reference and citation style

Choosing a target journal entails many considerations, including:

- The aim and scope of the journal
- The journal's audience
- The journal's impact factor and other metrics
- The possible costs of publication
- Online access options

37.2 Aim, Scope, and Audience

The most important consideration when identifying potential target journals is the fit of the research topic with the aims, scope, and audience of the journal. Some journals are very broad in focus, while others are very narrow and publish in only one subspecialty area. Some are international journals that publish research from around the world. Others have a very specific local or regional focus and publish only articles pertaining to that geographic area.

Determining whether an article is a fit with a specialty or regional journal is often straightforward. As an example, a journal focused on liver disease in Argentina will not be interested in a paper about osteoporosis in Mongolia, but it will review a manuscript on cirrhosis in Buenos Aires. A journal focused on nutrition in Southeast Asia would not review a manuscript on vision disorders in Sweden, but it would consider a paper on iodine deficiency in Cambodia. Knowing what topics fall within the scope of a general journal is a little harder. Some prestigious general journals will publish only articles expected to have a significant and nearly immediate impact on clinical practice. Some general journals in medicine, nursing, public health, and other health science fields will consider articles on just about any topic that is remotely related to the aims of the journal.

Considering the primary audience for a manuscript is also important. For example, if the article's message is targeted toward clinicians working in a focused geographic area, a journal sponsored by a regional professional society that provides a copy of each issue to all members of the organization might be the best venue. Publishing in such a journal will ensure that the paper reaches those who will most benefit from it. On the other hand, if the study has conclusions that are relevant to an international audience, then a journal known to have a global readership might be more appropriate. However, the expansion of the Internet is making regional and international journals less distinct. Libraries and researchers nearly anywhere in the world are able to acquire copies of even relatively obscure publications.

One way to identify journals likely to consider a paper for publication is to examine the manuscript's reference list. The journals cited most often in the manuscript are likely to be suitable target journals. Abstract databases and library holdings may also provide a sense of which journals are likely to be interested in a new manuscript.

37.3 Impact Factors and Indexing

A secondary consideration when selecting the target journal may be the impact factor, ranking, or reputation of the journal. The Thomson Reuter **impact factor** is based on the number of times a typical article in a journal is cited in its first year or two after publication. A few of the most prominent journals (like *Science, Nature, JAMA, The Lancet*, and the *New England Journal of Medicine*) have an impact factor of 10 or greater, but most journals in the health sciences have an impact factor closer to 1 or 2. Specialty journals may have an impact factor less than 1, but they can still be important within the specialty area. Impact factors are often listed on journal websites, and many universities subscribe to the annual ***Journal Citation Reports*** published by Thomson Reuter. Beware of fake impact factors and other misleading metrics placed on the websites of some low-quality journals.

It is also relevant to check which abstract databases index the journal. Some researchers prioritize journals indexed in Medline or in other disciplinary collections because being well indexed increases the likelihood that a published article will be read and cited.

37.4 Journal Characteristics

After identifying potential journals, a look at the journal's author guidelines reveals additional details that may be relevant to the selection of a target journal. For a review article, it may be necessary to confirm that the target journal will accept reviews. For a case report, a small case series, or an update to a previously published article, a brief report may be an appealing option. Some journals have a special section in each issue for short reports, and the author guidelines may highlight that information. Alternatively, a comprehensive report of a large study that will exceed the usual 3000- or 3500-word limit or the standard maximum of four tables and/or figures combined will require a journal that has more flexible word limits. In that situation, an online-only journal with generous word allowances may be the best option.

Some journals provide information about their average time from submission to first decision, their average time from submission to publication of accepted articles, and their overall acceptance rates. Many high-profile journals with very low acceptance rates have a turnaround time of only a few days because they send very few manuscripts out for external peer review. Specialty journals with higher acceptance rates may have a turnaround time of many months because three or more external referees review every manuscript.

Another consideration is the method of submission. Most journals have moved to online submission systems. These allow authors to upload manuscripts to a website and track the progress of their articles through the review process. Some journals only receive submissions via email. Some authors prefer online tracking systems because of the ability to monitor the status of their manuscripts.

Some authors have a preference about whether the article will appear on paper and/or online. Although the vast majority of print publications now also offer online access to subscribers (usually libraries), not all do. And a growing number of journals are online-only and do not print their issues. Although most online journals are likely to remain available on the Internet for many years to come, some researchers are wary about publishing in online journals that do not leave a paper trail, especially if those journals are new and unproven.

37.5 Publication Fees and Open Access

Although many journals are able to cover costs through subscriptions, advertising, and/or the support of a professional society, an increasing number are resorting to a variety of mechanisms that mandate that authors cover some or all of the costs of publishing.

A few journals require authors to pay a small **submission fee**, and they will not review an article until this payment is received. Some charge a small or large publication fee. The fee may be per article, sometimes called a **processing fee** or **processing charge**. Or the fee can be per article page, usually called a **page fee** or **page charge**. The number of pages is determined by the final ready-to-be-published article, not by the number of pages in the submitted manuscript. Some journals that are run by professional societies require the corresponding author of an accepted paper to become a member of the sponsoring society. In this situation, publication requires payment of a membership fee if the author is not already a society member.

Some journals require an **open-access fee**. The content of these journals is freely available to readers on the Internet, and no subscriptions to the journal are sold to libraries. This model of publishing, in which authors or their funders pay to make an article freely available to the public, is sometimes called **gold open access**. (This is contrasted with **green open-access** models in which authors are allowed to self-publish a version of the published article on their personal websites or in institutional repositories, usually after an embargo period of one year or longer.) A variety of copyright licenses are used when an author or publisher makes a copyrighted work available to others. **Creative Commons (CC) licenses** are one frequently used option, and they specify whether users of the work must give attribution to the author (indicated by "BY" or "CC-BY"), if users can distribute the work (indicated by "SA," for share-alike), if the work can be used only for noncommercial purposes (NC), and if no derivative products can be made from the original work (ND). Authors should carefully examine the copyright rules for journals before submitting their work.

Some journals give authors the choice of whether they want to pay for open access. These are usually subscription journals that put most articles behind a paywall. The open-access fee for these journals removes the paywall and makes the article freely available to all. Researchers sponsored by funding agencies that require articles written with their support to be publicly available may opt to pay for open access under this model. Authors without funding may publish at no cost, but their articles will be behind a paywall. A few journals that charge fees may allow authors to request waivers of some fees if the authors are from low-income countries and/or if the project was not supported by a contract or grant. These requests usually must be made before the paper is reviewed. Publication fees are usually disclosed in a journal's author guidelines or elsewhere on the journal's website. Authors are advised to look carefully for this information when considering publishing options. When authors are unable or unwilling to pay publication fees, it is important to confirm that there are no fees prior to submitting to a particular journal.

37.6 Predatory Journals

Authors must be aware of the growing number of dubious journals being launched by publication businesses that accept every submission upon receipt of payment by the author. Many open-access journals are well respected and regarded as having strong peer-review systems. However, a subset of open-access journals have a reputation for being pay-to-publish schemes. **Predatory open-access journals** do not follow good practices for editorial and peer review, and many are not transparent about their policies and fees. These journals should be avoided.

Before submitting to any journal, confirm that the journal is legitimate and respected. Watch out for journals that send unsolicited spam to email addresses, promise a very quick time to decision, have just launched or have published very few articles, and have poorly written author guidelines. Resources like *Beall's List*, a compendium of journals with problematic practices that is curated by academic librarian Jeffrey Beall, provide helpful guidelines for evaluating questionable journals.

CHAPTER 38

Manuscript Submission

Manuscripts should be formatted and submitted to one peer-reviewed journal as soon as the coauthors agree that the document is ready for external peer review.

38.1 Submission Timing

Publication is a priority for many health researchers because a project that has not been published is not contributing to advancing knowledge in their discipline. From the perspective of the broader scientific community, an unpublished project never happened. Submitting to a journal as soon as a revised and polished manuscript has been crafted and all the coauthors have signed off on it is critical. Procrastination can render the study useless because data in the health sciences quickly become obsolete and no longer publishable. Submission does not mean that a manuscript is perfect, just that it is ready to receive comments from external reviewers. Submission is not the end of the writing process. Additional revisions will likely be required, even if the first journal to which a manuscript is submitted accepts the paper. This is another incentive to submit as soon as possible: Revising a manuscript is easiest when the project is fresh in the minds of the coauthors.

38.2 Journal Selection

Once all coauthors are satisfied that the manuscript is ready to be submitted for peer review, one journal must be selected as the first journal for submission. Chapter 37 has suggestions for selecting an appropriate journal. A preliminary target journal may have been identified early in the research or writing process to serve as a guide. However, once a manuscript is completed, a variety of journals should again be considered. Only one can be selected as the first place to submit the completed manuscript.

Submitting to two or more journals at the same time is not permitted in the health sciences. Although editors of some popular magazines may compete for manuscripts from paid freelance authors, nearly all of the labor in the academic journal system is voluntary. Editors may receive little or no compensation for their time, and reviewers and authors are unpaid volunteers. It would be a major strain on the editorial and review system if every manuscript was sent to several journals at the same time. Thus, most journals require a statement with each submitted manuscript affirming that the manuscript is under consideration only by that one journal. This rule should be assumed to be true for all journals. Once a manuscript has been submitted to a journal, it cannot be submitted elsewhere until the authors are notified that it has been rejected or the authors formally withdraw the manuscript from consideration. The website of the **Committee on Publication Ethics (COPE)**, whose membership includes the editors of several thousand biomedical journals, provides additional information about appropriate conduct for authors and the repercussions for those who violate standard protocols.

38.3 Manuscript Formatting

Each journal provides **author guidelines** or **instructions for authors** that state how manuscripts should be formatted. The guidelines must be carefully followed. See **Figure 38-1** for examples of formatting preferences, which vary by journal.

FIGURE 38-1 Manuscript Formatting Requirements Addressed by Journals' Author Guidelines

Title Page	Should only the title be listed on the title page? Or should author names and affiliations, word counts, keywords, running headers (abbreviated versions of the title), or other information also be listed?
Blinding	Should authors' names be removed from the manuscript? Should other identifying information be blacked out in the manuscript, possibly including the citation information for references to previous works by the research team?
Abstract	Should the abstract be structured (showing subheadings for each section, such as "Objective... Methods... Results... Conclusion") or unstructured? If a structured abstract is expected, are there preferred subheadings? What is the word limit for the abstract? Should the abstract appear on its own page? Is an additional one-sentence summary or précis required? Are additional separate statements required about the contributions the paper will make to the literature?

FIGURE 38-1 (continued)

Keywords	How many keywords (search terms that will be linked to the article) should be provided? Must these be MeSH (medical subject heading) terms? Where should these be listed in the manuscript?
Sections	Is there a preference for how sections within the document are labeled and formatted?
Acknowledgments and Endmatter	Should acknowledgments of funding sources or personal assistance be included at the end of the manuscript? Is any additional endmatter to be included, such as information about the contributions of each coauthor, details about ethics committee review, declarations of potential conflicts of interest, or other disclosures?
In-Text Citation Style	How should in-text citations of works listed in the reference section be shown: as superscript numbers, as numbers within brackets, by the last name of the first author and the publication year in brackets or parentheses, by the names of several authors along with the publication year in brackets or parentheses, or by some other method? (Chapter 33 shows examples of these different citation styles.)
Reference List Order	Should the entries in the reference list be in alphabetical order (by the first author's last name) or in order of first appearance in the manuscript?
Reference Style	What specific style does the journal require for the reference list? For example, how many authors should be listed for articles with more than six coauthors? Should the full journal title be listed or an *Index Medicus* abbreviation provided for the title? Should the volume and issue be listed, or just the volume? Should any of the parts of the reference be in bold or italics? What types of punctuation should separate various components of the references?
Page Formatting	What margins and line spacing are required? Do the lines on each page need to be numbered?

FIGURE 38-1 Manuscript Formatting Requirements Addressed by Journals' Author Guidelines (continued)

Page Numbering	Should page numbers be shown at the bottom center of each page, the top right of each page, or elsewhere?
Fonts	Do particular fonts and font sizes need to be used? (For example, is Times New Roman 12 or Arial 11 recommended?)
Word and Page Limits	What is the word limit or page limit? Do these limits apply only to the main text of the article, or do they also include the abstract, references, and tables?
Tables and Figures	Is the number of tables and/or figures limited? Should tables and figures appear in the manuscript following the paragraph in which they are first mentioned, or should they all be placed at the end of the manuscript file after the references? Should each table and figure be saved as a separate file, or should tables be placed at the end of the manuscript file but figures saved as separate files?

Special attention should be paid to tables, figures, and other images when formatting the manuscript. The tables in the manuscript do not need to match the typographic style of the journal, but they should be relatively simple. Most journals will reformat the tables of all accepted manuscripts into their house styles when they convert the text into the single-spaced, small font, two-column format that is popular in health science journals. However, graphs, maps, and other illustrations are rarely reworked by a journal's graphic designer prior to publication, so all figures should be polished prior to submission. Journals may require image files in a specific electronic format, which may or may not be a standard file type. Most journals charge a fee for printing color images but not for grayscale images, so color should be used only when it is absolutely necessary. Alternatively, some journals charge for color in the print version but allow the online version of the manuscript to use color at no cost. In this situation, authors may submit a color version of the image but must make sure that the grayscale version of that color image has appropriate tones and adequate contrast. Also, because an image may be resized prior to publication, check that each image can be enlarged or reduced without distortion.

38.4 Cover Letter

Even though most submissions are made via computer instead of by postal delivery, most online submission systems still expect a **cover letter** to be uploaded. **Figure 38-2** summarizes the content of a cover letter. The letter should provide

FIGURE 38-2 Sample Cover Letter Content

Salutation	Address the letter to the editor(s) by name ("Dear Dr. ___") or, if names are not available, generically ("Dear editor").
Basic Information	Provide the title of the manuscript and, if the journal publishes different categories of articles, specify the type of article (such as original research, review, commentary, or short report).
Summary	Provide a short summary of the study design and key findings. Do not copy the abstract into the letter; write a new summary that emphasizes the key findings and implications of the study.
Importance and Fit	Briefly make the case for why the manuscript is important, significant, and original, and why the manuscript might be a good fit to the aims and scope of the journal.
Required Declarations	Some journals require the cover letter to affirm that the manuscript is not under review elsewhere and has not been previously published; to declare that all listed coauthors meet the ICMJE authorship criteria, including the approval of submitting the manuscript to the journal; and/or to disclose any potential conflicts of interest. Some journals may additionally require information about the funders of the research project and/or the specific contributions of each coauthor.
Thanks	Thank the editors for considering the manuscript for possible review and publication.
Names and Signatures	Some journals require the signatures of all authors to appear on the cover letter. When this is required, a signed letter can be scanned into a computer and uploaded on the journal's submission website, or it can be faxed to the journal office.

a brief description of the project and the major conclusions, and it should seek to convince the editor that the work is important, valid, original, and a good fit with the aims and scope of the journal. Once submitted, the editorial staff's decision about whether to consider the article for publication may be made solely on the basis of the abstract and the cover letter, so both of these items must be compelling.

38.5 Online Submission

Once the manuscript files have been prepared and all the required supplemental information has been compiled, the manuscript is ready to be submitted. The authors may need to email the manuscript and cover letter to the editor or send paper copies by postal mail, but most journals require online submission.

Creating an account with a journal's submission website usually takes only a few minutes. Only the **corresponding author**—the coauthor who will communicate with the journal and answer questions from readers after the paper is published—needs to register. The corresponding author may be the first author, the senior author, or the coauthor with the most stable email address and affiliation. In addition to facilitating submission of the manuscript, the online account enables the corresponding author to track the manuscript's progress through the review process. Most online systems will indicate when the editorial office is considering an article, when the article is undergoing external review, and when a decision is pending. Online submission usually takes about half an hour, although it may be faster or slower depending on the amount of information requested and the number of steps in uploading.

Most submission websites start by asking for basic information about the article, such as the title, abstract, and keywords. The keywords may be able to be typed or pasted in, or they might need to be selected from a list provided by the journal. Some journals will also ask for:

- The type of article (such as original research, review article, or letter)
- The word count
- The number of tables
- The number of figures (grayscale and color)
- Statements about ethics approval, funding, possible conflicts of interest, and author contributions
- Confirmation that the article is being submitted to only one journal

A second step asks for information about all contributing authors. The corresponding author should check ahead of time with coauthors about the preferred forms of their names. Most authors in the health sciences choose to use a middle initial when publishing, since PubMed and several other abstract databases list authors by their last names and their first and middle initials. Some journals also request a job title and affiliation, degrees earned, and contact information for all authors. These should be collected from all coauthors before beginning the submission process, just in case they might be required. The **affiliation** is usually the name of the school where a student coauthor is enrolled or the name of the employer of a coauthor who participated in the project as part of his or her job duties. Some journals allow multiple affiliations for each author, while others allow only one affiliation to be listed per author. When only one affiliation can be listed, many journals expect the listed organization to be the one where the coauthor was located when the bulk of the work on the project was being conducted, even if that is not the current institution. Other journals specifically request addresses and affiliations that are current at the time of submission.

There may be additional steps. For example, the journal may request the names and contact information for three or more potential reviewers. Some journals require a list of potential reviewers before a submission will be processed; some make this information optional. A senior author can usually offer guidance on how to select appropriate names to add to this list. They must not be people who have a conflict of interest that would prevent them from reviewing the manuscript. For example, journals may specify that the listed individuals cannot have written a paper with any of the coauthors within the past 5 years or may put other stipulations in place. The named individuals should not be contacted by the authors. If the editors select those individuals as reviewers, the editor will contact them directly. Some journals also allow the corresponding author to identify people who should not be reviewers because of a known conflict of interest, but it is not binding on the editor to respect this request.

The final step is uploading the manuscript files. The website will provide instructions about how various files should be attached. Some journals require the title page to be uploaded separately from the rest of the manuscript, especially if the journal uses double-blind review in which reviewers are not told the names of authors and authors are not told the names of reviewers. (Some journals use single-blind review, which means that reviewers are provided with the authors' names but authors are not provided with reviewers' names. Others use an open review process, and some even post reviewer comments on their websites alongside published articles.) Many journals require each table and figure to appear in a separate file. The file types acceptable for figures vary among journals. The journal may also request additional files, such as a publishing agreement signed by all authors or a checklist showing compliance with required contents and/or formats.

All of the manuscript files are typically combined into one PDF file during the submission process. Prior to finalizing the submission, the corresponding author should carefully review this file for completeness, page numbering, line numbering (if applicable), and the legibility of tables and figures. The author may also have an opportunity to review an HTML version of the uploaded paper and/or check the references for accuracy. Some systems automatically link manuscript references to abstract databases so that reviewers can easily access the abstracts of the cited articles, and incorrect references may be flagged as having errors. Once the manuscript and supporting files are confirmed to be correct, the author is usually prompted to click a link to approve submission to the editorial office. Once the submission is authorized by the corresponding author, the submission is complete.

CHAPTER 39

Review, Resubmission, and Publication

Manuscripts submitted to peer-reviewed journals are evaluated by external reviewers who provide feedback about how to improve a manuscript and by editors who make a decision about whether the paper is suitable for publication in a particular journal.

39.1 Initial Review

Once a manuscript is submitted, the journal's editorial staff does a preliminary review and decides whether to send the manuscript to external peer reviewers or to reject it without review. Although the organizational structures of journals vary, typically the editor in-chief who oversees the journal assigns new submissions to assistant editors for initial review. For manuscripts deemed worthy of review, the assistant editors identify *ad hoc* reviewers. These are reviewers who are not on the journal's editorial board who are asked to serve as peer reviewers because of their expertise on the paper's topic or methods. Some journals send nearly all manuscripts out to reviewers; others select only a small fraction of them for peer review.

Rejection without review (sometimes called a **desk rejection** or **bench rejection**) is often not a commentary on the quality of the manuscript. The decision to decline to review may be based solely on whether the cover letter, title, and abstract suggest that the paper is a good fit with the journal's current aim and scope. One of the advantages of the initial review process is that it allows authors whose submission is declined to quickly submit their work to a more suitable journal. If an article is rejected without review, the authors should identify a different journal that might be a better fit, update the manuscript to match the writing style and formatting requirements of the new target journal, and submit to the new journal as soon as possible.

Authors are often notified of a decision to reject without review within a few days or weeks of submission. When an article is selected for external review, notification of the first decision about the manuscript usually takes at least 2 or 3 months, if not longer. Authors should usually not contact editorial offices to inquire about the status of their manuscript until at least 3 or 4 months after submission. Even then, a request for an update should be made only if the status of the paper has not recently been updated in the online submission management system.

39.2 External Review Results

Decision letters sent after peer review are almost always accompanied by comments written by two or more reviewers. Reviewers usually provide two sets of comments to the journal.

- The first set of comments is on the quality of the manuscript. These observations are intended to be shared with the authors and often include specific points that the authors should address to strengthen their manuscript.
- The second set of comments is intended only for the editor. Reviewers may be asked to rate the manuscript's novelty, importance, and fit with the journal in addition to the quality of the work.

An external peer review can lead to three possible results: rejection, an opportunity to revise and resubmit, or acceptance (**Figure 39-1**). An article determined to be methodologically sound and well written may receive low scores in the areas of interest or relevance to the journal, so it is possible for a manuscript to be rejected even if all the comments shared with authors are very positive. Alternatively, an article deemed to be somewhat lacking in writing quality may receive high scores for the originality of the topic and the apparent significance of the work, and this

FIGURE 39-1 The Journal Review Process

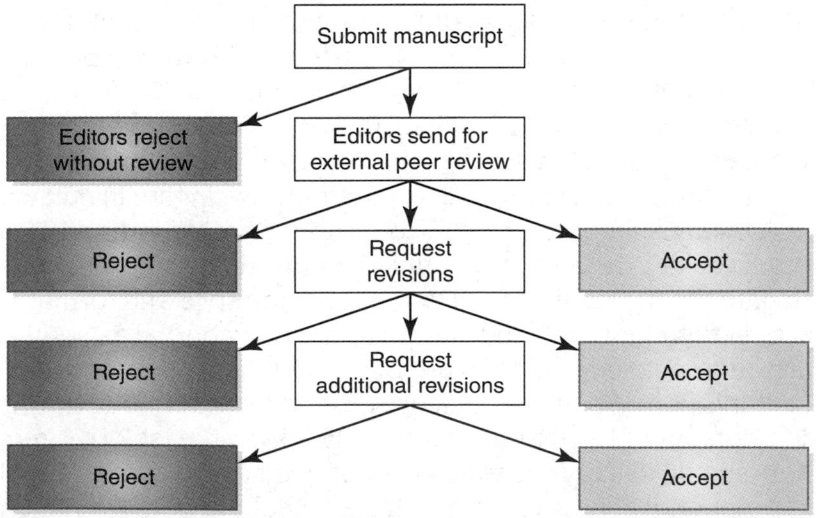

may result in an invitation to revise the manuscript and submit it to the same journal for another round of review. Often reviews are mixed, with one or more reviewers being very critical and one or more being quite positive. Mixed reviews may lead the editor to decide to reject the article, or they may lead the editor to offer the authors the opportunity to revise their manuscript and resubmit it to the journal for further consideration.

39.3 Rejection

Some manuscripts are rejected because they are poorly written, unsound, or of limited interest to those not directly involved in the project. However, many rejected manuscripts are well written, robust, and will be interesting to a wide audience. Many journals have low acceptance rates and routinely reject high-quality papers. An appeal to the editor to reconsider a rejected manuscript will almost never result in a different outcome. Rather than contesting a decision, authors should direct their energy into revising the manuscript for submission to another journal. A manuscript has a high likelihood of eventually being published if it is well written, if the study methods were valid and reasonably rigorous, and if the authors clearly link their results to broader applications or implications.

Rejection does not mean that the article has been rejected by all journals and will never be published anywhere. It simply means that one journal has decided that the paper is not suitable for its audience. Many authors find it helpful to take a few days to be disappointed about the rejection, to vent about some of the reviewer comments, and to complain to coauthors about the editorial decision. But one rejection—or even several of them—does not mean that a paper is not publishable. Each set of reviewer comments can be used to strengthen a paper. Most studies are not so badly designed and conducted that they are fatally flawed and cannot contribute to the scientific literature. Most papers can be made suitable for publication somewhere, although gaining acceptance may require several weeks or several months of additional work. As long as researchers are willing to learn from each set of reviewer comments, the manuscript will continue to become stronger with each submission.

It is usually best to begin work on revisions soon after receipt of a rejection letter. As time elapses after the completion of data collection and analysis, remembering the original aims, methods, and results becomes increasingly difficult. All reviewer comments should be read and carefully considered, with appropriate edits made. (The next section describes how to interpret reviewer comments.) Never submit to a second journal without taking advantage of the input provided by the first set of reviewers. The most important reason to make these updates is that the feedback from the reviewers will improve the paper. A secondary reason to take revisions seriously is that the new journal may send the manuscript to the same reviewers, and those reviewers will not be happy if their original evaluations were ignored. The revision process may require relatively little time, or it may demand significant reworking of entire sections of the manuscript. The background and discussion sections may need to be expanded to include more emphasis on the importance of the new paper and more citations of the relevant literature. The methods section may need to provide more details about the techniques used. The results section may need to show additional statistical output. Besides addressing all of the reviewer comments, the manuscript should be updated to match the writing style and formatting of the new target journal. Once the manuscript has been edited to the satisfaction of all coauthors, the manuscript should be submitted to the new journal.

Some journals are now offering a "**reject and resubmit**" option. These should usually be treated like a "revise and resubmit" opportunity. If the decision letter is not clear about whether a rejection is final or the authors are being invited to revise and resubmit their manuscript, the corresponding author should contact the editor to ask for clarification.

39.4 Revision and Resubmission

When authors are invited to **revise and resubmit (R&R)** their manuscript to the same journal, they need to prepare two documents. One is an edited version of the manuscript. The other is a file providing a response to each and every reviewer comment. Authors may be given a deadline for resubmission. If they miss the deadline, the revised manuscript may be treated as a new submission and be sent out to new reviewers, which may significantly extend the time to a final decision and decrease the likelihood of acceptance. Some journals make a distinction between a minor revision and a major revision. A **minor revision** might be reviewed solely by an editor after resubmission, whereas a **major revision** will likely be sent back to the original reviewers and perhaps also to new reviewers. A journal may allow only a very short time, often just a few weeks, for a minor revision to be returned. A major revision may be given a resubmission deadline of 3 months or longer.

Reviewers asked to examine a revised manuscript are provided with a copy of the authors' responses to the comments about the original submission. Accordingly, every response needs to be carefully constructed and respectful. Examples of responses to reviewer comments are shown in **Figure 39-2**. Some reviewer suggestions—often marked within their comments as "minor"—will be easy to respond to, such as correcting typos, reformatting tables, or adding a few more citations. Others—often marked as "major" or "compulsory"—may require more thought and time.

Responding to comments that are complimentary and to points that the authors agree strengthen their papers is fairly easy. Responding to negative comments is much more difficult. Authors who disagree with the suggestion of a reviewer are not obligated to change their paper to suit the reviewer, but they do need to write a thoughtful and courteous explanation of their point of view.

- Sometimes a reviewer's comments are hard to decipher or vague, such as "The entire manuscript is lacking focus and clarity." An appropriate response is to refer to exactly where and how the paper has been improved.

FIGURE 39-2 Sample Responses to Reviewer Comments

Sample Comment	Sample Response(s)
The specific aims of this paper should be clearly stated early in the manuscript.	We have edited the final paragraph of the introduction section to make it clear that the three specific aims of the paper are (1) to..., (2) to..., and (3) to....
The paragraph on ... is unclear.	We have rewritten this paragraph to improve clarity and to emphasize....
Did your survey include a question about...?	The data set we analyzed did not include a variable for.... However, even without that information, our analysis shows that....
	This would have been a helpful question to ask, but, unfortunately, it was not included in our questionnaire.
	We did not ask this question in the baseline survey presented in this paper, but we do plan to ask a question about ... in our follow up study next year. We agree that this will be an interesting question to explore.
	We did ask this question and found.... We have added this finding to the results section.
	We did ask this question and found....
The sample size seems too low to have adequate power for this study design.	We used ... software before initiating our study to estimate our required sample size. With expected inputs of ... and power of 80%, a sample size of ... was estimated to be required. In total we recruited ... participants. Based on the results of our study, and our estimates of power during data analysis, which showed..., our sample size is estimated to have sufficient power to yield significant results.
Table 3 seems incomplete. It should also report the results of the ... test for each row.	We have done the additional analysis requested and have added a new column to Table 3 that shows the results of the ... test. What we found was..., which is consistent with the results of our other statistical tests.
You used the ... test to analyze ..., but a ... test would be more appropriate.	The ... test that we used is the appropriate test because ... . The alternate ... test is not appropriate because....

FIGURE 39-2 Sample Responses to Reviewer Comments (continued)

Sample Comment	Sample Response(s)
In the discussion section, the authors claim…, but is it possible that … is happening instead?	Our assertion that … is happening is based on…. This interpretation is supported by several recent publications, including…. We have expanded our rationale for this conclusion in the discussion section and added additional references to previous literature.
	The reviewer raises a very interesting point. We agree that both of these interpretations are possible, and now discuss both perspectives in the discussion section.
The conclusion about … is not supported by the data.	We have removed this claim. Our primary conclusion, which is fully supported by our results, is….
You should include a discussion of….	Thank you for raising this interesting point. We have added commentary on … to the discussion section.
	We agree that this is an interesting topic, but since … is only tangentially related to our specific aims, we do not have space to discuss it in this paper.
You need to add a paragraph on the limitations of the study.	We have added a paragraph on limitations to the discussion section.
Several recent publications have addressed the themes of your work and should be cited, including…,…, and….	Thank you for bringing these articles to our attention. Both of the articles by … and … were helpful in supporting our findings and are now included as references.
I am not convinced that the study is important enough for publication in an international journal. It may be a better fit for a regional journal.	We have added an additional paragraph to the introduction that highlights what is new and significant about our findings. We have also added an additional paragraph to the discussion section that discusses the implications of our findings for other settings. We believe that our paper is important because … .
There are typos in lines … and … of page….	Thank you for catching these typos. We have corrected both of them.

- Sometimes a reviewer's comments exhibit a lack of comprehension. Although it is tempting (and sometimes accurate) to assume that the reviewer was reading carelessly, the authors should consider how that part of the manuscript might be revised to promote clarity.
- Sometimes two reviewers offer conflicting advice. The responses to both of the comments should summarize both reviewers' perspectives and explain how the authors decided to address the underlying issue in the manuscript.

The responses to the reviewers' comments should be prepared in a separate file from the revised manuscript. Additionally, some journals require a version of the manuscript that highlights or tracks all of the changes made in the document between the original submission and revised submission. Once all of the documents associated with the revision have been compiled, a new cover letter, the revised manuscript, and the responses to reviewer comments can be uploaded to the journal submission website. The cover letter should thank the editors for the opportunity to revise and resubmit, thank the reviewers for their comments and their advice that improved the paper, and affirm that each reviewer comment has been addressed and responded to.

The time needed for second review varies widely among journals, ranging from a few days to several months, depending on how many parties are involved in the re-review. Journal editors rarely promise authors that revisions will be accepted. However, the likelihood of acceptance is usually strong. The editors would not request a revision unless they were seriously considering accepting and publishing the edited version. Some journals may ask for third or even fourth or more revisions, with each round strengthening the paper's arguments. This can be frustrating to authors, but it is also evidence of the editor's intention to accept the paper for publication. Unless there is a very good reason to move on to another journal, the best option is to revise and resubmit to any journal that offers an R&R.

39.5 After Acceptance

Some initial acceptances are **provisional acceptances** with final acceptance pending until a few minor adjustments to the manuscript are submitted. If a provisional acceptance is offered, journals will often ask that the required updates be made within a short period of time, sometimes in as little as a few days or 1 week. After the journal receives the corrected manuscript, a final acceptance letter will be sent to the corresponding author, usually by email.

Once a paper is formally accepted, it may be sent to a copyeditor, who checks the paper carefully for grammar, spelling, and adherence to the journal's style. (Some journals have a style manual for copyeditors that specifies the preferred phrases, terms, abbreviations, and spellings for articles published in that journal.) The paper is then sent to a layout specialist, who formats the document to look like all the other articles published in the journal. The **page proofs** (or **galley proofs**) are then sent to the corresponding author for review, usually as a PDF file. Authors are usually given only 1 to 3 days to meticulously check the document, respond to any queries from the editor, and make any final requests for corrections. This is not the time to make any substantive changes. Requests for modifications should be limited to new problems, like formatting errors and copyedits that have changed the meaning of the text. However, authors should read every line carefully, examine every figure for clarity and crispness, and check details like the spelling of authors' names, the contact information provided for the corresponding author, and the references. This is the last opportunity to catch errors.

After the authors return the page proofs, the time to publication of the article depends on the journal. Some journals will post a PDF file of the corrected page proofs on their websites as an **advance access article** or **preprint**. Others will not post the article online until it has been assigned to an issue and published in print form. An article may be published in an issue mere weeks after acceptance or many months after the page proofs are approved. Soon after the article is published, the abstract will be added to the databases that index the journal. The published article may be cited for the first time in another article about a year or so after publication. At this point, the full research cycle is complete.

Glossary

Abstract A paragraph-length summary of an article, chapter, or book.

Abstract database An online collection of abstracts that allows researchers to search for articles using keywords or other search terms.

Accuracy In a survey instrument, diagnostic test, or other assessment tool, a condition that is established when the responses or measurements are shown to be correct; also called *validity*.

Action research Qualitative research that is designed to allow participants to work together to solve a problem.

Advance access The availability of a research manuscript on a journal's website prior to the assignment of that article to a particular issue of the journal.

Adverse event A negative reaction to an intervention during an experimental study or another bad outcome of research; these must be immediately reported to the appropriate institutional review board (IRB).

Affiliation The name of the school where an author is enrolled or the name of the employer of an author who participated in the project as part of his or her work responsibilities.

Age adjustment Methods used to improve the accuracy of comparisons of two populations with very different age distributions; similar methods can be used to statistically adjust for other important differences between comparison populations.

Agent-based modeling Modeling that uses computers to simulate the actions and interactions of various individuals (agents) in a population; sometimes called *agent-based simulation* or *individual-based modeling*.

Aggregate study A study that analyzes population-level data and does not include any individual-level data; also called a *correlational study*.

Allocation bias Bias that occurs as a result of non-random assignment of participants to experimental study groups.

Allowable costs Expenses that are approved for a funded grant or contract as opposed to items that are not acceptable according to the terms of the grant or contract.

Alpha A Greek letter (α) used to indicate the *p*-value at which a statistical result is considered statistically significant.

Alternative hypothesis A statement describing the expected result if there is a difference between the populations being compared.

AMA style The citation and reference style recommended by the American Medical Association, which is widely used by medical and health science journals; a variation of this style is called *Vancouver style*.

ANCOVA Acronym for analysis of covariance, which is used to control for confounding variables when comparing the means of two or more groups.

Annotated bibliography A bibliography that includes, at the minimum, a full reference for the document being reviewed and a brief summary.

Anonymity The inability of the identity of a participant to be identified from his/her responses to a survey instrument or records in a database.

Anonymized data set A data file that has been stripped of all potentially identifying information, such as names, contact information, national identity numbers, health insurance information, or facial photographs.

ANOVA Acronym for analysis of variance, which compares the mean values of a continuous variable among three or more independent populations.

Anthropometry The measurement of the human body, such as the measurement of height, weight, waist circumference, and hip circumference.

APA style The citation and reference style recommended by the American Psychological Association, which is widely used by social science and nursing journals.

AR% (Attributable risk percent) Acronym for attributable risk percent, which is the proportion of incident cases among the exposed people in a cohort study that are due to the exposure.

Ascertainment bias Bias that occurs when a study population is not representative of the source population.

Assent The expressed willingness to participate in a study by a child (or another person who is deemed not legally competent to provide his or her own consent).

Association A relationship between two variables; this term does not indicate anything about whether the relationship is or is not causal.

Attributable risk The absolute difference between the incidence rates in two independent populations (often an exposed group and an unexposed group in a cohort study); also called *excess risk*.

Attributable risk percent (AR%) Acronym for attributable risk percent, which is the proportion of incident cases among the exposed people in a cohort study that are due to the exposure.

AUC An acronym for the area under the curve of an ROC curve that displays the diagnostic accuracy of a test; AUC values range from 0 to 1, with 1 indicating a perfect test.

Audit A formal checking of financial records.

Author guidelines Instructions from a journal that state how manuscripts should be formatted prior to submission; also called *instructions for authors*.

Autocorrelation A pattern in which a variable measured over time has values influenced by its own past values as per a Durbin-Watson test or another test statistic or, in spatial analysis, a measurement of how similar one location is to nearby places.

Autonomy An ethical principle requiring that only the individual (or his or her legal guardians) is authorized to make a decision about whether to volunteer to participate in a research study.

Back translation A translation approach in which one person translates a questionnaire from the original language to a new language and a second person then translates the survey instrument in the new language back into the original language to ensure that the correct meanings were conveyed in the translation; also called *double translation*.

Background section The first section of a scientific report, which presents foundational theories, provides critical definitions, and spells out the study goals; also called an *introduction section*.

Bar chart A graph that presents categorical data using rectangular bars with lengths proportional to the values they represent.

Before-and-after study A non-randomized experimental study that measures the same individuals before and after an intervention so that participants can serve as their own controls.

Belmont Report A report published by the U.S. National Commission for the Protection of Human Subjects of Biomedical and Behavioral Research in 1979 that defined the key research principles of beneficence, respect for persons, and distributive justice.

Bench rejection The rejection of a manuscript from a journal without external peer review; also called *desk rejection*.

Beneficence A research ethics principle that requires a study to do good.

Beta A Greek letter (β) used to indicate power ($1 - \beta$) or to indicate the coefficients of predictor variables in a regression model.

Bias A systematic error in the design, conduct, or analysis of a study that causes the results in a study population not to accurately reflect the truth about the source population; many types of bias can be prevented with careful study design and implementation.

Big data Data sets that are so large and complex that they require powerful hardware and special statistical software applications to analyze them.

Bioinformatics The use of computer technologies to manage biological information.

Bimodal A numeric variable with a two-peaked distribution.

Binomial test A statistical test used to compare the proportion expressed by a binomial variable to a selected value.

Binomial variable A categorical variable that has only two possible responses.

Biosketch A brief summary of a person's professional and educational accomplishments.

Bivariable analysis Statistical analyses such as rate ratios, odds ratios, and other comparative statistical tests that examine the relationship between two variables.

Blinding An experimental design that keeps participants (and sometimes some members of the research team) from knowing whether a participant is in the active intervention group or the control group; also called *masking*.

Block randomization An allocation method that randomly assigns groups of people to an intervention group and other groups of people to a control group; randomization occurs at the group rather than individual level.

Boolean operators Mathematical and logical search operators such as AND, OR, and NOT.

Boxplot A graphical depiction of a numeric variable that displays the median, the interquartile range, and any outliers; also called a *box-and-whisker plot*.

Bradford Hill criteria A set of conditions that provide support for the existence of a causal relationship between an exposure and an outcome.

Brainstorming A process of gathering long lists of spontaneous ideas about possible research questions.

Breslow-Day test A test for assessing the homogeneity of the odds ratios across strata (that is, across independent populations from within the same data set, such as when separate 2×2 tables are created for males and for females or separate 2×2 tables are created for several age groups).

Callout A reference in a text that points readers to an element like a figure or table.

Canonical analysis A statistical method that identifies the set of ratio/interval and/or nominal variables that most accurately predict group membership in a model with a two ratio/interval and/or nominal dependent variables.

Carryover effects Residual effects from the first part of an experimental study that may bias the results of the second part of a crossover study if a sufficient washout period between the two arms of the study is not implemented.

Case A study participant with the infectious or parasitic disease, noncommunicable disease, neuropsychiatric condition, injury, or other disease, disability, or health condition of interest.

Case definition A list of the inclusion and exclusion criteria for being considered a person with the disease of interest in a case series, case–control study, or other type of study.

Case fatality rate The proportion of persons with a particular disease who die as a result of that condition.

Case report A report that describes one patient.

Case series A report that describes a group of individuals who have the same disease or who have undergone the same procedure.

Case–control study A study that compares the exposure histories of people with disease (cases) and people without disease (controls).

Categorical variable A variable that has responses that represent groups, usually groups with no inherent rank or order; also called a *nominal variable*.

Causation A relationship in which an exposure directly causes an outcome; the presence of causality is usually determined with both quantitative analysis and a qualitative consideration of causal theory using the Bradford Hill criteria or other guidelines.

CBPR Acronym for Community-Based Participatory Research, in which academicians and community representatives work together to identify research priorities and conduct applied research in a community.

CEA Acronym for cost-effectiveness analysis.

Censoring Ensuring that participants in a prospective or longitudinal study who leave the study early do not make further contributions to the person-time denominator used in survival analysis and other outcome evaluations.

Central tendency The average value for numeric variables, such as a mean or median.

Certificate of confidentiality A legal document that protects the identity of participants in a study of sensitive topics from being subject to court orders and other legal demands for information.

Chi-square goodness-of-fit test A statistical test used to compare the proportion of responses to a nominal variable to a selected value.

Chi-square test A statistical test used to compare the value of a nominal variable in two or more independent populations.

Closed-ended questions Questions that allow a limited number of possible answers.

Closeout (of a grant) The process by which it is determined that all applicable administrative actions and all required work for an award have been completed by the grantee.

Coauthorship Jointly authoring a research report with one or more collaborators.

Cochran's Q statistic A statistical test used in meta-analysis to examine the heterogeneity (statistical differences) among the included studies.

Cochran's Q test A statistical test used to compare the values of a binomial or nominal variable in two or more individually matched populations.

Codebook A guide written for a particular study that describes each variable and specifies how the collected information will be entered into a computer database.

Coding (of qualitative data) The use of words or short phrases to briefly summarize the contents, attitudes, processes, or other aspects of each item in a transcript or other qualitative document.

Coefficient of determination (r^2) A statistic that shows how strong a correlation is without indicating the direction of the association; r^2 values range from 0 to 1, with 1 indicating perfect correlation.

Coercion Compelling an individual to participate in a research study; this is a violation of the principles of autonomy and respect for persons.

Cohort A group of similar people followed through time together.

Cohort study An observational study that follows people forward in time so that the rate of incident (new) cases of disease can be measured.

COI An acronym for a conflict of interest.

Common knowledge Information that a typical person in the discipline knows, so it does not require citations and references in a research report; also called *general knowledge*.

Common Rule The current U.S. federal policy for protecting human research participants.

Comparative statistics Tests that categorize study participants into two or more groups and then compare the characteristics of those groups.

Compartmental model A mathematical model in which each "individual" in the simulated population exists in only one of several states at one time, but over time these individuals can move between states.

Concept A theory informed by observations.

Concept mapping A visual method for listing ideas and then grouping them to reveal relationships; this technique can be useful when identifying a study question and as part of narrative analysis of qualitative data.

Conceptual framework A model that a researcher sketches out using boxes and arrows to illustrate the various relationships that will be evaluated during a study.

Concordance Agreement.

Concrete validity Survey instrument validity demonstrated when an established test is used as a standard for confirming the utility of a new test that examines a similar theoretical construct; also called *criterion validity*.

Concurrent validity Survey instrument validity demonstrated when participants in a pilot study complete both an existing test and a new test and the correlation between the test results is strong.

Conditional probability The probability of an event (B) occurring given that some prior event (A) has already occurred; for example, the probability of surviving to age 95 (B) given that one has already survived to age 90 (A).

Conference papers Article-length research reports published in the proceedings of a conference.

Confidence interval (CI) A statistical estimate of the range of likely values of a statistic in a source population based on the value of that statistic in a study population; a narrow CI indicates more certainty about the value than a wide CI.

Confidentiality The protection of personal information provided to researchers.

Conflict of interest (COI) A financial or other relationship could influence the design, conduct, analysis, or reporting of the study, or could appear to have caused bias.

Confounder A third variable that may make the association between an exposure variable and an outcome variable appear more or less significant than it truly is.

CONSORT An acronym for the writing checklist for Consolidated Standards of Reporting Trials (for randomized controlled trials).

Construct A theory informed by complex abstractions and not merely by observations.

Construct validity Survey instrument validity demonstrated when a test measures the theoretical construct the test is intended to assess.

Constructivism A qualitative research paradigm in which researchers have a relativist perspective that considers reality for each individual to be a function of that person's lived experiences.

Content validity Survey instrument validity demonstrated when subject matter experts agree that a set of survey items captures the most relevant information about the study domain; also called *logical validity*.

Contingency table A row-by-column table that displays the counts of how often various combinations of events happen; also called a *crosstab*.

Continuous variable A numeric variable that can take on any value within a range.

Contract Research funding that requires the researcher to deliver an agreed-upon product to the funder.

Control A participant in a case–control study who does not have the disease being examined or a participant in an experimental study assigned not to receive the active intervention.

Control definition A list of the eligibility criteria for inclusion in a comparison population.

Controlled trial An experiment in which some of the participants are assigned to an intervention group and some are assigned to a non-active comparison group.

Convenience population A nonprobability-based source population selected due to ease of access to those individuals, schools, workplaces, organizations, or communities.

Convergent validity Survey instrument validity demonstrated when two indicators that the underlying theory says should be related are shown to be correlated.

COPE The Committee on Publication Ethics, which provides guidance on how to avoid research misconduct during the dissemination phase of a research project.

COREQ An acronym for the writing checklist for Consolidated Criteria for Reporting Qualitative Research.

Correlation A statistical measure of the degree to which changes in the value of one variable predict changes in the value of another; a correlation can be present even when the relationship is not causal.

Correlational study A study that uses population-level data to look for associations between two or more group characteristics.

Corresponding author The coauthor who will take the lead on communicating with journal editors and answering questions from readers after a paper is published.

Cost-effectiveness analysis (CEA) An economic analysis that compares the health gains from an intervention to the financial costs of that intervention.

Cover letter A letter that accompanies a submitted proposal or manuscript.

Cox proportional hazards regression A type of regression model used for survival analysis that estimates a hazard ratio comparing the duration of times to an event in two populations.

CPT codes Acronym for Current Procedural Terminology codes.

Cramér's V A statistical measure of the degree to which changes in the value of one categorical variable predict changes in the value of another categorical variable.

Creative Commons (CC) license One option for allowing a research article to be freely available for others to use while the authors retain the copyright and are credited for their work.

Criterion validity Survey instrument validity demonstrated when an established test is used as a standard for confirming the utility of a new test that examines a similar theoretical construct; also called *concrete validity*.

Critical theory A qualitative research paradigm that considers reality to be dependent on social and historical constructs and assumes that reality can be uncovered by identifying and challenging power structures.

Cronbach's alpha A measure of the internal consistency among questionnaire items.

Crossover design An experimental study design in which each participant serves as his or her own control; some participants are assigned first to the active intervention and then the control, and others are assigned first to the control and then to the active intervention.

Cross-sectional survey A study that measures the proportion of a population with a particular exposure or disease at a particular time by recruiting a representative sample of the source population; also called a *prevalence study*.

Crosstab A row-by-column table that displays the counts of how often various combinations of events happen; also called a *contingency table*.

Crude statistic A raw or unadjusted statistic.

Cumulative probability The probability of an event occurring by the end of a particular observation period.

Cutpoint The threshold for recoding a numeric variable into categories; for example, a systolic blood pressure of 140 mm Hg could be defined as the cutpoint for defining the presence or absence of hypertension.

DALY An acronym for disability-adjusted life year, which is the sum of years of life lost (YLL) to premature death and years lived with disability (YLD) in burden of disease studies.

Data cleaning The process of correcting any typographical or other errors in data files.

Data management The entire process of record keeping before, during, and after a research study.

Data mining The process of examining big data sets to identify patterns and new knowledge.

Database An organized collection of data created using a specialized software program.

Data security The process of protecting computer files with passwords and other mechanisms for restricting unauthorized access and use.

Deciles The division of a data set into 10 ordered parts of equal size.

Declaration of Helsinki A document written by the World Medical Association in 1964 to provide ethical guidelines for clinicians conducting experimental studies.

Degrees of freedom (df) The number of values in the final calculation of a statistic that are free to vary.

Deidentification The process of removing potentially identifying information from a data file in order to create an anonymized data set.

Deliverable A term used to describe a tangible or intangible object produced by a contract-funded research project.

Delphi method A structured consensus-building method in which experts complete questionnaires, a facilitator summarizes and shares the responses, and panelists reconsider their perspectives after reflecting on the opinions expressed by others.

Demography The study of populations and population dynamics, such as birth and death rates.

Denominator The bottom number in a ratio; that is, the "B" in the ratio "A/B."

Dependent variable A variable in a statistical model that represents the output or outcome for which the variation is being studied; also called an *outcome variable*.

Derived variables A new variable created during data analysis from existing variables in the data file; derived variables may be recoded based on the categories of the original variable or may be calculated from numeric original variables.

Descriptive statistics Statistics that describe the basic characteristics of quantitative data, such as means and proportions.

Desk rejection The rejection of a manuscript from a journal without external peer review; also called *bench rejection*.

Deterministic model A mathematical model in which the outcomes will be the same every time the model is run with the same inputs.

Diagnostic accuracy The percentage of individuals who a diagnostic test correctly classifies as true positives or true negatives.

Dichotomous variable A categorical variable with only two possible answers, usually "yes" and "no".

Direct age adjustment A method of age adjustment that can be conducted when age-specific health data are available for the populations being compared.

Direct costs The specific monetary expenses associated with a particular research project.

Discordant In disagreement.

Discourse analysis Analysis of qualitative data using the tools of linguistics to evaluate the written, spoken, or nonverbal language used by participants.

Discrete variable A numeric variable that is not continuous.

Discriminant analysis A statistical method that identifies the set of ratio/interval and/or nominal variables that most accurately predicts group membership in a model with a nominal dependent variable; also called *discriminant function analysis*.

Discriminant function analysis A statistical method that identifies the set of ratio/interval and/or nominal variables that most accurately predicts group membership in a model with a nominal dependent variable; also called *discriminant analysis*.

Discriminant validity Survey instrument validity demonstrated when two indicators that the construct says should not be related are shown not to be associated.

Discrimination The ability of a statistical model to distinguish between independent groups.

Discussion section The final section of a typical four-part scientific report, which compares the new findings to the prior literature on the topic, acknowledges the limitations of the study, and summarizes the implications and conclusions of the study.

Disease Illness in general, or the particular adverse health outcome that is the focus of a health science study.

Dispersion A measure that describes the variability and distribution of responses to a numeric variable; also called *spread*.

Distributive justice A principle of research ethics that requires the benefits and burdens of research to be equitable.

Double-blind An experimental study design in which neither the participants nor the persons assessing the participants' health status know which participants are in the active and control groups.

Double-entry A method for ensuring the accuracy of a data file by having two individuals enter the same data into separate computer files, comparing the two files for agreement, and resolving any discrepancies.

Double translation A translation approach in which one person translates a questionnaire from the original language to a new language and a second person then translates the survey instrument in the new language back into the original language to ensure that the correct meanings were conveyed in the translation; also called *back translation*.

Dummy variables Derived variables created by recoding a variable with n categorical responses into a series of $n - 1$ dichotomous (0/1) variables.

Dynamic population A study population with rolling enrollment; also called an *open population*.

Ecological fallacy The incorrect assumption that individuals follow the trends observed in population-level data.

Ecological study A correlational study that explores an environmental exposure, such as distance from the equator or level of air pollution.

EDPs Acronym for exposures, diseases/outcomes, and populations, which can be combined to form study questions using a standard format of "Is [exposure] related to [disease/outcome] in [population]?"

Effect modifier A third variable that represents biologically distinct groups of individuals who might experience different responses to various exposures.

Effect size The point estimate of a statistical measure like an odds ratio, rate ratio, efficacy, correlation coefficient, or difference in means.

Effectiveness A measure of the success of an intervention under real-world conditions.

Efficacy A measure of the success of an intervention that calculates the proportion of individuals in the control group who experienced an unfavorable outcome but could have been expected to have a favorable outcome if they been in the active group instead.

Efficiency An evaluation of the cost-effectiveness of an intervention that is based on both its effectiveness and resource considerations.

EHRs An acronym for electronic health records.

Eligibility criteria A set of inclusion criteria that must be present for an individual (or, for a systematic review, a research manuscript) to be allowed to participate in a study along with a set of exclusion criteria that would remove an individual from the study population

Emic perspective In ethnography, a study that aims to develop an insider's view.

EMRs An acronym for electronic medical records.

Endmatter The acknowledgments of funders, disclosures about possible conflicts of interest, author and contributor information, and other details that some journals place between the end of the main text of an article and the start of the reference list.

Epidemiology The study of the distribution and determinants of health and disease in human populations.

Epistemology The study of knowledge and the nature of how an investigator knows what is real and true.

Equipoise A research principle that requires experimental research to be conducted only when there is genuine uncertainty about which treatment will work better.

Equivalence trial An experimental study that aims to demonstrate that a new intervention is as good as some type of control.

Erratum A published correction to a minor error in an article, sometimes called a *corrigendum* (*printer's error*).

Ethnography The systematic study of people and cultures.

Etic perspective In ethnography, a study that aims to develop an outsider's view.

Etiology The cause of a disease or other health disorder.

Evaluation An assessment process that includes a variety of approaches for examining the goals, processes, and/or outcomes of projects, programs, or policies.

Excess risk The absolute difference between the incidence rates in two independent populations (often an exposed group and an unexposed group in a cohort study); also called *attributable risk*.

Exemption from review A determination by an institutional review board (IRB) that a research protocol does not require full IRB review because it involves the analysis of existing data, documents, or records or existing biological specimens that cannot be linked to individuals.

Expedited review A determination by an institutional review board (IRB) that a full review by the committee is not required because a minor change to a previously approved protocol is being requested or because a new proposal will not expose participants to risks greater than those encountered in ordinary daily life or during routine clinical examinations or procedures.

Experimental study A study that assigns participants to receive a particular exposure; also called an *intervention study*.

Exposure An intervention, environmental encounter, behavior, or personal characteristic that might change the likelihood of developing a health condition.

External grants Grants funded by organizations outside the researcher's institution.

External validity The likelihood that the results of a study with internal validity can be generalized to other populations, places, and times.

Extraneous variable A potential confounder that may make the association between an exposure variable and an outcome variable appear more or less significant than it truly is; also called *third variable*.

F&A costs An acronym for facilities and administrative costs, the general costs associated with maintaining a research environment, such as the costs of maintaining research infrastructure, operating research facilities, purchasing library resources, and administering research functions such as ethics reviews and compliance reports.

Fabrication A form of research misconduct involving the creation of fake data, such as creating fictitious rows of data in a spreadsheet for people who never completed a questionnaire or participated in an experiment.

Face validity Survey instrument validity demonstrated when content experts and users agree that a survey instrument will be easy for study participants to understand and correctly complete.

Factor analysis A statistical method for identifying interrelationships among variables intended to measure different aspects of the same construct.

Factorial design An experimental design that tests several different interventions in various combinations within one trial.

Falsification The misrepresentation of research results, such as modifying extreme data values to improve the results of statistical tests, manipulating photographs or other images collected during laboratory work, or intentionally misreporting a study's methods to make the study look more rigorous than it was.

Figure In a research report, the visual presentation of key findings in the form of a photograph, map, flowchart, or other image.

FINER An acronym reminding a researcher that a good research plan is feasible, interesting, novel, ethical, and relevant.

First author Typically, the person who was the most involved in writing a manuscript; also called the *lead author*.

Fisher's exact test A statistical test used to compare the values of a binomial variable in two independent populations.

Fixed effects model A statistical model that can be used for meta-analysis when there is little variability between the included studies.

Fixed population A prospective or longitudinal study design that requires all participants to start the study at the same time and does not allow anyone to join later.

Focus groups A qualitative data gathering technique in which groups of about 8 to 10 people spend 1 or 2 hours participating in a moderated discussion.

Forest plot A graphical display of the results of the studies included in a meta-analysis and the pooled statistic calculated from those results.

Formal sources Peer-reviewed journal articles and reports that are appropriate to cite in formal research reports.

Free-response questions Survey or interview questions that allow an unlimited number of possible answers; also called *open-ended questions*.

Frequency matching A sampling design that is used to assure that cases and controls in a case–control study or exposed and unexposed participants in a cohort study have similar demographic characteristics; also called *group matching*.

Friedman test A statistical test used to compare the values of an ordinal/ratio variable in two or more individually matched populations.

F-test A statistical test used to compare the mean values of an interval/ratio variable in three or more independent populations; also called a *one-way ANOVA*.

Full review A determination by an institutional review board (IRB) that the full committee must discuss a study protocol in order to ensure that the requirements for the protection of human subjects are met.

Funnel plot A graphical display of the results of the studies included in a meta-analysis that reveals the likelihood that publication bias has kept relevant studies with null results out of the formal literature.

FWA An acronym for federal-wide assurance, a status that applies to institutional review boards that are registered with the U.S. federal government.

Galley proofs The copyedited version of a manuscript sent to an author for review prior to publication; also called *page proofs*.

Gantt chart A type of bar chart that visually displays the research timeline and marks critical calendar dates and deadlines.

Gaps in the literature Missing pieces of information in the scientific body of knowledge that a new study proposes to fill.

Gaussian distribution A histogram with a bell-shaped curve with one peak in the middle; also called *normal distribution*.

General knowledge Information that a typical person in the discipline knows, so it does not require citations and references in a research report; also called *common knowledge*.

Generalizability The external validity of a study that allows its results to be considered applicable to a target audience.

Ghost authorship Failure to include as a coauthor a contributor who has made a substantial intellectual contribution to a research project.

Gift authorship Inclusion as a coauthor of someone who has not earned authorship according to disciplinary standards, such as those spelled out in the ICMJE authorship criteria.

GIS An acronym for geographic information system, a computer-based geographic data set that allows for the mapping of the locations of events, the identification of disease clusters, and the testing of complex spatial associations.

Gold open access A publishing model in which authors pay a fee to make their journal articles freely available to readers on the Internet.

Goodness-of-fit A statistical test for how well real data match the values predicted by a model.

GPS An acronym for global positioning system, which uses satellites to collect data about the latitude, longitude, and sometimes the altitude of locations.

Grant continuation An extension of a grant that provides additional funding to continue the research project and expand it in new directions; also called *grant renewal*.

Grant renewal An extension of a grant that provides additional funding to continue the research project and expand it in new directions; also called *grant continuation*.

Graph A scatterplot, timeline, or other diagram that visually displays quantitative results.

Gray literature Research reports that are available but have not been peer-reviewed and formally published.

Green open access A publishing model in which after an embargo period of 1 year or longer authors are allowed to post on their personal websites or in institutional repositories a version of an article they wrote and had published in a subscription journal.

Grounded theory A qualitative research approach that uses an inductive reasoning process to develop general theories that explain observed human behavior.

Group matching A sampling design that is used to assure that cases and controls in a case–control study or exposed and unexposed participants in a cohort study have similar demographic characteristics; also called *frequency matching*.

Habituation An error that occurs when participants completing a questionnaire or interview become so accustomed to giving a particular response (like "agree… agree… agree…") that they continue to reply with the same response even when that does not reflect their true perspective.

Hand searching A literature review technique that involves looking at every article in the table of contents of selected volumes of journals known to publish research reports in a particular area of interest.

Hawthorne effect A type of bias that occurs when participants in a study change their behavior for the better because they know they are being observed.

Hazard ratio The ratio of two hazard functions, such as a comparison of the durations of time to an event (such as death) in two populations.

Health informatics The application of advanced techniques from information science and computer science to the compilation and analysis of health data.

Health research Investigation of biological, socioeconomic, environmental, and other factors that contribute to the presence or absence of physical, mental, and social health and well-being.

Heterogeneity Dissimilarity.

Heteroscedasticity The heterogeneity of variance among the variables in a linear regression model that is demonstrated when the distribution of residuals from a regression model across the length of the best-fit line is uneven.

Hierarchical linear model A multilevel regression model that adjusts for different levels of exposure, such as for both census tract and county.

HIPAA An acronym for the Health Insurance Portability and Accountability Act, a set of regulations about patient protection that apply in the United States.

Histogram A graphical representation of the distribution of ratio/interval data in which the *x*-axis shows the values of responses and the *y*-axis displays the count of the number of times each response was given.

Historic cohort study A cohort study that recruits participants based on data about their exposure status at some point in the past and typically also measures outcomes that have already occurred (but happened after the baseline exposures were established); also called *retrospective cohort studies*.

Homogeneity Similarity.

Homoscedasticity The homogeneity of variance among the variables in a linear regression model that is demonstrated by the even distribution of residuals from a regression model across the length of the best-fit line.

House style The style sheet or guide used by a particular journal or publisher to dictate the requirements for spelling, citation style, and other formatting details.

HRQOL An acronym for health-related quality of life.

I^2 statistic A statistic used to examine heterogeneity in the studies included in a meta-analysis that adjusts the Q statistic based on the number of studies being pooled.

IACUC An acronym for Institutional Animal Care and Use Committee.

ICD codes An acronym for International Classification of Diseases codes, known more formally as the *International Statistical Classification of Diseases and Related Health Problems*.

ICMJE An acronym for the International Committee of Medical Journal Editors, which provides guidelines about manuscript formatting and authorship criteria that are widely used in the health sciences.

Impact factor An annual determination by the Thomson Reuter company about the number of times a typical article in a particular journal is cited in its first year or two after publication.

Incidence rate The number of new cases of disease in a population during a specified period of time divided by the total number of persons in the population who were at risk during that period.

Incidence rate ratio (IRR) The most common measure of association for cohort studies, this ratio compares the incidence rate among the exposed to the incidence rate in the unexposed.

Independent populations Populations in which each individual can be a member of only one of the groups being compared; for example, in a case–control study, each participant can only be a case or a control so the case and control populations are independent.

Independent variable A variable in a statistical model that is used to predict the value of some outcome variable; also called *predictor variable*.

Independent-samples *t*-test A statistical test used to compare the mean values of a ratio/interval variable in two independent populations; also called *2-sample t-test*.

In-depth interview A qualitative research technique in which an interviewer spends one or two hours interviewing a key informant using open-ended questions and then transcribes the interview so that the content can be coded.

Indirect age adjustment A method of age adjustment that can be conducted when age-specific health data are not available for the populations being compared.

Indirect costs The general costs to an institution of supporting a research environment, as opposed to the direct costs of conducting one particular study.

Individual matching A study in which each case is personally linked to a particular individual control, such as a genetic sibling; also called *matched-pairs matching*.

Inferential statistics Evidence-based assumptions in which generalizations are made about a population based on a study population that is a subset of the larger group.

Informal sources Websites, factsheets, newspapers, and other source of information that are not peer-reviewed and should generally not be cited in formal research reports.

Informed consent The voluntary decision of an individual to participate in a research study after reviewing essential information about the project.

Instructions for authors Instructions from a journal that state how manuscripts should be formatted prior to submission; also called *author guidelines*.

Intention-to-treat analysis Analysis of experimental data that includes all participants even if they were not fully compliant with their assigned intervention; also called *treatment-assigned analysis*.

Interaction term A third variable that might alter the relationship between two other variables in an additive or multiplicative way.

Intercorrelation A situation in which two or more related items in a survey instrument measure various aspects of the same concept.

Internal consistency A measure of how well the items in a survey instrument measure various aspects of the same concept; internal consistency can be assessed with Cronbach's alpha, KR-20, and other tests.

Internal grants Research funds provided by the researcher's school or employer.

Internal validity Evidence that a study measures what it intended to measure.

Inter-observer agreement The degree of concordance among independent raters assessing the same study participants; also called *inter-rater agreement*.

Inter-rater agreement The degree of concordance among independent raters; also called *inter-observer agreement*.

Interval variable A numeric variable for which "0" does not mean "nothing" (such as 0°F not meaning the complete absence of heat, since it is possible to measure a temperature lower than 0°F).

Intervention study A study in which participants are assigned to receive a particular exposure; also called *experimental study*.

Interview The process of a researcher verbally asking a participant questions and recording that person's responses.

Introduction section The first section of a scientific report, which presents foundational theories, provides critical definitions, and spells out the study goals; also called a *background section*.

IQR An acronym for interquartile range, which is the range for the 25th to 75th percentiles, which captures the middle 50% of responses.

IRBs An acronym for Institutional Review Boards, the research ethics committees responsible for protecting human subjects who participate in research studies.

Journal Citation Reports An annual publication by Thomson Reuters that offers critical evaluations of peer-reviewed journals based on their impact factors and other metrics.

KAP survey A common type of survey that asks participants about their **K**nowledge, **A**ttitudes (or beliefs or perceptions), and **P**ractices (or behaviors).

Kaplan-Meier plot A time graph that displays cumulative survival rates in a study population.

Kappa statistic A statistical measure of the agreement between two assessors who are evaluating the same study participants.

Kendall's tau (τ) A statistical measure of the degree to which changes in the value of one rank/order variable predict changes in the value of another rank/order variable.

Key informants A selected group of participants in a qualitative study who have been identified through purposive sampling.

Keyword A word, MeSH term, or short phrase used in a database search.

KR-20 An acronym for the Kuder-Richardson Formula 20, which is a measure of the internal consistency among questionnaire items.

Kruskal-Wallis *H* test A statistical test used to compare the median values of an ordinal/rank variable in three or more independent populations.

Kurtosis A description of how peaked or flat a normal distribution is.

Last author An experienced researcher who guides the work of a newer investigator and chooses to be listed last in the order of authors in the resulting scientific manuscript.

Lead author Typically, the person who was the most involved in writing a manuscript; also called the *first author*.

Lead researcher Typically, the researcher who will do the majority of the work on a project.

Leptokurtic A numeric distribution curve that is very peaked.

Letter of inquiry A letter to a funding agency presenting a preliminary research plan so that the funder can review the initial plan before deciding whether to invite a full proposal to be written and submitted.

Letter of intent A letter to a funding agency presenting a preliminary research plan and stating the intention to submit a full proposal.

Levene's test A statistical test of the homogeneity of the variances across different groups.

Life table An actuarial table that displays conditional and cumulative survival rates in a population.

Likelihood ratio (LR) tests Probability ratios used to evaluate the accuracy of diagnostic tests.

Likert scale A scale of ranked/ordered response items that ask participants to indicate preferences like "On a scale from 1 to 5, with 1 indicating strong disagreement and 5 indicating strong agreement,...."

Logical validity Agreement by subject matter experts that a set of survey items captures the most relevant information about the study domain; also called *content validity*.

Logistic regression model A regression model used when the outcome variable is dichotomous; also called *logit regression models*.

Logit regression model A regression model used when the outcome variable is dichotomous; also called *logistic regression models*.

Log-rank test A statistical test that determines whether survival rates are longer in one population than another.

LOINC codes An acronym for Logical Observation Identifiers Names and Codes, which are often used in laboratory records.

Longitudinal cohort study A study that follows a group of individuals who are representative members of a selected population forward in time; also called a *panel study*.

Loss to follow-up Inability to continue tracking a participant in an prospective or longitudinal study because the person drops out, relocates, dies, or stops responding to study communication for another reason.

LR+ An acronym for the positive likelihood ratio test, which examines whether a diagnostic test is good at predicting the presence of disease.

LR– An acronym for the negative likelihood ratio test, which examines whether a diagnostic test is good at predicting the absence of disease.

Lurking variable A potential confounder that may make the association between an exposure variable and an outcome variable appear more or less significant than it truly is; also called *third variable*.

M&E An acronym for monitoring and evaluation.

Machine learning A method of data analysis derived from artificial intelligence in which a computer "learns" more about a data set by running and re-running many rounds of analysis.

Major revision An invitation by a journal to significantly update a manuscript in response to reviewer comments and then to resubmit it for another round of review.

MANCOVA Acronym for multivariate analysis of covariance, which controls for potential confounders when comparing multiple dependent variables.

Mann-Whitney *U* test A statistical test used to compare the median values of an ordinal/rank variable in two independent populations; also called a *Wilcoxon rank sum test*.

MANOVA Acronym for multivariate analysis of variance, which is used to test for differences in group means when there are multiple dependent variables.

Mantel-Haenszel A weighting method used to adjust measures of association.

Masking An experimental design that keeps participants (and sometimes also some members of the research team) from knowing whether a participant is in the active intervention group or the control group; also called *blinding*.

Matched-pairs matching A study in which each case is personally linked to a particular individual control, such as a genetic sibling; also called *individual matching*.

Matched-pairs OR A special kind of odds ratio that compares the number of matched-pairs in a study for which the case had the exposure and the control did not (in the numerator) to the number of pairs for which the control had the exposure and the case did not (in the denominator).

Matched-pairs *t*-test A statistical test used to compare the values of an interval/ratio variable in one population measured twice or in two paired groups.

Matching Protocols for recruiting one or more controls who are demographically similar to each case in a case–control study or recruiting one or more unexposed individuals who are demographically similar to each exposed person in a cohort study.

Maximum The greatest (highest) numeric value for a variable in a data set.

McNemar's test A statistical test used compare the values of a binomial or nominal variable in one population measured twice or in two paired groups.

Mean A measure of the average value of a variable that is calculated by adding up the values of all responses provided to a question and dividing that sum by the total number of individuals who answered the question.

Median A measure of the average value of a variable that is calculated by putting all the responses in order from least to greatest and finding the middle number.

Mentorship A formal or informal relationship in which an experienced mentor offers professional development advice and guidance to a less experienced mentee.

MeSH Acronym for Medical Subject Headings, a dictionary used for searches in MEDLINE.

Meta-analysis The calculation of a pooled statistic that combines the results of similar studies identified during a systematic analysis.

Methods section The second section of a scientific report, which presents details about the processes used for data collection and analysis.

Minimum The least (lowest) numeric value for a variable in a data set.

Minor revision An invitation by a journal to make a limited set of manuscript updates in response to reviewer comments and then to resubmit the paper for editorial review and a final decision about acceptance.

Misclassification bias Bias that occurs when participants are not correctly categorized, such as when some controls in a case–control study are incorrectly classified as cases.

Mixed methods The use of both quantitative and qualitative techniques in one research study.

MLE An acronym for maximum likelihood estimation, which can be used in regression modeling to find the coefficient values that best explain the outcome.

Mode The most common answer given by respondents to a particular question.

Monitoring Ongoing assessment to ensure that a project or program is staying on track.

Morbidity Illness.

Mortality Death.

Mortality rate The proportion of members of a population who die of any condition during a specified time period.

Multicollinearity A problem that occurs when two or more predictor variables in a multiple regression model are highly correlated, and that redundancy means that the coefficients for one or more of those variables are highly inaccurate.

Multilevel model A statistical model that adjusts for different levels of exposure, such as for both census tract and county.

Multiple linear regression A statistical method that examines the relationships between several ratio/interval and/or nominal predictor variables and the value of one ratio/interval outcome variable.

Multiple logistic regression A statistical method that examines the relationships between several ratio/interval and/or nominal predictor variables on the value of one nominal outcome variable.

Multivariable analysis Statistical tests such as multiple regression models that examine the relationships between three or more variables.

Narrative analysis A qualitative analysis method that uses established theories to understand personal stories.

Narrative inquiry Qualitative research that examines autobiographies, personal letters, family stories, and other records to understand how people frame their identities and social relationships.

Narrative review A tertiary analysis that uses evidence from the literature to support the "plot" but does not involve a systematic search of the literature.

Natural experiment An experiment in which the independent variable is not manipulated by the researcher but instead changes due to external forces.

Natural language processing A machine learning algorithm that is used in the analysis of qualitative and social media data to examine how people speak and write in real-life situations.

Negative predictive value (NPV) The proportion of people who test negative with a diagnostic test who actually do not have the disease (according to a reference standard).

NNH An acronym for number needed to harm, which is the number of people who would need to receive a particular treatment in order to expect that one of them would have a particular adverse outcome.

NNT An acronym for number needed to treat, which is the expected number of people who would have to receive a treatment to prevent an unfavorable outcome in one person.

No-cost extension An extension of the timeline for spending grant money in which the closing date moved to a later time but no additional funding is provided.

Nominal variable A categorical variable for which the responses have no inherent order or ranking.

Noninferiority trial An experimental study that aims to demonstrate that a new intervention is no worse than some type of control.

Nonmaleficence Something that does not harm.

Nonparametric tests Statistical tests that do not make assumptions about the distributions of responses.

Non-random-sampling bias Bias that occurs when each individual in the source population does not have an equal chance of being selected for the sample population.

Nonrecursive model A causal analysis model in which causal pathways can be bidirectional.

Nonresponse bias Bias that occurs when the members of the sample population who agree to be in the study are systematically different from nonparticipants.

Normal distribution A histogram with a bell-shaped curve with one peak in the middle; also called a *Gaussian distribution*.

Null hypothesis A statement describing the expected result of a statistical test if there is no difference between the two or more values being compared.

Numerator The top number in a ratio; that is, the "A" in the ratio "A/B."

Nuremburg Code One of the first codes of research ethics, which in 1947 mandated voluntary consent for experimental studies of humans.

Observational study A non-experimental study in which participants are not asked to change their behavior; by contrast, an interventional study assigns participants to an exposure.

Observer bias Bias that occurs when an observer (a researcher) intentionally or unintentionally evaluates participants differently based on their group membership, such as systematically evaluating cases and controls in a case–control study differently.

Odds A ratio of the likelihood of an event happening and the likelihood of that event not occurring; for example, when a person has a 25% likelihood of developing a particular disease and a 75% likelihood of not developing that disease, the odds are 25%/75% = 0.33.

Odds ratio (OR) A ratio of odds in which the denominator represents the reference group; for a case–control study, the OR is the ratio of the odds of exposure among cases (in the numerator) to the odds of exposure among controls (in the denominator).

ODE An acronym for ordinary differential equations, which can be used to describe the flows between compartments in mathematical models.

OLS An acronym for ordinary least squares, a model-fitting approach typically used to find the best-fit line in linear regression.

One-sample *t*-test A statistical test used to compare the mean value of a ratio/interval variable to a selected value.

One-sided *p*-value The probability value that is used for a statistical test when a direction is specified in the alternative hypothesis.

One-way ANOVA A statistical test used to compare the mean values of an interval/ratio variable in three or more independent populations; also called an *F-test*.

Ontology The study of the nature of being, becoming, existence, reality, or truth.

Open-access fee A charge that authors pay to journals in order to make their articles freely available to online readers.

Open-ended questions Survey or interview questions that allow an unlimited number of possible answers; also called *free-response questions*.

Open population A study population with rolling enrollment; also called a *dynamic population*.

OR An acronym for *odds ratio*.

Oral consent Informed consent for participation in a study that is spoken and witnessed rather than requiring a participant's signature; also called as *verbal consent*.

Oral presentations Spoken presentations, which at conferences usually are about 15 minutes in duration.

Ordinal variables Variables for which responses are ranked from best to worst, most to least, or other scales.

Originality The aspects of a new research project that are novel and will allow it to make a unique contribution to the health science literature.

Outcome The measured endpoint in an experimental study or an observed event such as the onset of incident disease in a cohort study.

Outcome variable A variable in a statistical model that represents the output or outcome whose variation is being studied; also called a *dependent variable*.

Outlier A value in a numeric data set that is distant from other observations and outside the expected range of values.

Overhead The indirect costs of research, such as the institutional costs of maintaining research infrastructure and administering compliance activities.

Overmatching Recruiting challenges and possible statistical bias resulting from matching cases and controls, or exposed and unexposed participants, on too many characteristics.

Page charge A charge that some journals mandate based on the number of pages in the final PDF of an article accepted for publication; also called *page fee*.

Page fee A charge that some journals mandate based on the number of pages in the final PDF of an article accepted for publication; also called *page charge*.

Page proofs The copyedited version of a manuscript sent to an author for review prior to publication; also called *galley proofs*.

Panel study A study that follows a group of individuals who are representative members of a selected population forward in time; also called a *longitudinal cohort study*.

Parametric tests Tests that assume the variables being examined have particular distributions, often requiring the variables to have normal or approximately normal distributions.

Participant observation A method of qualitative field observation in which a trained viewer enters the group under analysis as a member.

Path analysis A causal analysis strategy that uses regression models to examine causal patterns among variables, assuming a recursive model in which all causality is unidirectional.

PCA An acronym for principal component analysis, which can provide information about which items in an assessment tool might be redundant or unnecessary and can be removed.

Pearson correlation coefficient (*r*) A statistical measure of the degree to which changes in the value of one numeric variable predict changes in the value of another numeric variable.

Person-time A way of accounting for different individuals in the study population being observed for different lengths of time using units like person-years or person-months.

Phenomenology A qualitative research approach that seeks to understand how participants understand, interpret, and find meaning in their own unique life experiences and feelings.

Phi coefficient (ϕ) A statistical measure of the degree to which changes in the value of one binomial variable predict changes in the value of another binomial variable.

Photovoice A qualitative research technique in which participants take photographs that they feel represent their communities and then they share what aspects of their lived experiences they intended to capture in those images.

PICOT An acronym for Patient/Population, Intervention, Comparison, Outcome, Timeframe, a framework that is helpful for developing clinical research questions and designing intervention studies.

Pie chart A circle in which each wedge or slice displays the percentage of participants who provided a particular answer to one question; the sum of the percentages for the slices must add up to 100%.

Pilot test A small-scale preliminary study conducted to evaluate the feasibility of a full-scale research project.

Placebo An inactive comparison used in an experimental study, such as a sugar pill used as a control for a pill with an active medication, a saline injection used as a control for an injection of an active substance, and a sham procedure that is designed to look and feel like a real clinical procedure used as a control for that active procedure.

Plagiarism The use of other people's ideas, words, or images without proper attribution.

Platykurtic A distribution curve for a histogram that is relatively flat.

Point estimate The value of a statistic in a study population, which is typically presented along with a corresponding 95% confidence interval that provides additional information about the likely value of the statistic in the source population.

Population A group (or subgroup) of individuals, communities, or organizations; research studies usually carefully identify a target population, source population, sample population, and study population.

Population-based study A cross-sectional study, longitudinal cohort study, or other type of study that uses a random sampling method to generate a sample population that is representative of a general population; studies that use convenience samples or recruit from a patient or occupational population are usually not considered to be population-based studies.

Population health research Health research that focuses on humans as the unit of investigation rather than examining molecules, genes, cells, or other smaller biological components.

Positive predictive value (PPV) The proportion of people who test positive with a diagnostic test who actually have the disease (according to a reference standard).

Poster sessions Designated times at an academic or professional conference when researchers are available to talk about their posters with other attendees.

Post-positivism A qualitative research paradigm in which researchers aim to experimentally test theories about how the world works, but they acknowledge that the unpredictability of human behavior limits the validity of some empirical methods.

Power (statistical) The ability of a statistical test to detect significant differences in a population when differences really do exist; the power of tests is increased when the number of participants included in the analysis is large.

PPTs Acronym for person, place, and time, which are essential components of case definitions and descriptive epidemiology studies.

Pragmatism A qualitative research paradigm in which researchers assume that reality is situational, and it is acceptable to use any and all research tools and frameworks to try to understand a particular problem so it can be solved.

Précis A concise one- or two-sentence summary of a research study's key finding.

Precision In a survey instrument, diagnostic test, or other assessment tool, a quality that is demonstrated when consistent answers are given to similar questions and when an assessment yields the same outcome when repeated several times; also called *reliability*.

Predatory open-access journals Exploitative journals that charge authors hidden publication fees without providing the quality editorial and publishing services associated with legitimate journals.

Predictive validity Survey instrument validity demonstrated when a new test is correlated with subsequent measures of performance in related domains.

Predictor variable A variable in a statistical model that is used to predict the value of some outcome variable; also called *independent variable*.

Preprint A PDF file of the corrected page proofs posted by a journal on their website prior to assigning the article to a particular issue of the journal.

Pre-proposal A brief research plan requested or required by funders who want to confirm that there is a reasonable match between the sponsor and the proposed research plan before inviting a full proposal to be written and submitted.

Pretest A small-scale preliminary study conducted to evaluate the utility of a new survey instrument; also called a *pilot test*.

Prevalence rate The percentage of the population with a given trait at the time of a study.

Prevalence rate ratio (PRR) Compares the prevalence rates for the same variable in two independent populations by taking a ratio of them; the bottom number in the ratio is the reference population.

Prevalence study A study that measures the proportion of a population with a particular exposure or disease at a particular time by recruiting a representative sample of the source population; also called a *cross-sectional survey*.

Primary investigator (PI) The researcher who accepts principal responsibility for a research project, guaranteeing that the protocol is being followed, the budget is properly managed, and any adverse outcomes are immediately reported to the institution's research ethics committee; the PI for a project conducted by a new researcher is often a professor or senior employee.

Primary study The collection of new data from individuals.

PRISMA An acronym for the writing checklist for Preferred Reporting Items for Systematic Reviews and Meta-Analyses.

Privacy The assurance that research participants get to choose what information they reveal about themselves.

Probability-based sampling Methods for ensuring that members of a source population have an equal likelihood of being invited to participate in a research study.

Processing charge A per-article charge that some journals mandate prior to an accepted article being published; this may or may not make the article open access; also called a *processing fee*.

Processing fee A per-article charge that some journals mandate prior to an accepted article being published; this may or may not make the article open access; also called a *processing charge*.

Program An group of projects.

Program evaluation The systematic collection and analysis of information to answer questions about the effectiveness and efficiency of a project, program, or policy.

Project A specific, time-limited activity.

Project narrative The research goals and methods spelled out in a research plan or proposal.

Propensity score matching A statistical technique for predicting the probability of group membership while adjusting for covariates.

Proportionate mortality rate The proportion of deceased members of a population whose death was attributable to a particular cause.

Proposal A written request for approval of or funding for a research project.

Prospective cohort study A cohort study that recruits participants because they have or do not have an exposure of interest and then follows them forward in time to look for incident cases of disease.

Prospective study A study that follows participants forward in time.

Protected health information (PHI) Information about an individual's health history or health status that by law is required to be kept confidential.

Protocol A detailed written research plan that describes all the processes and procedures that will be used during participant recruitment (if relevant), data collection, and analysis.

Provisional acceptance Notification from a journal that a final acceptance will be granted once minor adjustments to the manuscript are submitted.

Publication bias Bias that occurs when articles with statistically significant results are more likely to be published than those with null results.

PubMed A service of the U.S. National Library of Medicine that provides access to more than 25 million abstracts.

Purposive sampling A nonprobability-based sampling method that recruits participants for a qualitative study based on the special insights they can provide.

***p*-Value** A probability value that indicates the likelihood that a test statistic as extreme as or more extreme than the one observed would occur by chance if the null hypothesis was true; a very small *p*-value means that the observed test result is highly unlikely to have occurred by chance.

QALY An acronym for quality-adjusted life year, which is commonly used in health economics to quantify population-level gains in health status.

QOL An acronym for quality of life.

Q statistic A statistical test used in meta-analysis to examine the differences among the included studies; also called *Cochran's Q statistic*.

Qualitative research An unstructured or semi-structured approach for using participant observations, in-depth interviews, focus group discussions, and textual data to identify themes and patterns and to formulate new theories.

Quantitative research A structured survey-based approach for statistically testing hypotheses.

Quartiles The division of a data set into four ordered parts of equal size.

Quasi-experimental designs Experimental studies that assign participants to an intervention or control group using a non-random method.

Questionnaire A series of questions used as a tool for systematically gathering information from study participants; also called a *survey instrument*.

R&R An acronym for revise and resubmit, which is a term used by journals when authors are invited to edit their manuscript in response to reviewer comments and then send it back to the journal for another round of consideration.

Random effects model A statistical model that can be used for meta-analysis when there is considerable variability (that is, heterogeneity) between the included studies.

Random-digit dialing Calls made to a computer-generated list of unscreened telephone numbers.

Randomization Assignment of participants to an exposure group in an experimental study using a method that minimizes bias.

Range The difference between the minimum and the maximum values of a variable.

Ranked variables The type of variable used when categorical variables are ordered from best to worst, most to least, or other scales; also called *ordinal variables*.

Rate ratio (RR) A ratio of two rates, with the reference (comparison) group in the denominator; may also be called the *relative rate*, the *risk ratio*, or the *relative risk*.

Ratio variable A numeric variable that can be plotted on a scale on which a value of zero indicates "nothing" (such as 0 inches meaning no height).

RCR An acronym for responsible conduct of research, a common component of research ethics training that emphasizes professionalism and best practices for collaborative research.

RCT An acronym for randomized controlled trial, one of the most common experimental study designs in the health sciences.

Realist synthesis A qualitative analysis technique that uses a systematic process to find and interpret evidence for the complex reasons some programs succeed and others fail.

REC An acronym for a research ethics committee, often referred to as an *institutional review board (IRB)*.

Recall bias Bias that occurs when cases and controls in a case-control study systematically have different memories of the past.

Recoding The process of using one (or more) variable in a database to create a new derived variable.

Reconciliation The process of resolving any discrepancies between the researcher's financial records and the reports produced by the institution hosting the researcher's grant/contract accounts.

Recursive model A causal analysis model in which all causal pathways are unidirectional.

Reference standard The existing "gold standard" test that is used as a comparison for a new diagnostic test.

Regression model A statistical model that seeks to understand the relationship between one or more independent (predictor) variables and one dependent (outcome) variable.

Reject and resubmit A rejection letter from a journal editor that invites the authors to revise a manuscript and resubmit it to the same journal for consideration as a "new" article; most rejection letters specify that a different version of the same manuscript will not be considered by the journal, but this unusual outcome is akin to a "revise and resubmit" offer.

Reliability In a survey instrument, diagnostic test, or other assessment tool, a quality that is demonstrated when consistent answers are given to similar questions and when an assessment yields the same outcome when repeated several times; also called *precision*.

Repeated cross-sectional study A study that re-samples representatives from the same source population at two or more different time points; this is different from a longitudinal study that follows the same people forward in time, since a new set of participants in a repeated cross-sectional survey is recruited for each round of data collection.

Repeated-measures ANOVA A statistical test used to compare the values of an interval/ratio variable in two or more individually matched populations.

Replication studies Studies that repeat a study in a new population as part of attempting to confirm that the original findings were not due to chance.

Representativeness The degree to which the participants in a study are similar to the source population from which they were drawn.

Request for applications (RFA) A notice distributed by a funding organization seeking applications from researchers who want to conduct research on topics of interest to the funder.

Request for proposals (RFP) A notice distributed by a funding organization to inform researchers of their desire to receive grant proposals for research on topics of interest to the funder.

Research The process of systematically and carefully investigating a subject in order to discover new insights about the world.

Residual The vertical distance of a data point in a linear regression model to the best-fit line.

Respect for persons A research principle that emphasizes participant autonomy.

Results section The third section of a typical four-part scientific report, which contains key findings with text as well as tables and/or figures.

Retraction Removal of a published article from the accepted scientific literature due to major errors or author misconduct.

Retrospective cohort study A cohort study that recruits participants based on data about their exposure status at some point in the past and typically also measures outcomes that have already occurred (but happened after the baseline exposures were established); also called *historic cohort studies*.

Revise and resubmit (R&R) A term used by journal editors when authors are invited to edit a manuscript in response to reviewer comments and then send it back to the journal for another round of consideration.

Risk factor An exposure that increases an individual's likelihood of subsequently experiencing a particular disease or outcome.

ROC curve An acronym for receiver operating characteristic curve, which is a graphical plot of the true positive rate against the false positive rate for the different possible cutoff points of a diagnostic test.

RR An acronym for *rate ratio*.

Sample population Individuals from the source population who are invited to participate in a research study.

Sample size In statistics, the number of observations in a data set (that is, the number of individuals in the study population).

Sample size calculator A tool used to identify an appropriate number of participants to recruit for a quantitative study; this is more accurately called a *sample size estimator* because the range of suggested sample sizes is based on a series of guesses about the expected characteristics of the sample population.

Sampling frame A well-defined subset of individuals from the target population from which potential study participants will be sampled; also called a *source population*.

Secondary study The analysis of an existing data set or existing health records.

Selection bias Bias that occurs when the members of the study population are not representative of the source population from which they were drawn.

Self-administered surveys Survey forms that participants complete for themselves, either using a paper-and-pencil version or an online version.

SEM An acronym for structural equation modeling, a causal analysis strategy that uses maximum likelihood estimation regression models to examine complex causal patterns.

Semi-structured interview A qualitative conversation with a key informant that covers a range of preselected topics using open-ended questions, probing for clarifications about verbal responses, and observations of body language and other nonverbal communication.

Senior author An experienced researcher who guides the work of a newer investigator and may choose to be listed last in the order of authors in the resulting scientific manuscript.

Senior researcher An experienced researcher who guides the work of a newer investigator.

Sensitivity The proportion of people who actually have a disease (according to a reference standard) who test positive with a diagnostic test.

Sensitivity analysis Tests of the robustness of statistical methods and results.

Significance level The *p*-value (usually $p = 0.05$) at which the null hypothesis is rejected and a statistical result is considered statistically significant.

Significant figures The number of digits in a number that are presented after a decimal point.

Simple linear regression A model that examines whether there is a linear relationship between one predictor variable and an outcome variable.

Simple randomization The use of a coin toss, a random number generator, or some other simple mechanism to randomly assign each individual in an experimental study to one of the exposure groups.

Simultaneous multiple regression A model that includes all predictor variables in the model rather than fitting the model using a stepwise approach.

Single-blind An experimental study design in which the participants do now know whether they are in the active group or a control group.

SIR model A mathematical model of infection transmission that describes how the susceptible (S) individuals in a population may become infected (I) and then eventually recover (R) with immunity.

Skewness An asymmetric distribution in which a histogram extends farther from the peek on one side than the other, exhibiting left-skewness or right-skewness.

Skips Non-applicable questions that are jumped over in interviews because of the response to a previous question; for example, participants in a study who indicate that they have never used tobacco products could be prompted to skip a series of questions about smoking habits.

Snowballing A literature review technique that involves looking up every article cited by eligible articles in order to identify new sources that might be relevant but not widely indexed.

Solicited proposal A request for funding submitted by a researcher after a funder has contacted the researcher to invite that person to submit a proposal.

Source population A well-defined subset of individuals from the target population from which potential study participants will be sampled; also called a *sampling frame*.

Spearman rank-order correlation (ρ) A statistical measure of the degree to which changes in the value of one rank/order variable predict changes in the value of another rank/order variable.

Specific knowledge Information that is specific to a particular study, such as a particular statistic or a particular laboratory report; specific knowledge derived from the literature requires citations and references in a research report.

Specificity The proportion of people who do not have a disease (according to a reference standard) who test negative with a diagnostic test.

Spread A measure that describes the variability and distribution of responses to a numeric variable; also called *dispersion*.

Spreadsheet An interactive computer application that organizes and stores data in table form.

Standard deviation A measure of the narrowness or wideness of a normal distribution, which is calculated as the square root of the variance; in a normal distribution, 68% of the responses will fall within one standard deviation above or below the mean and 95% of the responses will fall within two standard deviations above or below the mean.

Standard error A measure of the narrowness or wideness of a normal distribution, which is calculated by dividing the variance by the sample size and then taking the square root of the resulting number.

Standard of care An existing therapy (such as the best therapy currently available or the therapy that is used most often in the location where the study is being conducted) that is used as a comparison for a new therapy being experimentally tested.

Stepwise multiple regression A model that systematically adds or removes predictor variables to a regression model to find the model that provides the best fit.

Stochastic model A mathematical model with inputs that vary according to a probability distribution so the outcomes differ slightly every time the model is run.

Stratified randomization The division of a population into subgroups prior to randomly assigning each individual within each subgroup to one of the exposure groups in an experimental study; this method is better than simple randomization at ensuring that the members of a subpopulation are distributed evenly across treatment arms of a trial.

STROBE An acronym for the writing checklist for Strengthening the Reporting of Observational Studies in Epidemiology.

Structured abstract An abstract that uses subheadings like Objective, Methods, Results, and Conclusion.

Study goal The main research question that a research project seeks to answer; the study goal is typically accomplished by answering a series of specific objectives, aims, or hypotheses.

Study population The individuals who participate in a study.

Submission fee A charge that some journals mandate for all manuscripts prior to review; paying the submission fee is not a guarantee of acceptance, and it is not refunded if a manuscript is rejected.

Superiority trial An experimental study that aims to demonstrate that a new intervention is better than some type of control, not merely as good as the control.

Survey instrument A series of questions used as a tool for systematically gathering information from study participants; also called a *questionnaire*.

Survival analysis Statistical evaluations of the distribution of the durations of time that individuals in a study population experience from an initial time point (such as the time of enrollment in a study or the time of diagnosis of a particular condition) until some well-defined event, which can be death, discharge from a hospital, or some other outcome.

SWOT An evaluation method that identifies the strengths, weaknesses, opportunities, and threats of a program.

Systematic review The use of a predetermined and comprehensive searching and screening method to identify relevant articles during a literature review.

Table In a research report, the concise presentation of key findings in a grid.

Talk-aloud protocol Participants in a qualitative study are asked to describe their thoughts and actions while they complete a task; also called *think-aloud protocol*.

Target journal The journal a researcher intends to submit a manuscript to first.

Target population The broader population to which the results of a study should be applicable.

Tertiary study A research analysis that reviews and synthesizes the existing literature on a topic; examples include narrative reviews, systematic reviews, and meta-analyses.

Tertiles The division of a data set into three ordered parts of equal size.

Test statistic A value calculated from study data for a hypothesis test, such as the t-stat used for t-tests or the F-stat used for one-way ANOVA.

Testability The ability of a research question to be measured and examined.

Test-retest reliability In a survey instrument or other assessment tool, a condition that is demonstrated when people who complete a baseline assessment and then re-take the test later have about the same scores each time they are tested.

Theoretical framework A set of established models in the published literature that can inform the components and flows of the conceptual framework for a new research study.

Think-aloud protocol Participants in a qualitative study are asked to describe their thoughts and actions while they complete a task; also called *talk-aloud protocol*.

Third variable A potential confounder that may make the association between an exposure variable and an outcome variable appear more or less significant than it truly is.

Time series study A research study that measures participants or samples at multiple points in time.

Transformative paradigm A qualitative research framework in which researchers assume that reality can be changed when research addresses a social justice issue.

Treatment-assigned analysis Analysis of experimental data that includes all participants even if they were not fully compliant with their assigned intervention; also called *intention-to-treat analysis*.

Treatment-received analysis Analysis of experimental data that includes only the participants who were fully compliant with their assigned intervention.

TREND An acronym for the writing checklist for Transparent Reporting of Evaluations with Nonrandomized Designs.

Two-by-two (2×2) table A row-by-column table that displays the counts of how often various combinations of events happen; in epidemiological analysis, the columns typically display disease status (yes/no) and the rows typically display exposure status (yes/no).

Two-sample *t*-test A statistical test used to compare the mean values of a ratio/interval variable in two independent populations; also called *independent-samples t-test*.

Two-sided *p*-value The probability value that is used for a statistical test when a direction is not specified in the alternative hypothesis.

Two-way ANOVA A test that compares the mean values of a continuous variable among independent groups across two factors (such as both sex and smoking status).

Type 1 error An error that occurs when a study population yields a significant statistical test result even though a significant difference or association does not actually exist in the source population.

Type 2 error An error that occurs when a statistical test of data from the study population finds no significant result even though a significant difference or association actually exists in the source population.

Understood consent Evidence that a potential study participant comprehends the study benefits, risks, and procedures and his/her rights as a study prior to agreeing to participate.

Uniform distribution A distribution of responses to a variable in which approximately equal numbers of people provided each allowable answer.

Unimodal A numeric variable with a one-peaked distribution.

Univariate analysis Statistical analysis that describes one variable in a data set.

Unstructured abstract An abstract that does not list section titles like Objective, Methods, Results, and Conclusion.

Validity In a survey instrument, diagnostic test, or other assessment tool, a condition that is established when the responses or measurements in a study are shown to be correct; also called *accuracy*.

Variable A characteristic that can be assigned more than one value.

Variance A measure of the narrowness or wideness of a normal distribution, which is calculated as the sum of the squares of the differences between each observation and the mean divided by the sample size.

Variance inflation factor (VIF) A test for whether the independent variables in a regression model have reasonably independent errors and are not too intercorrelated.

Vital signs Physiological measurements such as body temperature and blood pressure.

Vital statistics Population-level measurements related to births, deaths, and other demographic indicators.

Voluntariness A choice being made of a person's own free will.

Vulnerable populations At-risk populations, such as young children and people in prison, whose members might have limited ability to make an autonomous decision about volunteering to participate in a research study.

Waiver (of consent documentation) Permission from an institutional review board not to collect signed consent forms from participants because they could be harmed by being able to be linked to participation in a study on a sensitive topic.

Washout period A period during an experimental study during which patients receive no treatment.

Weighting Statistical methods used to adjust for sampling methods, for demographic differences between a population and a source population, for varying sample sizes in a meta-analysis, or for other circumstances.

White space Blank areas between printed content on a page.

Wilcoxon rank sum test A statistical test used to compare the median values of an ordinal/rank variable in two independent populations; also called a *Mann-Whitney U test*.

Wilcoxon signed-rank test A statistical test used to compare the values of an ordinal/rank variable in one population measured twice or in two paired groups.

Writer's block Sustained struggles with writing that an author might experience due to fear of failure or other barriers to productivity.

YLD An acronym for years lived with disability in a population, a commonly used metric in burden of disease studies.

YLL An acronym for years of life lost to premature death in a population, a commonly used metric in burden of disease studies.

***z*-Score** A score that indicates how many standard deviations away from the sample mean an individual participant's response is.

Index

A

B

C

D

E

J

K

L

M

N

O

P

Q

R

S

T